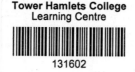

Introduction to
HUMAN ANATOMY
and PHYSIOLOGY

Third Edition

Eldra Pearl Solomon, PhD

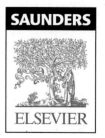

SAUNDERS

ELSEVIER

SAUNDERS
ELSEVIER

11830 Westline Industrial Drive
St. Louis, Missouri 63146

INTRODUCTION TO HUMAN ANATOMY AND PHYSIOLOGY,   ISBN: 978-1-4160-4405-5
THIRD EDITION

Notice

Neither the Publisher nor the Author assumes any responsibility for any loss or injury and/or damage to persons or property arising out of or related to any use of the material contained in this book. It is the responsibility of the treating practitioner, relying on independent expertise and knowledge of the patient, to determine the best treatment and method of application for the patient.

The Publisher

Library of Congress Control Number 2007940910

ISBN: 978-1-4160-4405-5

Editor: Jeff Downing
Developmental Editor: Karen C. Maurer
Publishing Services Manager: Deborah L. Vogel
Project Manager: Pat Costigan
Book Designer: Kimberly Denando

Printed in the United States of America

Last digit is the print number: 9 8 7 6 5 4 3

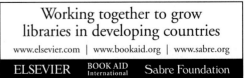

Working together to grow
libraries in developing countries

www.elsevier.com | www.bookaid.org | www.sabre.org

ELSEVIER   BOOK AID International   Sabre Foundation

ELSEVIER

evolve

REVIEWERS

I am grateful to the reviewers, who took the time to read the manuscript and provide valuable suggestions for improving it. Their input has contributed to this third edition.

Donna J. Burleson, RN, MS, MSN
Cisco Junior College
Abilene, Texas

Susan Mary Caley-Opsal, MS
Illinois Valley Community College
Oglesby, Illinois

Joyce Harris, RN, MA
Butler Technology and Career
  Development Schools
Hamilton, Ohio

Patricia Laing-Arie, RN
Meridian Technology Center
Stillwater, Oklahoma

Robert R. Smith, PhD
Meramec Community College
St. Louis, Missouri;
St. Charles Community College
St. Peters, Missouri

ACKNOWLEDGMENTS

The author wishes to acknowledge the support and valuable input received from family, friends, editors, students, and colleagues. I especially thank Dr. Kathleen M. Heide and Dr. Amy Solomon for their support and for critically reading selected portions of the manuscript. I appreciate the help of Mical and Karla Solomon in developing the new edition of the Study Guide and the help of Rebecca Hickey for contributing to the Evolve website.

I appreciate the support of my editors at Elsevier, especially Editor Jeff Downing, who was there to help with every aspect of this project. I thank Project Manager Pat Costigan for expertly keeping the process flowing. I also want to acknowledge the help of Developmental Editor Karen Maurer with the Study Guide and other facets of this project. I am also grateful for the help of Publishing Services Manager Deborah Vogel and Designer Kim Denando.

I appreciate the contributions of Science Illustrator Suzannah Alexander, who helped us develop many new illustrations and updated many existing figures. Her talent, eye for detail, and consistency greatly contributed to this new edition. All of these dedicated professionals provided the skills needed to produce this third edition of *Introduction to Human Anatomy and Physiology*. I thank them for their help and support throughout this project.

DEDICATION

To the many educators and students who have used Introduction to Human Anatomy and Physiology . . .

And to the students preparing for careers in the health-related professions who use this new edition.

And to my colleagues, friends, and family who have supported and encouraged me as I developed this book.

PREFACE

This third edition of *Introduction to Human Anatomy and Physiology* builds on the strengths of the first two editions. We have developed a book that makes learning about the complexities of human structure and function both manageable and interesting. The numerous terms, facts, and principles of this fascinating subject are presented clearly and accurately. Through the years, students have told us that this book is enjoyable to read and that they appreciate its excellent learning aids. This new edition continues in that tradition and emphasizes **Tools for Learning**, a toolbox of integrated strategies designed to help the student succeed.

Introduction to Human Anatomy and Physiology focuses on the human body as a living, functioning organism. A principal goal in preparing this book has been to share a sense of excitement about the body's elegant structure and function. The emphasis is on how tissues, organs, and body systems work together to carry out complex activities such as maintaining body temperature, regulating blood pressure, learning, and responding to stress. As each of the body's many parts is described, its interaction with other structures and its role in maintaining the conditions necessary for life are discussed.

TOOLS FOR LEARNING

In addition to the conversational tone of the text, we have developed the following learning strategies to help students master the major concepts of *Introduction to Human Anatomy and Physiology*:

1. A **Chapter Outline** at the beginning of each chapter provides an overview of the material covered in the chapter.
2. **Learning Objectives** specify how to demonstrate mastery of the material covered in the chapter. Beginning with this edition, Learning Objectives are now integrated into the text. After each major heading, we include the Learning Objectives to help the student identify the goals of that section of the chapter.
3. **Quiz Yourself questions** are included at the end of each major section of the chapter. New to this edition, these questions help the student gauge how well he or she is mastering the material.
4. **Concept-statement headings** within each chapter introduce the key idea in the information that follows.
5. **Sequence summaries** within the text simplify information presented in paragraph form. For example, paragraphs describing blood flow through regions of the body are followed by a sequence summary that lists in order the structures through which the blood flows.
6. The **Summary** at the end of each chapter is organized around the Learning Objectives. The Summary provides a quick review of the material presented. Selected key terms are boldfaced in the Summary to help the reader

learn the vocabulary within the context of related concepts.
7. **Chapter Quizzes** and **Review Questions** at the end of each chapter provide an opportunity to evaluate mastery of the material in each chapter. Answers to Chapter Quizzes are provided in Appendix A.
8. The **Glossary** at the end of the book provides definitions for terms and includes pronunciations.
9. An appendix on **Dissecting Terms** teaches how to analyze new terms to discover their meaning.

In addition, boldfaced terms emphasize new words, often accompanied by phonetic pronunciations in parentheses. Numerous tables—many of them illustrated—summarize and organize material presented in the text. Accurate, carefully drawn illustrations support ideas covered in the text. We include many new and revised illustrations in this new edition.

The *Study Guide for Introduction to Human Anatomy and Physiology* highlights concepts in the text and provides testing exercises and answers. Questions are provided for each section of a chapter, and figures are included for you to label. A chapter test is included for each chapter. Crossword puzzles test your knowledge of terminology.

evolve

http://evolve.elsevier.com/Solomon/introAP/

This edition of *Introduction to Human Anatomy and Physiology* is supported by an Evolve Resources website for instructors and students. Instructors can take advantage of:

- Detailed lesson plans
- Lesson outlines
- Electronic test bank

Students can access additional study and research help with:

- Audio glossary
- *Body Spectrum Electronic Anatomy Coloring Book*
- Exercises and activities on the *Panorama of Anatomy and Physiology*
- WebLinks

TO THE STUDENT

You may be reading this book purely because you want to understand how the human body works, or you may also be meeting a requirement for beginning your career in one of the health-related professions. Whatever your motivation, learning about the complexities of the human body is a challenging endeavor. You will need to learn the language in order to understand the concepts. For example, you must know the meaning of words like *cardiac output, peripheral resistance,* and *aldosterone* in order to understand how the body regulates blood pressure. *Introduction to Human Anatomy and Physiology,* Third Edition, has been written to help you achieve your goal of succeeding in your course—and to enjoy the process. The **Tools for Learning** just described will guide you in your journey through this book.

Here are some additional suggestions that will contribute to your success. When you begin a new chapter in the book, read the Chapter Outline in order to gain an overview of the material that will be discussed in the chapter. Use the Learning Objectives, keeping them in mind as you make your way through each section of the chapter.

Pay attention to the tables. We have condensed and organized a great deal of material into tables, especially in Chapters 4 (The Skeletal System) and 5 (The Muscular System).

After you read the chapter, test your knowledge by taking the Chapter Quiz and answering the Review Questions. Pay close attention to the new terms. Remember that you must know the vocabulary to understand the concepts. Remember to use the Glossary and Appendix B (Dissecting Terms).

Make a study schedule and adhere to it. There is far too much material to learn the night before your test. Review the lecture material after each class. Many students find it helpful to type their lecture notes; the process of figuring out what they wrote and then typing it facilitates learning.

Answering the questions in the Study Guide is a convenient way to gauge your knowledge before each test. Some students find small study groups helpful for reviewing material.

TO THE INSTRUCTOR

Each chapter in this new edition of *Introduction to Human Anatomy and Physiology* has been carefully updated so that the material presented is accurate and current. The emphasis is on concepts and relationships, particularly the relationships between structure and function. The excellent art program supports the text, and the numerous tables and other **Tools for Learning** help the student master the material.

Students learn best when they can relate what they are studying to familiar issues, problems, and experiences. For this reason we use examples that are easily recognized. Suntan and sunburn help explain melanin and pigment cells. Normal body functioning is made clearer by showing what happens when its balance is upset by disease-causing organisms or by such conditions as diabetes mellitus.

In this new edition, we have made changes that reduce concept density. We have integrated the Learning Objectives into the text and provided questions (Quiz Yourself) after each major section. We have integrated part captions into illustrations so that descriptions and explanations are included with each part of the figure. We have also added numbered steps to help students navigate complex figures.

To help you in your evaluation of student mastery, we have revised the Test Bank and made it available electronically on the Evolve Instructor's website. This Test Bank provides two tests for each chapter and also provides final examinations.

At the end of a successful course in human anatomy and physiology, the student should be able to demonstrate mastery of the concepts by responding to the following Course Learning Outcomes:

- Describe how each organ system contributes to homeostasis.
- Compare the major types of tissues and describe how each contributes to the function of the body.
- List the functions of the skeletal system and describe the bones of the axial and appendicular skeletons.
- Trace the events that take place during muscle contraction and describe the interaction of each of the four functional groups of muscles.
- Describe the sequence of events that must take place before you can make a conscious, adaptive response to a sudden event, such as a child running out in front of your car. Include the major regions of the brain that might be involved.
- Trace the transmission of light through the eye and sound through the ear.
- Describe how specific hormones regulate metabolic rate, glucose concentration, blood pressure, and response to stress.
- Trace a drop of blood through the pulmonary and systemic circulations, listing in sequence the heart chambers and principal blood vessels through which it must pass on its journey from one organ in the body to another (e.g., from brain to liver).
- Contrast antibody-mediated immunity with cell-mediated immunity.
- Trace a breath of air through the respiratory system from the moment it is inspired until oxygen from that breath enters a capillary.
- Trace the journey taken through the body by a bite of food from ingestion to absorption or elimination, describing how the body processes it along the way.
- Trace a drop of filtrate as it passes through the urinary system from glomerulus to urethra and describe how the kidneys produce urine and help maintain fluid balance.
- Summarize the interaction of the hypothalamus, pituitary gland, and ovaries that maintains the menstrual cycle.

1 Introducing the Human Body

Chapter Outline

I. **Anatomy and physiology are the studies of structure and function**

II. **The body has several levels of organization**

III. **The body is composed of inorganic compounds and organic compounds**

IV. **Metabolism is essential to maintenance, growth, and repair of the body**

V. **Homeostatic mechanisms maintain an appropriate internal environment**

VI. **The body has a basic plan**

  A. Directions in the body are relative
  B. The body has three main planes
  C. We can identify specific body regions
  D. The body has two main body cavities
  E. It is important to view the body as a whole

The human body is an amazingly complex mechanism. It consists of billions of atoms, molecules, and cells that interact in precise, coordinated ways. No machine known, not even the most sophisticated computer, begins to rival the complexity of the human body. Hans Moravec, a research professor at the Robotics Institute of Carnegie Mellon University, recently calculated that the human brain has a processing capacity of 100 trillion instructions per second!

What is the structure of the body's components? And how do all of these parts communicate and work together to maintain a functioning human? These questions are the fascinating subject matter of this book.

ANATOMY AND PHYSIOLOGY ARE THE STUDIES OF STRUCTURE AND FUNCTION

LEARNING OBJECTIVE

1. **Define anatomy and physiology.**

This book is an introduction to **anatomy** (ah-**nat′**-ah-me), the science of body structure, and to **physiology** (fiz′-ee-ol′-oh-jee), the study of body function. The anatomy and physiology of the body are closely related. Each body part is precisely adapted for carrying out its specific job. For example, the stomach has muscular walls well suited for churning and breaking down food. Its lining produces substances that break down food chemically. As you study the human body, look for the relationships between the structure and function of the body parts you are learning about. Notice how the size, shape, and structure of each part is related to the job it performs.

Anatomy and physiology are broad fields with many sub-disciplines. For example, **gross anatomy** focuses on structures that can be studied by dissection. **Microscopic anatomy** focuses on structures that must be studied with microscopes. **Cell biology** is the study of the structure, function, and interaction of cells.

The health sciences are applied fields of anatomy and physiology. You may choose a career in one of the health sciences such as nursing, medicine, dentistry, physical therapy, occupational therapy, nuclear medicine technology, or radiation therapy technology. The basic concepts you learn in this book provide the foundation for careers in the health sciences.

ⓘ *Quiz Yourself*

- A student is studying the structure of each bone in the body. Is this an example of anatomy or of physiology?
- A student is learning about how the systems of the body interact to maintain normal blood pressure. Is this an example of anatomy or of physiology?

THE BODY HAS SEVERAL LEVELS OF ORGANIZATION

LEARNING OBJECTIVES

2. **Describe the levels of biological organization in the human body, from the simplest (the chemical level) to the most complex (the organism).**
3. **Describe the principal organ systems.**

The body is highly organized. Its simplest level of organization is the **chemical level** (Figure 1-1). All matter is composed of **chemical elements**—pure chemical substances such as iron, calcium, or oxygen. About 98% of the body is composed of only six elements—oxygen, carbon, hydrogen, nitrogen, calcium, and phosphorus. Table 1-1 lists the elements that are most abundant in the human body and explains why each is important.

An **atom** is the smallest amount of a chemical element that has the characteristic properties of that element. Atoms can combine chemically, forming **molecules.** For example, two atoms of hydrogen chemically combine with one atom of oxygen to produce water (H_2O).

The next level of organization above the chemical level is the **cellular level.** In living things, atoms and molecules associate in specific ways to form **cells,** the building blocks of the body. The human body is composed of about 100 trillion cells of many types, such as bone cells, blood cells, and muscle cells. Although cells vary in size and shape according to their function, most are so small that they can be seen only with a microscope. Each cell consists of specialized cell parts called **organelles** (or-gah-**nells′**). One organelle, the **nucleus,** serves as the information and control center of the cell. Several other kinds of organelles scattered throughout the cell perform specific functions, such as manufacturing needed substances or breaking down fuel molecules to provide energy.

The next highest level of organization above the cellular level is the **tissue level.** A **tissue** is a group of closely associated cells specialized to perform particular functions. The four main types of tissue in the body are muscle tissue, nervous tissue, connective tissue, and epithelial tissue. Cells and tissues are discussed in Chapter 2.

Tissues are organized into **organs,** such as the brain, stomach, or heart. Although the heart consists mainly of muscle tissue, it is covered by epithelial tissue and also contains connective and nervous tissue.

A group of tissues and organs that work together to perform specific functions makes up a body system, or **organ system.** The circulatory system, for example, consists of the heart, blood vessels, blood, lymph structures, and several other organs. Each organ system contributes to the dynamic, carefully balanced state of the body. Table 1-2 summarizes and Figure 1-2 illustrates the 11 main systems of the human body. Working together with great precision and complexity, the body systems make up the living organism (or′-guh-nizm)—for example, you.

ⓘ *Quiz Yourself*

- What are tissues? Organelles?
- List the levels of organization in sequence from simplest to most complex.
- What are the functions of the endocrine system? The circulatory system?

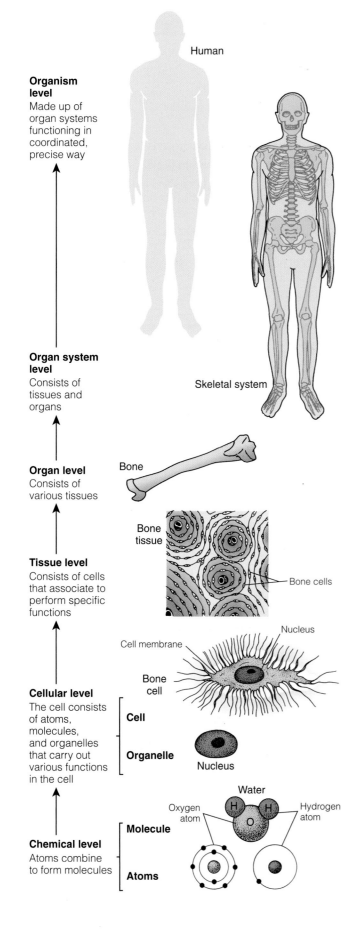

Organism level
Made up of organ systems functioning in coordinated, precise way

Human

Skeletal system

Organ system level
Consists of tissues and organs

Organ level
Consists of various tissues

Bone

Tissue level
Consists of cells that associate to perform specific functions

Bone tissue

Bone cells

Nucleus

Cell membrane

Bone cell

Cellular level
The cell consists of atoms, molecules, and organelles that carry out various functions in the cell

Cell

Organelle

Nucleus

Water

Molecule

Oxygen atom

Hydrogen atom

Chemical level
Atoms combine to form molecules

Atoms

THE BODY IS COMPOSED OF INORGANIC COMPOUNDS AND ORGANIC COMPOUNDS

LEARNING OBJECTIVE

4. **Distinguish between inorganic and organic compounds and briefly describe four important groups of organic compounds.**

The body is made up of atoms, ions, and molecules; life processes depend on the organization and interaction of these chemical units. An **ion** (eye′-on) is an electrically charged atom or group of atoms. For example, an electrically charged hydrogen atom is called a hydrogen ion (H^+). When placed in water, hydrochloric acid (HCl) has a tendency to separate into hydrogen ions (H^+) and chloride ions (Cl^-). Sodium chloride (NaCl) is table salt. When placed in water, it has a tendency to separate into sodium (Na^+) and chloride (Cl^-) ions. Because of their electric charges, ions are very important in many life processes, including energy transformations, transmission of nerve impulses, and muscle contraction.

A **chemical compound** is a molecule that consists of two or more different elements combined in a fixed proportion. Water is a chemical compound consisting of two atoms of hydrogen chemically combined with one atom of oxygen (H_2O). The simple sugar glucose consists of 6 carbon atoms combined with 12 hydrogen atoms and 6 oxygen atoms ($C_6H_{12}O_6$).

Chemical compounds can be classified in two broad groups—inorganic and organic. **Inorganic compounds** are relatively small, simple compounds such as water, salts, simple acids (e.g., hydrochloric acid), and simple bases (e.g., ammonia). These substances are required for fluid balance and for many cell activities such as transporting materials through cell membranes.

Organic compounds are large, complex compounds containing carbon. They are the chemical building blocks (structural components) of the body and also serve as fuel molecules that provide energy for body activities. Organic compounds also regulate and participate in thousands of chemical reactions necessary for life. Four important groups of organic compounds are carbohydrates, lipids, proteins, and nucleic acids.

Carbohydrates (kar′-bow-**hi**′-drates) are sugars and starches. They are used by the body as fuel molecules and to store energy. Glucose is a simple sugar that is a main source of energy for the body. The liver and muscles can link glucose molecules into long chains, producing glycogen, a large molecule that can be stored.

Among the biologically important groups of **lipids** are the fats, compounds that store energy, and phospholipids, which are components of cell membranes. Steroids, another

---

FIGURE 1-1 • Levels of organization in the human body. Note the progression from simple to complex.

TABLE 1-1	ELEMENTS THAT MAKE UP THE HUMAN BODY		
Name	Chemical Symbol	Approximate Composition by Mass (%)	Function
Oxygen	O	65	Required for cellular respiration; present in most organic compounds; component of water
Carbon	C	18	Backbone of organic molecules
Hydrogen	H	10	Present in most organic compounds; component of water
Nitrogen	N	3	Component of all proteins and nucleic acids
Calcium	Ca	1.5	Structural component of bones and teeth; important in muscle contraction, conduction of nerve impulses, and blood clotting
Phosphorus	P	1	Component of nucleic acids; structural component of bone; important in energy transfer
Potassium	K	0.4	Principal positive ion within cells; important in nerve function; affects muscle contraction
Sulfur	S	0.3	Component of most proteins
Sodium	Na	0.2	Principal positive ion in interstitial (tissue) fluid; important in fluid balance; essential for transmission of nerve impulses
Magnesium	Mg	0.1	Needed in blood and other body tissues
Chlorine	Cl	0.1	Principal negative ion of interstitial fluid; important in fluid balance; component of sodium chloride
Iron	Fe	Trace amount	Component of hemoglobin and myoglobin; component of certain enzymes
Iodine	I	Trace amount	Component of thyroid hormones

Other elements found in very small amounts in the body include manganese (Mn), copper (Cu), zinc (Zn), cobalt (Co), fluorine (F), molybdenum (Mo), selenium (Se), and a few others. They are called *trace elements.*

important group of lipids, include several hormones, for example, male and female sex hormones.

Proteins (**pro'**-teens) are large, complex molecules composed of subunits called **amino acids.** Some proteins serve as **enzymes** (**en'**-zimes)—catalysts that regulate chemical reactions. Other proteins are important structural components of cells and tissues. The kinds and amounts of proteins in a cell determine to a large extent what a cell looks like and how it functions. For example, muscle cells have large amounts of the proteins *myosin* and *actin,* which are responsible for their appearance and their ability to contract.

Nucleic (new-**klee'**-ik) **acids,** like proteins, are large, complex compounds. Two very important nucleic acids are DNA (deoxyribonucleic acid) and RNA (ribonucleic acid). **DNA** makes up the genes—the hereditary material; it contains the instructions for making all the proteins needed by the cell. **RNA** is important in the process of manufacturing proteins.

Quiz Yourself

- How are organic compounds different from inorganic compounds?
- What are two functions of proteins?

METABOLISM IS ESSENTIAL TO MAINTENANCE, GROWTH, AND REPAIR OF THE BODY

LEARNING OBJECTIVE

5. Define metabolism and contrast anabolism and catabolism.

All the chemical processes that take place within the body are referred to as its **metabolism** (meh-**tab'**-oh-liz-um). Two phases of metabolism are catabolism and anabolism. **Catabolism** (kah-**tab'**-oh-liz-um), the breaking-down phase of metabolism, provides the energy needed to carry on activities necessary for life (Figure 1-3). For example, catabolism generates the energy needed for muscle contraction and for growth. Cells obtain energy from food molecules by a complex series of catabolic chemical reactions referred to as **cellular respiration.** During this process, certain nutrients are used as fuel and are slowly broken down. As the energy stored in these nutrients is released, it is packaged within a special energy-storage molecule called **ATP (adenosine triphosphate).** Cellular respiration requires oxygen as well as nutrients.

TABLE 1-2	THE ORGAN SYSTEMS	
System	**Components**	**Functions**
Integumentary	Skin, hair, nails, sweat glands	Covers and protects body; helps regulate body temperature; receives information about touch, pressure, temperature, and pain
Skeletal	Bones, cartilage, ligaments	Supports and protects body; muscles attach to bones; stores calcium; produces blood cells
Muscular	Skeletal muscle, cardiac muscle, smooth muscle	Moves parts of skeleton, locomotion; pumps blood; moves internal materials
Nervous	Nerves and sense organs; brain and spinal cord	Principal regulatory system; receives stimuli from external and internal environment; transmits impulses to muscles and glands
Endocrine	Pituitary, adrenal, thyroid, and other ductless glands	Works with nervous system in regulating metabolic activities and body chemistry; secretes hormones
Cardiovascular	Heart, blood vessels, blood	Transports nutrients, gases, hormones, wastes, and other materials from one part of the body to another; helps maintain fluid balance
Lymphatic (immune system)	Lymph, lymphatic vessels, lymph nodes, and other lymph structures	Collects and transports tissue fluid to blood; absorbs lipids from digestive tract and transports them to cardiovascular system; defends body against organisms that cause disease
Respiratory	Lungs, trachea, and other air passageways	Exchanges gases between blood and external environment; maintains appropriate oxygen content; helps regulate acid-base balance of blood
Digestive	Mouth, esophagus, stomach, intestine, liver, pancreas, salivary glands	Ingests and digests foods; absorbs nutrients into blood
Urinary	Kidney, bladder, and associated ducts	Excretes metabolic wastes; helps regulate volume and composition of blood and other body fluids
Reproductive	Testes, ovaries, and associated structures	Reproduction; maintains sexual characteristics

Anabolism (a-**nab′**-oh-liz-um) is the building, or synthetic, phase of metabolism. In anabolism, energy is used to manufacture needed chemical compounds from the nutrients provided by food. These chemical compounds are needed for growth, maintenance, and repair of the body.

Quiz Yourself

- How is anabolism different from catabolism?

HOMEOSTATIC MECHANISMS MAINTAIN AN APPROPRIATE INTERNAL ENVIRONMENT

LEARNING OBJECTIVE

6. **Define homeostasis and contrast negative and positive feedback mechanisms.**

Metabolic activities occur continuously in every living cell, and they must be carefully regulated to maintain **homeostasis** (ho-me-oh-**stay′**-sis), an appropriate internal environment. The body maintains its internal environment, for example body temperature, within narrow limits, which we call a steady state. The body maintains a balanced concentration of nutrients, oxygen and other gases, ions, and various chemical compounds.

Homeostatic mechanisms, the self-regulating control systems that maintain homeostasis, are remarkably sensitive and efficient. Homeostasis must be maintained even though conditions may continuously change in the external environment. A **stressor** is a stimulus that disrupts homeostasis and causes **stress** in the body. For example, eating a bag of candy is a stressor that raises the blood sugar concentration above the homeostatic level. This stress activates homeostatic mechanisms that bring the blood sugar concentration back to the normal range. When homeostatic mechanisms are unable to manage stress, the steady state is not restored. The stress may then lead to a malfunction, which can cause disease or even death.

How do homeostatic mechanisms work? Most are **negative feedback systems** like the thermostat in your furnace or air conditioning system. In a negative feedback system, a change

Text continues on p. 8.

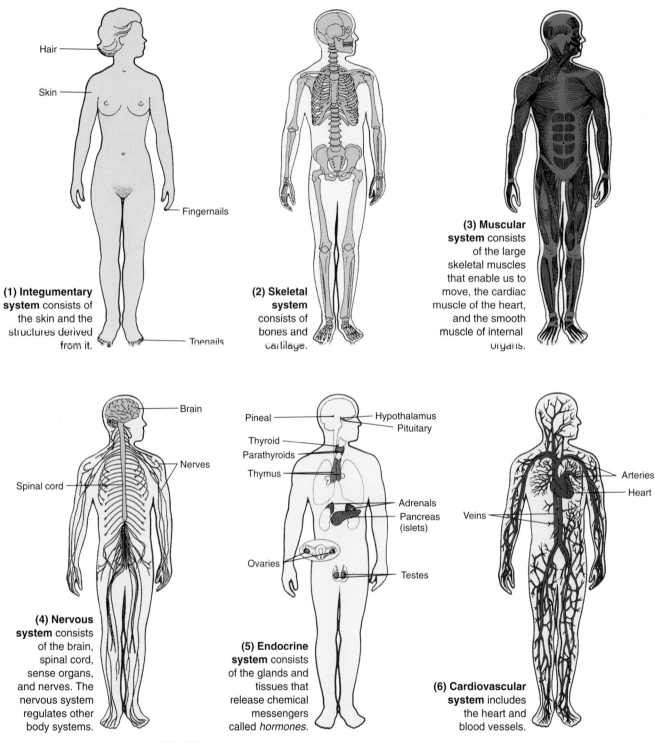

Hair

Skin

Fingernails

(1) Integumentary system consists of the skin and the structures derived from it.

Toenails

(2) Skeletal system consists of bones and cartilage.

(3) Muscular system consists of the large skeletal muscles that enable us to move, the cardiac muscle of the heart, and the smooth muscle of internal organs.

Brain

Nerves

Spinal cord

(4) Nervous system consists of the brain, spinal cord, sense organs, and nerves. The nervous system regulates other body systems.

Pineal

Thyroid
Parathyroids

Thymus

Hypothalamus
Pituitary

Adrenals
Pancreas (islets)

Ovaries

Testes

(5) Endocrine system consists of the glands and tissues that release chemical messengers called *hormones*.

Arteries

Heart

Veins

(6) Cardiovascular system includes the heart and blood vessels.

FIGURE 1-2 • The principal organ systems of the human body.

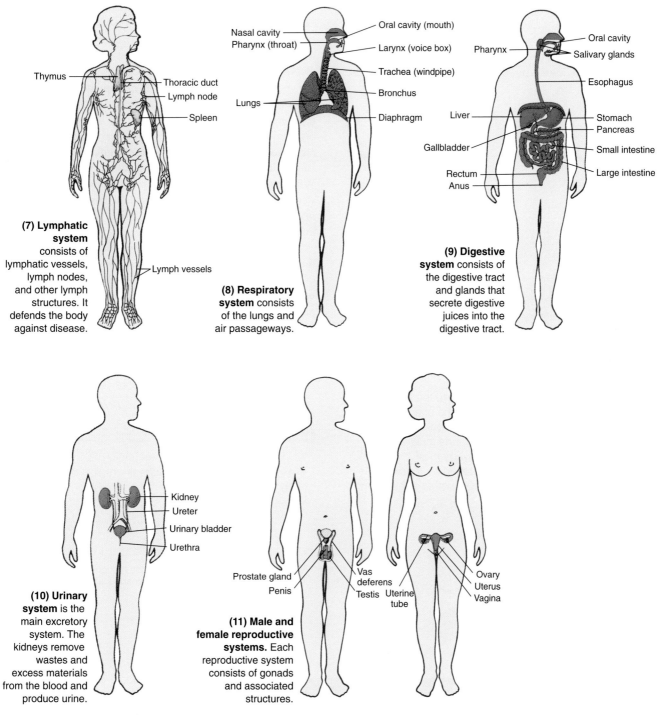

(7) Lymphatic system consists of lymphatic vessels, lymph nodes, and other lymph structures. It defends the body against disease.

Thymus
Thoracic duct
Lymph node
Spleen
Lymph vessels

(8) Respiratory system consists of the lungs and air passageways.

Nasal cavity
Pharynx (throat)
Oral cavity (mouth)
Larynx (voice box)
Trachea (windpipe)
Bronchus
Lungs
Diaphragm

(9) Digestive system consists of the digestive tract and glands that secrete digestive juices into the digestive tract.

Pharynx
Oral cavity
Salivary glands
Esophagus
Liver
Stomach
Pancreas
Gallbladder
Small intestine
Rectum
Large intestine
Anus

(10) Urinary system is the main excretory system. The kidneys remove wastes and excess materials from the blood and produce urine.

Kidney
Ureter
Urinary bladder
Urethra

(11) Male and female reproductive systems. Each reproductive system consists of gonads and associated structures.

Prostate gland
Penis
Vas deferens
Testis
Ovary
Uterus
Vagina
Uterine tube

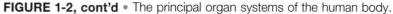

FIGURE 1-2, cont'd • The principal organ systems of the human body.

in some steady state triggers a response that is *opposite* (negative) to the change.

First, a sensor detects a change, a deviation from the steady state (e.g., a change in temperature). The sensor signals a regulator, or control center (in this case, the thermostat). The regulator can control the process (temperature regulation). For example, when temperature increases too much, the thermostat shuts off the furnace. In this way the temperature is kept within the desired range.

Note that in a negative feedback system the response of the regulator *counteracts* the inappropriate change, thus restoring the appropriate state. The response of the regulator reverses the stimulus (Figure 1-4). Many homeostatic mechanisms in the body are negative feedback systems, for example, regulation of body temperature, regulation of glucose (sugar) level in the blood, and regulation of blood pressure. When some condition varies too far from the appropriate state (either too high or too low), a control system uses negative feedback to bring the condition back within normal limits.

The body also has a few **positive feedback systems.** In these systems the variation from the steady state sets off a series of events that *intensify* the changes. A positive feedback system operates in the delivery of a baby. As the head of the baby pushes against the cervix (the lower part of the uterus), a reflex action causes the uterus to contract. The contraction forces the baby's head against the cervix again, resulting in another contraction, and the positive feedback cycle is repeated again and again until the baby is delivered.

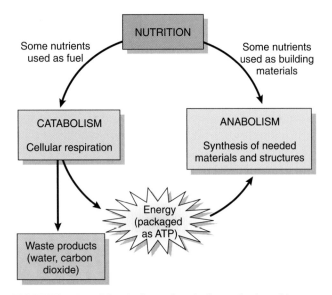

FIGURE 1-3 • Metabolism. Catabolism, the breaking-down phase of metabolism, provides the energy for anabolism, the phase of metabolism in which molecules, cells, and tissues are manufactured. Energy is also needed for muscle contraction, movement of material into and out of cells, growth, maintenance, repair, reproduction, development, and many other activities. *ATP,* Adenosine triphosphate.

ⓐ *Quiz Yourself*

- What are homeostatic mechanisms?
- How is positive feedback different from negative feedback?

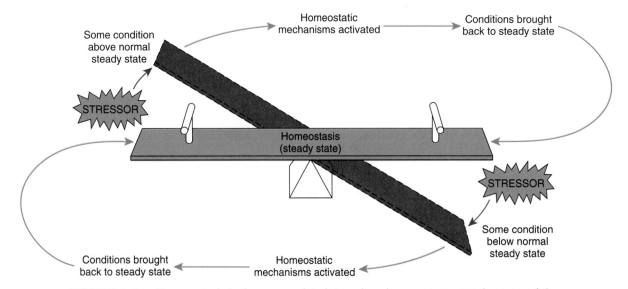

FIGURE 1-4 • Homeostasis is the appropriate internal environment, or steady state, of the body. Stressful stimuli, called *stressors,* disrupt homeostasis, causing stress. Any deviation from the steady state is regarded as stress. Stress activates homeostatic mechanisms that bring conditions back toward the steady state.

THE BODY HAS A BASIC PLAN

LEARNING OBJECTIVES

7. **Describe the anatomical position of the human body.**
8. **Define and use properly the principal directional terms used in human anatomy.**
9. **Recognize sagittal, transverse, and frontal sections of the body and of body structures.**
10. **Define and locate the principal regions and cavities of the body.**

The body consists of right and left halves that are mirror images; that is, it has **bilateral symmetry.** Two of the structures that characterize humans as vertebrates are the **cranium** (**kray′**-nee-um), or brain case, and the backbone, or **vertebral column.** Humans are also mammals and so have hair, mammary (milk) glands, and teeth that are differentiated into types (incisors, canines, premolars, and molars).

Directions in the Body Are Relative

To identify the structures of the body, it is useful to learn some basic terms and directions. Directional terms in human anatomy are relative, somewhat like directional terms in geography. Thus you could say that New York City is north of Washington, DC, but south of Boston or that Chicago is west of Philadelphia but east of San Francisco. Bear this in mind as you learn the anatomical directional terms. Directional terms are applied to the body when it is in the **anatomical position,** which means that the body is standing erect, eyes looking forward, arms at the sides, and palms and toes directed forward (Figure 1-5).

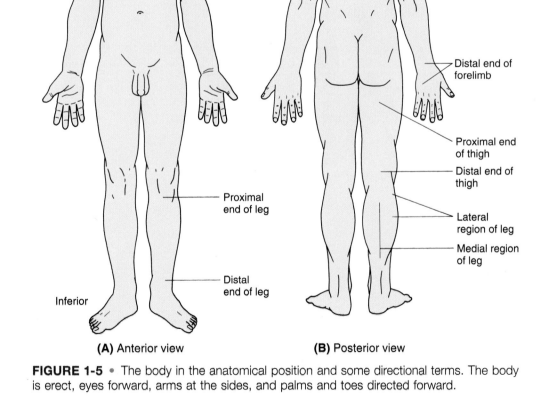

(A) Anterior view   **(B)** Posterior view

FIGURE 1-5 • The body in the anatomical position and some directional terms. The body is erect, eyes forward, arms at the sides, and palms and toes directed forward.

1. **Superior/Inferior.** The "North Pole" of the human body is the top of the head—its superior point. Its "South Pole" is represented by the soles of the feet—its most inferior part (Figure 1-5). Thus the heart is superior to the stomach because it is closer to the head. The heart is inferior to the brain. The stomach is inferior to the heart. The terms **cephalic** (seh-**fal′**-ik) and **cranial** (toward the skull) are sometimes used instead of the word *superior*. The term **caudal** (toward the tail) is sometimes used instead of the word *inferior*.

2. **Anterior/Posterior.** The front (belly) surface of the body is anterior, or **ventral.** The stomach is anterior to the vertebral column. The back surface of the body is posterior, or **dorsal.** The vertebral column is posterior to the stomach.

3. **Medial/Lateral.** A structure is said to be medial if it is closer to the midline of the body than to another structure. The navel is medial to the hip bone. A structure is lateral if it is toward one side of the body. Thus the hip bone is lateral to the navel.

4. **Proximal/Distal.** When a structure is closer to the body midline or point of attachment to the trunk, it is described as proximal. This term is used especially in locating limb structures. Thus the wrist is proximal to the fingers. Distal means farther from the midline or point of attachment to the trunk. The fingers are distal to the wrist.

5. **Superficial/Deep.** Structures located toward the surface of the body are superficial. Blood vessels in the skin are superficial to those lying beneath in the muscle. Structures located farther inward (away from the body surface) are deep. Blood vessels in the muscle are deep to those in the skin.

The Body Has Three Main Planes

The body has three axes, each at right angles to the other two: an anterior-posterior axis extending from head to the most caudal part of the body; a dorsoventral axis extending from back to belly; and a left-right axis extending from side to side. In studying anatomy, and in clinical practice, it is often helpful to view internal structures by dividing the body into sections,

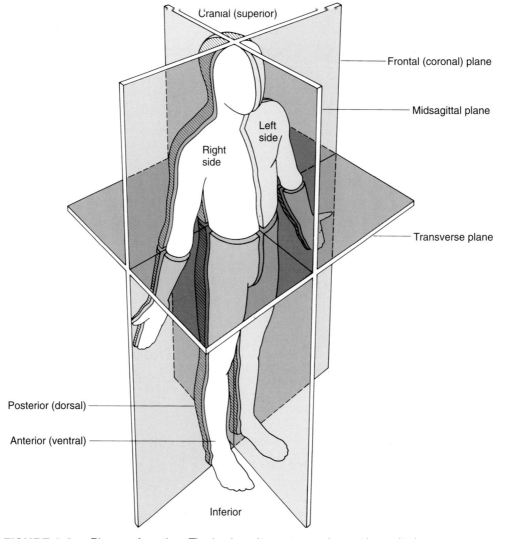

FIGURE 1-6 • Planes of section. The body or its parts can be cut in sagittal, transverse, or frontal sections.

or slices. We can distinguish three sections, or planes (imaginary flat surfaces), that divide the body into specific parts (Figure 1-6):

1. **Sagittal** (**sadj′**-ih-tul) **plane.** A sagittal plane divides the body into right and left parts. A midsagittal (or median) plane passes through the main body axis and divides the body into two (almost) mirror image halves.
2. **Transverse (cross) plane.** This plane is at right angles to the body axis. It divides the body into superior and inferior parts.
3. **Frontal (coronal) plane.** This plane divides the body into anterior and posterior parts.

We Can Identify Specific Body Regions

The body can be subdivided into an **axial** portion, consisting of the head, neck, and trunk, and an **appendicular** (ap-pen-**dik′**-u-lar) portion, consisting of the limbs. The trunk, or

torso, consists of the thorax, abdomen, and pelvis (Figure 1-7).

Some of the terms used to indicate specific body regions or structures follow.

Region	Part of the Body Referred to
Abdominal	Portion of trunk below the diaphragm
Arm	Technically, the part of the upper limb between the shoulder and the elbow, as distinguished from the forearm. (Popularly, the term *arm* refers to the entire upper limb.)
Axillary (**ak′**-sih-lar-ee)	Armpit area
Brachial (**bray′**-kee-al)	Arm
Buccal (**buk′**-al)	Inner surfaces of the cheeks
Carpal (**kar′**-pal)	Wrist
Celiac (**see′**-lee-ak)	Abdomen
Cephalic	Head
Cervical	Neck
Costal (**kos′**-tal)	Ribs

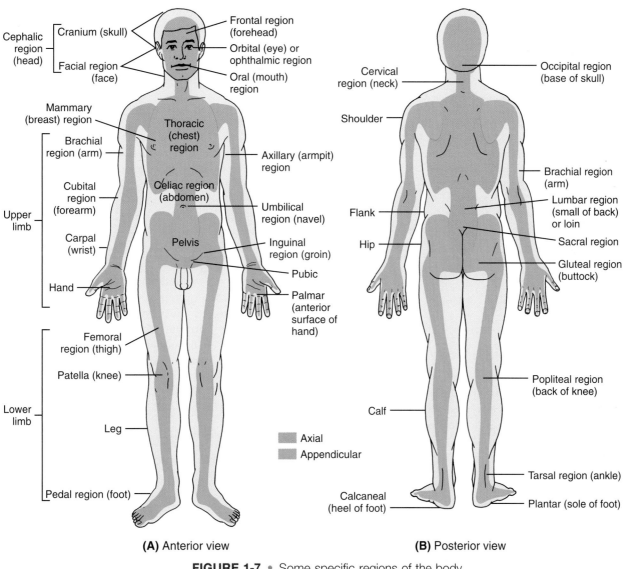

(A) Anterior view   **(B)** Posterior view

FIGURE 1-7 • Some specific regions of the body.

Region	Part of the Body Referred to
Cranial	Skull
Cubital	Elbow or forearm
Cutaneous (ku-**tay**'-nee-us)	Skin
Femoral (**fem**'-or-al)	Thigh; the part of the lower extremity between the hip and the knee
Forearm	Upper extremity between the elbow and the wrist
Frontal	Forehead
Gluteal (**gloo**'-tee-al)	Buttock
Groin	Depressed region between the abdomen and the thigh
Inguinal (**ing**'-gwih-nal)	Groin
Leg	Lower limb; especially the part from the knee to the foot
Lumbar	Loin, the region of the lower back and side, between the lowest rib and the pelvis
Mammary	Breasts
Occipital (ok-**sip**'-ih-tal)	Back of the head
Ophthalmic (ahf-**thal**'-mik)	Eyes
Oral	Mouth
Orbital	Bony cavity containing the eyeball
Palmar	Palm
Patellar	Knee
Pectoral (**pek**'-tow-ral)	Chest
Pedal	Foot
Pelvic	Pelvis; the bony ring that girdles the lower portion of the trunk
Perineal (per'-ih-**nee**'-al)	Region between the anus and the pubic arch; includes the region of the external reproductive structures
Plantar	Sole of the foot
Popliteal (pop-**lit**'-ee-al)	Behind the knee
Sacral	Base of spine
Tarsal	Ankle
Thoracic	Chest; the part of the trunk below the neck and above the diaphragm
Umbilical	Navel; depressed scar marking the site of entry of the umbilical cord in the fetus

The Body Has Two Main Body Cavities

The spaces within the body, called **body cavities,** contain the internal organs, or **viscera** (**vis**'-ur-uh). The two principal body cavities are the **dorsal cavity** and the **ventral cavity** (Figure 1-8). The bony dorsal cavity is located near the dorsal (posterior) body surface. The dorsal cavity is subdivided into the **cranial cavity,** which holds the brain, and the **vertebral** (or **spinal**) **canal,** which contains the spinal cord. The ventral cavity is located near the ventral (anterior) body surface. It is subdivided into the **thoracic** (or **chest**) **cavity** and the **abdominopelvic** (ab-dom'-ih-no-**pel**'-vik) **cavity.**

The thoracic and abdominopelvic cavities are separated by a broad muscle, the **diaphragm** (**die**'-ah-fram), which forms the floor of the thoracic cavity. Divisions of the thoracic cavity

are the **pleural cavities,** each containing a lung, and the **mediastinum** (me'-dee-as-**tie**'-num) between them. Within the mediastinum lies the heart, thymus gland, and parts of the esophagus and trachea. The heart is surrounded by yet another cavity, the **pericardial** (per'-ee-**kar**'-dee-al) **cavity.**

The upper portion of the abdominopelvic cavity is the **abdominal cavity,** which contains the stomach, small intestine, much of the large intestine, liver, pancreas, spleen, kidneys, and ureters. Although not separated by any kind of wall, the lower portion of the abdominopelvic cavity is the **pelvic cavity,** which holds the urinary bladder, part of the large intestine, and, in the female, the reproductive organs. In males, the pelvic cavity has a small outpocket called the *scrotal cavity,* which contains the testes.

To help describe the location of internal organs or locate pain, health professionals divide the abdominopelvic cavity into four quadrants: right upper, right lower, left lower, and left upper (Figure 1-9, *A*). These quadrants are established by a midsagittal and a transverse plane that pass through the umbilicus. Another system divides the abdominopelvic cavity into nine regions according to two transverse and two sagittal planes. These nine regions of the abdomen are indicated in Figure 1-9, *B*.

It Is Important to View the Body as a Whole

This chapter has introduced you to the organization of the body and its systems. You have examined the principal regions and cavities of the body and have learned to follow anatomical directions and to visualize body planes and sections. Now you can begin to integrate all these bits of knowledge and view the body as a whole functioning organism.

Figure 1-10 shows some of the major organs of the body so that you can view them in relation to one another and to the body as an integrated, functioning organism. Anterior structures have been progressively removed in Figures 1-11 and 1-12 so that you can study the relationship of the deeper organs. Figure 1-13 is a posterior view.

A different perspective is provided in Figure 1-14. There, transverse sections through the head, mediastinum, and abdomen give you the opportunity to study the relationships between anterior and posterior structures within each of these body regions.

Quiz Yourself

- Using anatomical directional terms, locate the heart in relation to the brain and the kidney in relation to the heart.
- What are the three main planes of the body?
- To which part of the body does each of the following terms refer: (a) orbital, (b) plantar, (c) tarsal?
- What are the subdivisions of the ventral cavity?

Text continues on p. 20.

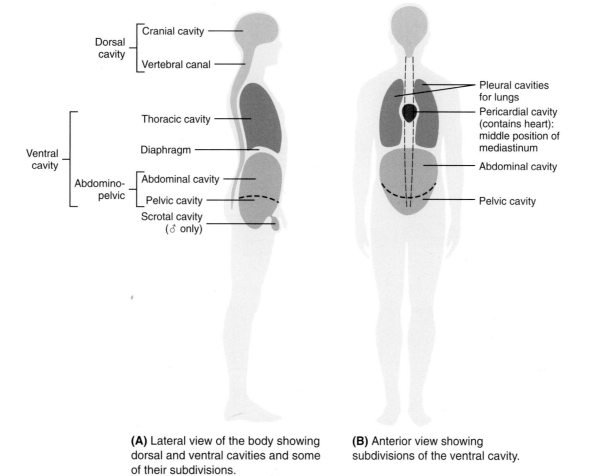

(A) Lateral view of the body showing dorsal and ventral cavities and some of their subdivisions.

(B) Anterior view showing subdivisions of the ventral cavity.

FIGURE 1-8 • Principal cavities of the human body.

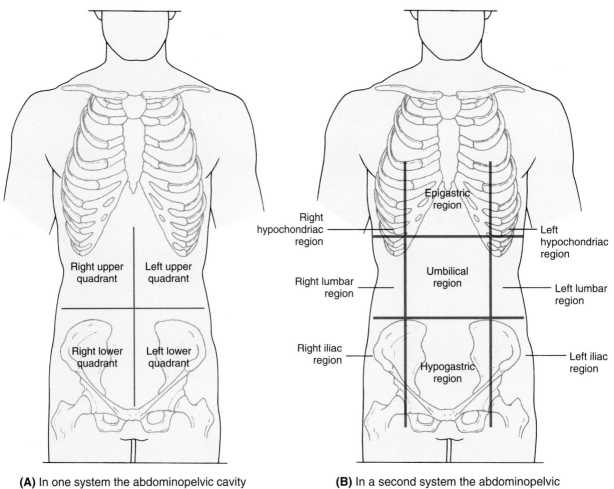

(A) In one system the abdominopelvic cavity is divided into four quadrants by drawing imaginary transverse and sagittal lines through the umbilicus (navel).

(B) In a second system the abdominopelvic cavity is divided into nine regions using two transverse and two sagittal planes.

FIGURE 1-9 • The abdominopelvic cavity can be divided into regions that can be used clinically to locate internal organs.

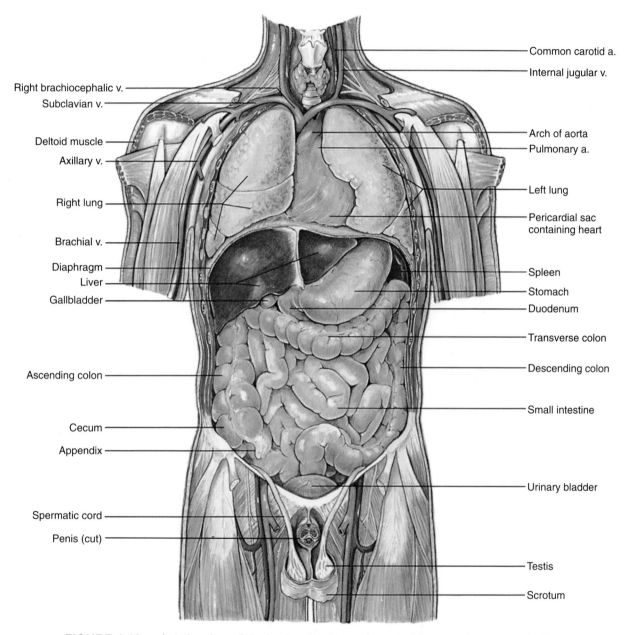

Right brachiocephalic v.
Subclavian v.
Deltoid muscle
Axillary v.
Right lung
Brachial v.
Diaphragm
Liver
Gallbladder
Ascending colon
Cecum
Appendix
Spermatic cord
Penis (cut)

Common carotid a.
Internal jugular v.
Arch of aorta
Pulmonary a.
Left lung
Pericardial sac containing heart
Spleen
Stomach
Duodenum
Transverse colon
Descending colon
Small intestine
Urinary bladder
Testis
Scrotum

FIGURE 1-10 • Anterior view of the body with skin and most of the muscles removed. The rib cage and the fatty membrane that hangs down from the stomach have also been removed. The scrotum has been opened to expose the testes, and the penis has been cut transversely to show its inner structure. *v.,* Vein; *a.,* artery. Many of the structures shown here and in Figures 1-11 through 1-14 are discussed in later chapters.

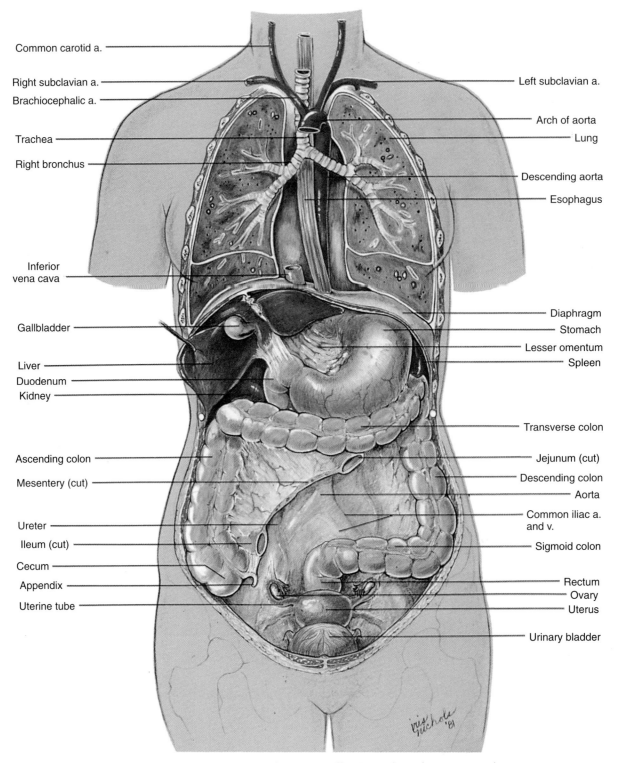

Common carotid a.

Right subclavian a.
Brachiocephalic a.

Trachea

Right bronchus

Inferior
vena cava

Gallbladder

Liver
Duodenum
Kidney

Ascending colon

Mesentery (cut)

Ureter
Ileum (cut)
Cecum
Appendix
Uterine tube

Left subclavian a.

Arch of aorta
Lung

Descending aorta
Esophagus

Diaphragm
Stomach
Lesser omentum
Spleen

Transverse colon

Jejunum (cut)
Descending colon
Aorta
Common iliac a.
and v.
Sigmoid colon

Rectum
Ovary
Uterus

Urinary bladder

FIGURE 1-11 • Deeper anterior view of the body. The lungs have been cut to show internal structure, and the heart and small intestine have been removed. *v., Vein; a.,* artery.

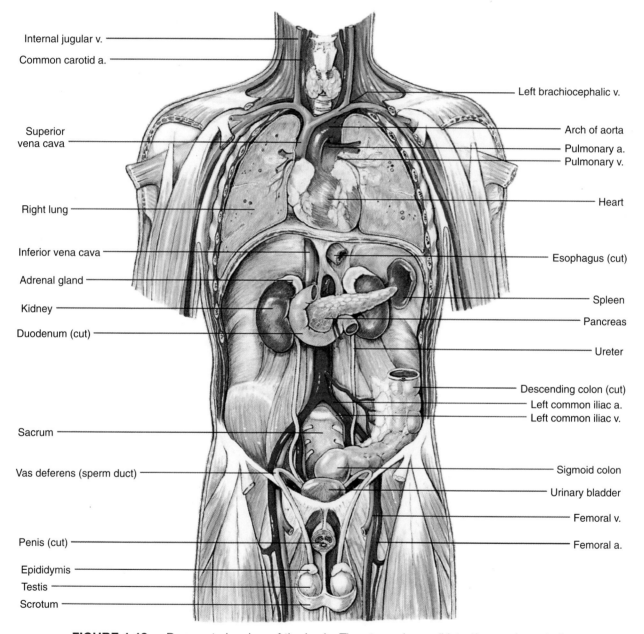

Internal jugular v.

Common carotid a.

Left brachiocephalic v.

Superior
vena cava

Arch of aorta

Pulmonary a.

Pulmonary v.

Right lung

Heart

Inferior vena cava

Esophagus (cut)

Adrenal gland

Spleen

Kidney

Pancreas

Duodenum (cut)

Ureter

Descending colon (cut)

Left common iliac a.

Left common iliac v.

Sacrum

Vas deferens (sperm duct)

Sigmoid colon

Urinary bladder

Femoral v.

Penis (cut)

Femoral a.

Epididymis

Testis

Scrotum

FIGURE 1-12 • Deep anterior view of the body. The stomach, small intestine, and most of the large intestine have been removed. The kidneys, pancreas, and other deep structures are visible. *v.*, Vein; *a.*, artery.

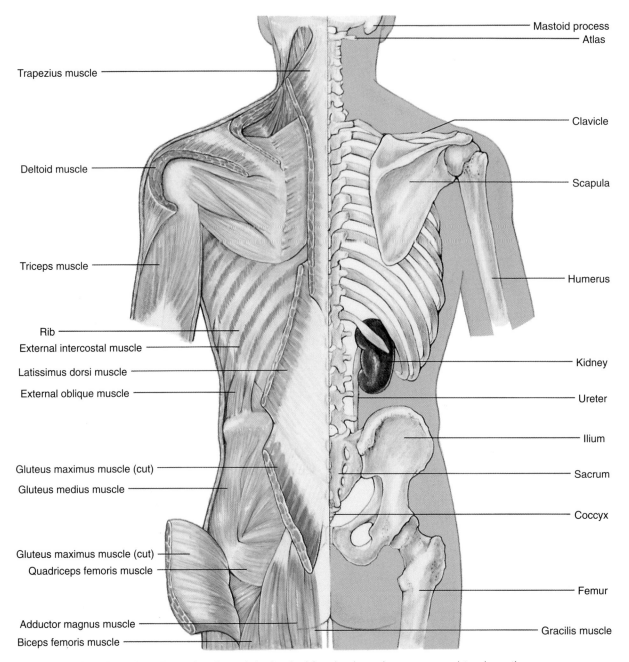

FIGURE 1-13 • Posterior view of the body. Muscles have been removed to show the skeletal structures and position of the kidneys.

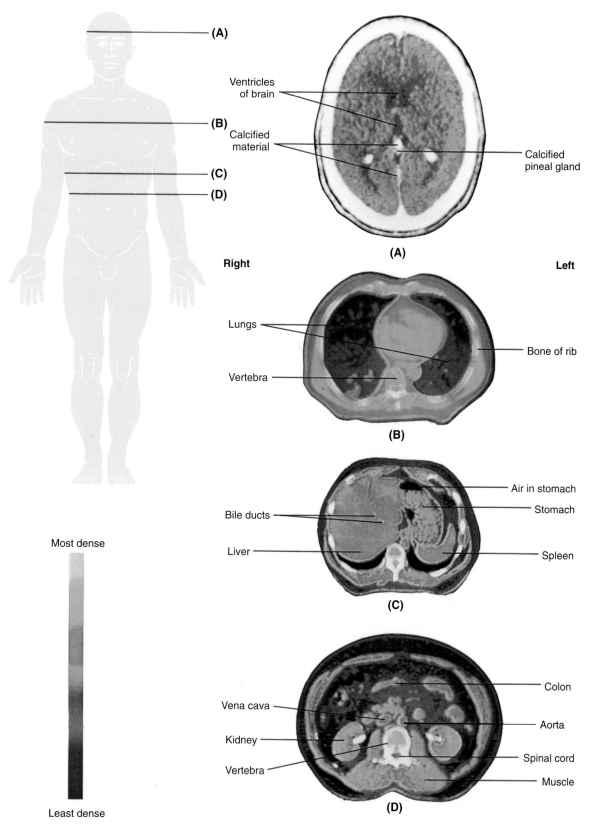

FIGURE 1-14 • A series of computed tomography scans through various regions of the body. The level of the scan is indicated on the figure of the body. The color spectrum bar indicates the gradient of structure density as represented by color. The most dense structures, such as bone, appear white in the scans. The least dense structures appear red. (Computed tomography scans courtesy Professor Jon H. Ehringer.)

SUMMARY

LO 1. Define anatomy and physiology.
- **Anatomy** is the science of body structure; **physiology** is the study of function, or how the body works.

LO 2. Describe the levels of biological organization in the human body, from the simplest (the chemical level) to the most complex (the organism).
- The simplest level of organization is the **chemical level,** consisting of **atoms** and **molecules.**
- Atoms and molecules associate to form the **organelles** and **cells** of the **cellular level.**
- Cells associate to form **tissues** such as muscle or bone tissue, and tissues may be organized to form **organs** such as the brain or heart.
- Certain tissues and organs function together to make up an **organ system,** or **body system.** The body systems work together to make up the human **organism.**

LO 3. Describe the principal organ systems.
- The human organism is made up of 11 main organ systems that work together to maintain life.
- The **integumentary system** provides a protective covering for the body and helps to regulate body temperature. The **skeletal system** helps support and protect the body and works with the **muscular system** to carry out effective movement.
- The **nervous system** is the principal regulatory system. The nervous system works with the **endocrine system** to regulate metabolic activities. The endocrine system secretes chemical messengers called **hormones.**
- The **digestive system** breaks down food and absorbs nutrients into the blood. The **respiratory system** delivers oxygen to the blood and removes carbon dioxide from the body.
- The **cardiovascular system** transports nutrients, oxygen, hormones, and other substances to the body cells and carries wastes from the cells to the excretory organs. The **lymphatic system** collects excess tissue fluid and returns it to the blood and defends the body against organisms that cause disease. The **urinary system** functions to excrete metabolic wastes and helps regulate fluid balance and acid-base balance.

LO = Learning Objective

- The **reproductive system** of the male produces and delivers sperm; the reproductive system of the female produces ova and incubates the developing offspring. Both systems release hormones that establish and maintain sexuality.

LO 4. Distinguish between inorganic and organic compounds and briefly describe four important groups of organic compounds.
- **Inorganic compounds** are relatively small, simple **chemical compounds** such as water, salts, and simple acids and bases. **Organic compounds** are large, complex compounds containing carbon.
- Four important groups of organic compounds are carbohydrates, lipids, proteins, and nucleic acids.
- **Carbohydrates** are sugars and starches. They are used as fuel and to store energy.
- **Lipids** include fats, compounds that store energy; phospholipids, which are components of cell membranes; and steroids, which include several hormones.
- **Proteins** are complex compounds composed of **amino acids;** some serve as enzymes and others function as structural components of cells.
- **Nucleic acids** are large, complex compounds. Two important nucleic acids are **DNA,** which makes up the genes, and **RNA,** which is important in making proteins.

LO 5. Define metabolism and contrast anabolism and catabolism.
- The chemical activities that take place in the body are its **metabolism.**
- During **anabolism** energy is used to make chemical compounds and structures needed by the cell.
- **Catabolism,** the breaking-down phase of metabolism, provides the energy required for anabolism, the building phase of metabolism. **Cellular respiration** is a catabolic process in which nutrients are broken down and their energy packaged for use by the cell.

LO 6. Define homeostasis and contrast negative and positive feedback mechanisms.
- Metabolic activities are carefully regulated to maintain **homeostasis**—an appropriate internal environment, or steady state.

- **Homeostatic mechanisms** are the self-regulating control systems that maintain homeostasis. **Stressors,** stimuli that disrupt homeostasis, cause **stress** that activates homeostatic mechanisms.
- Many homeostatic mechanisms are **negative feedback systems,** in which the response of the regulator (control center) is opposite (negative) to the change.
- Some homeostatic mechanisms are **positive feedback systems,** in which variation from the steady state sets off a series of events that intensify the change.

LO 7. **Describe the anatomical position of the human body.**
- Anatomical directional terms are applied to the body when it is in the **anatomical position.** In this position the body is standing erect, eyes looking forward, arms at the sides, and palms and toes directed forward.

LO 8. **Define and use properly the principal directional terms used in human anatomy.**
- The principal directional terms are the following:

Term	Orientation
Superior (cephalic)	Upward; toward the head
Inferior (caudad)	Downward; toward the feet
Anterior (ventral)	Belly surface; toward the front of the body
Posterior (dorsal)	Back surface; toward the back of the body
Medial	Toward the midline
Lateral	Toward the side
Proximal	Toward the midline or point of attachment to the trunk
Distal	Away from the midline or point of attachment to the trunk
Superficial	Toward the body surface
Deep	Within the body

LO 9. **Recognize sagittal, transverse, and frontal sections of the body and of body structures.**
- We can distinguish three main sections, or planes (imaginary flat surfaces), that divide the body into specific parts. A **sagittal plane** divides the body into right and left parts. A **transverse** (or **cross**) **plane** divides the body into superior and inferior parts. A **frontal** (or **coronal**) **plane** divides the body into anterior and posterior parts.

LO 10. **Define and locate the principal regions and cavities of the body.**
- The body may be divided into **axial** and **appendicular regions.** The axial portion consists of the head, neck, and trunk. The appendicular portion consists of the limbs. The **torso,** or trunk, consists of the thorax, abdomen, and pelvis.
- Terms such as **abdominal, pectoral,** and **lumbar** are used to refer to specific body regions or structures (see pp. 11 and 12).
- Two principal **body cavities** are the dorsal cavity and the ventral cavity. The **dorsal cavity** includes the **cranial cavity** and the **vertebral canal.**
- The **ventral cavity** is principally subdivided into the **thoracic cavity** and the **abdominopelvic cavity.** The two cavities are separated by the **diaphragm,** a broad muscle.
- The thoracic cavity includes the **pleural cavities** that hold the lungs and the **mediastinum,** where the heart is located. The upper part of the abdominopelvic cavity is the **abdominal cavity;** the lower part is the **pelvic cavity.**

CHAPTER QUIZ

Fill in the Blank

1. The science of body structure is called _____; the study of body function is called _____.

2. The chemical processes that take place in the body are collectively referred to as its _____.

3. The breaking-down part of metabolism is called _____.

4. _____ refers to the balanced, appropriate internal environment.

5. Atoms combine chemically to form _____.

6. The basic building blocks of the body are called _____.

7. Various types of tissues may be organized to form _____.

8. Chemical messengers released by endocrine glands are called _____.

Multiple Choice

9. The body's principal regulatory system is the: a. endocrine system; b. integumentary system; c. cardiovascular system; d. nervous system.

10. The organ system that defends the body against disease organisms is the: a. endocrine system; b. integumentary system; c. lymphatic system; d. respiratory system.

11. The organ system that supports and protects the body is the: a. skeletal system; b. muscular system; c. respiratory system; d. nervous system.

12. The transportation system of the body is the: a. endocrine system; b. integumentary system; c. cardiovascular system; d. urinary system.

13. The organ system that maintains adequate blood oxygen content is the: a. endocrine system; b. integumentary system; c. respiratory system; d. urinary system.

14. Ductless glands that release hormones are part of the: a. endocrine system; b. integumentary system; c. lymphatic system; d. urinary system.

Matching

Select the most appropriate match in column B for each item in column A.

Column A	Column B
15. Heart in relation to lung	a. superficial
16. Wrist in relation to elbow	b. medial
17. Knee in relation to ankle	c. lateral
18. Skin in relation to muscle	d. deep
19. Stomach in relation to backbone	e. proximal
	f. distal
	g. anterior
	h. posterior

Matching

Select the most appropriate match in column B for each item in column A.

Column A	Column B
20. Head	a. cervical
21. Skull	b. cephalic
22. Skin	c. cranial
23. Chest	d. cutaneous
24. Neck	e. pectoral
25. Armpit	f. axillary

REVIEW QUESTIONS

1. Describe the position of each of the following using anatomic terms: (a) navel; (b) ear; (c) great toe; (d) elbow; (e) backbone.

2. Define homeostasis, and give an example. Describe how your example is regulated by negative feedback mechanisms.

3. List in sequence the levels of organization within the human organism, from atom to organism.

4. What are the functions of each body system?

5. Define anatomical position.

6. Identify the body cavities described in this chapter and identify an organ or structure found in each.

7. Define each of the following: (a) cephalic; (b) cervical; (c) cranial; (d) abdominal; (e) sagittal; (f) proximal; (g) distal; (h) bilateral symmetry.

8. Label the diagram. (See Figure 1-10 to check your answers.)

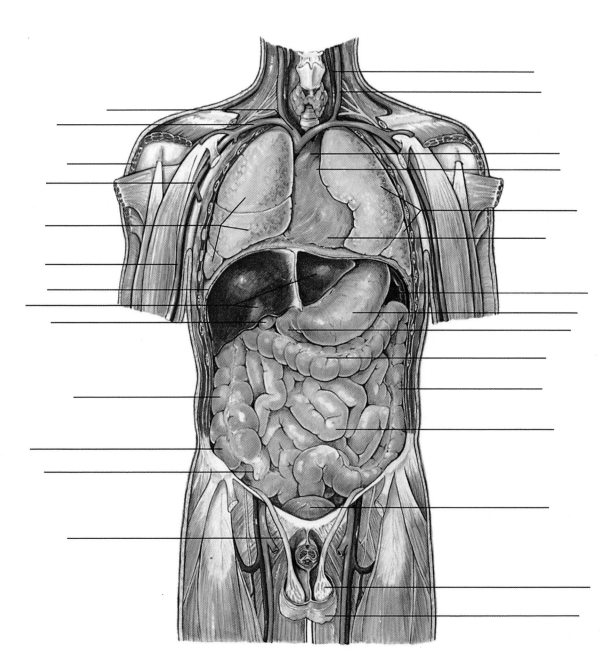

2

Cells and Tissues

Chapter Outline

In Chapter 1 we learned that cells are the living building blocks of the body and that cells associate to form tissues. Each of us began life as a single cell—the fertilized egg. That cell gave rise to the millions of cells that make up the complex tissues, organs, and systems of the body. In this chapter we examine more closely the structure and function of cells and tissues.

THE CELL CONTAINS ORGANELLES THAT PERFORM SPECIFIC FUNCTIONS

LEARNING OBJECTIVES

1. Describe the general characteristics of cells.
2. State three functions of cell membranes and describe the structure of the plasma membrane.
3. Describe the structure and functions of the cell nucleus.
4. Describe, locate, and list the functions of the principal cytoplasmic organelles and label them on a diagram.

The cell is an amazingly complex structure. It has a control center, internal transportation system, power plants, factories for making needed materials, and packaging plants. Despite their complexity, most cells are so small that they can be studied only under a microscope.

The microscope is one of the biologist's most important tools for studying the internal structure of cells. Most cell structures were first identified with an ordinary **light microscope,** which uses visible light as the source of illumination. (This is the kind of microscope used by students in most college laboratories.) The development of the **electron microscope,** which came into widespread use in the 1950s, enabled researchers to study the fine detail (ultrastructure) of cells and their parts. The electron microscope uses an electron beam of energized electrons.

Although the ordinary light microscope can magnify a structure about a thousand times, the electron microscope can magnify it 250,000 times or more. The electron microscope also has much greater resolving power—the ability to distinguish fine detail in an image. Two main types of electron microscopes are the transmission electron microscope, which images thin cross sections of cells, and the scanning electron microscope, which views the surface of a specimen. Photographs taken with the light microscope are referred to as **light photomicrographs (LMs),** whereas those taken with the electron microscope are **electron micrographs (EMs).**

The size and shape of a cell are related to the specific functions it must perform (Figure 2-1). For instance, sperm cells are tiny cells with long, whiplike tails (called *flagella*). The tail is used to move toward the ovum, or egg. The ovum is one of the largest cells in the human body, but even it is only about as large as a period on this page. Epithelial cells, which look like little building blocks, cover body surfaces and line body cavities. Muscle cells are elongated and specialized for contraction. Nerve cells have long extensions that permit them to transmit messages over long distances within the body. Lymphocytes, a type of white blood cell, change their shape as they move through the tissues of the body, destroying invading bacteria.

The jellylike material of the cell is called **cytoplasm** (sy′-toe-plazm). A great variety of substances needed by the cell are dissolved within the cytoplasm. For example, amino acids found in the cytoplasm are used as subunits of proteins. Scattered throughout the cell are specialized **organelles** (little organs)—structures that perform jobs within the cell (Figure 2-2).

Membranes Surround the Cell and Divide It Into Compartments

Many of the organelles within the cell are enclosed by membranes that partition the cytoplasm into different compartments. Specific cell activities can be localized within these compartments, and different processes can take place in different compartments. Membranes also serve as work surfaces. For example, many types of enzymes (proteins that speed specific chemical reactions) are bound to membranes.

Every cell is surrounded by a thin **plasma membrane** that protects the cell and regulates the passage of materials into and out of the cell. The plasma membrane consists of a double layer (bilayer) of lipids in which a variety of proteins are embedded (Figure 2-3, *A*, p. 28). Many of the lipids are **phospholipids,** lipids that contain phosphorus. The positions of the proteins change as they move about like icebergs in a fluid sea of phospholipids. Some of the proteins form channels that selectively permit the passage of certain substances through the membrane (Figure 2-3, *B*, p. 28).

The Nucleus Controls Cell Activities

The **nucleus,** a large, rounded organelle, is the control center of the cell. In a cell that is not in the process of dividing, the nucleus contains loosely coiled material called chromatin (**krow′**-muh-tin). When a cell prepares to divide, the chromatin becomes more tightly coiled and condenses to form rod-shaped bodies, the **chromosomes** (**krow′**-mah-sowms). Each chromosome contains hundreds or thousands of **genes**—units of hereditary information that govern the structure and activity of the cell. The genes, which are arranged in a specific linear order, are composed of the chemical compound **DNA.** We can think of the chromosomes as a chemical cookbook for the cell, and each gene is a recipe for making a specific protein.

The complete set of genes that make up the human genetic material is the human **genome** (jee′-nome). The **Human Genome Project,** completed in 2003, mapped the 30,000 or so genes that make up the human genome. Researchers continue to study the proteins coded by the genes. Genome research is providing knowledge that can be applied to prevention and treatment of many human disorders.

The **nucleolus** (new-**klee′**-oh-lus) (little nucleus) is a specialized region within the nucleus. The nucleolus assembles ribosomes, organelles that help manufacture proteins.

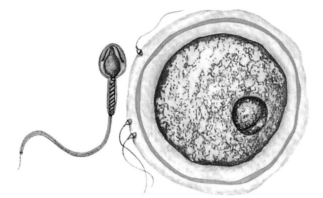
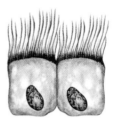

(A) Ova (eggs) are among the largest cells in the body. Sperm cells are among the smallest. Note the long tail (called a flagellum), which is used by the sperm cell in locomotion.

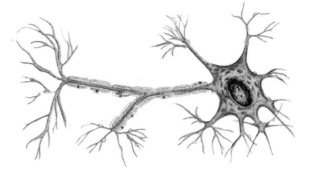

(B) Epithelial cells join to form tissues that cover body surfaces and line body cavities.

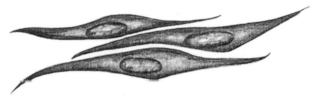

(C) Smooth muscle fibers form the involuntary muscle tissues of the internal organs. For example, smooth muscle in the wall of the digestive tract moves food through the intestine.

(D) Nerve cells (neurons) are specialized to transmit messages from one part of the body to another.

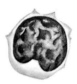

(E) Lymphocytes are a type of white blood cell. They move through the tissues of the body and destroy invading disease organisms.

FIGURE 2-1 • The size and shape of cells are related to their functions.

The Cytoplasm Contains Many Types of Organelles

The **endoplasmic** (en'-doe-**plaz'**-mik) **reticulum** (reh-**tik'**-yoo-lum) **(ER)** is a system of membranes that extends throughout the cytoplasm of many cells. The ER is somewhat like a complex tunnel system through which materials can be transported from one part of the cell to another.

Two types of ER can be distinguished: smooth and rough. **Rough ER** has a granular appearance that results from the presence of organelles called **ribosomes** (**rye'**-bow-sowms) along its outer walls. Ribosomes function as factories where proteins are manufactured. **Smooth ER** is the main site of steroid, phospholipid, and fatty acid synthesis. In liver cells, enzymes in the smooth ER break down many drugs, including alcohol and amphetamines. These enzymes also break down

many toxic chemicals, including some agents that cause cancer.

Looking somewhat like stacks of pancakes, the **Golgi** (**goal'**-jee) **complex** is composed of layers of platelike membranes. This organelle functions as a protein processing and packaging plant. An important function of the Golgi complex is to produce **lysosomes** (**lye'**-so-sowms). These little sacs contain about 40 different digestive enzymes that destroy bacteria and other foreign matter. Under some conditions, lysosomes break down organelles; the components of these organelles can then be recycled or used as an energy source.

Cells contain power plants called **mitochondria** (my'-tow-**kon'**-dree-ah). These organelles carry on **cellular respiration,** the process of breaking down fuel molecules and releasing their energy. Some of the energy is temporarily stored in **ATP**

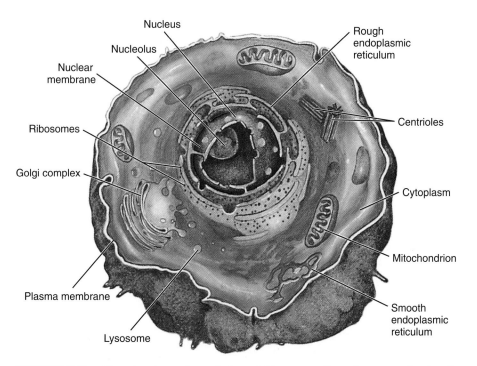

Nucleus

Nucleolus

Nuclear membrane

Ribosomes

Golgi complex

Plasma membrane

Lysosome

Rough endoplasmic reticulum

Centrioles

Cytoplasm

Mitochondrion

Smooth endoplasmic reticulum

FIGURE 2-2 • The structure of a cell. An artist's conception of a generalized cell.

(adenosine triphosphate), a chemical compound that can be used to power a variety of chemical reactions in the cell. Mitochondria can affect health and aging by leaking electrons that form **free radicals.** These toxic, highly reactive compounds interfere with normal cell function. Mitochondria also play an important role in programmed cell death, referred to as **apoptosis** (ap-oh-**toe′**-sis). Apoptosis is a normal part of development and maintenance. For example, cells in the outer layer of the human skin and in the intestinal wall are continuously destroyed by apoptosis and replaced by new cells.

A **vesicle** is a small membrane-enclosed structure that holds or transports some type of cargo within the cell. A **vacuole** (**vac′**-you-ole) is a larger membrane-enclosed sac found in the cytoplasm. Vacuoles form when a cell ingests a large particle such as a bacterium (see discussion of phagocytosis later in this chapter).

The shape of a cell and its ability to move are determined in large part by its **cytoskeleton,** a dense network of protein filaments (tiny fibers). The cytoskeleton is also important in cell division and in transporting materials within the cell. The cytoskeleton is composed of three types of protein filaments: microtubules, microfilaments, and intermediate filaments. **Microtubules** are tiny hollow tubes.

Cilia and flagella, two types of organelles important in movement, are composed of microtubules. **Cilia** (**sil′**-ee-ah), tiny hairlike organelles projecting from the surfaces of some types of cells, help to move materials outside the cell. For example, the cells lining the respiratory passages are equipped with cilia, which continuously beat a layer

of mucus away from the lungs. The mucus traps particles of dirt that are inhaled. Each human sperm cell is equipped with a whiplike tail, or **flagellum** (flah-**jel′**-um), that is used in locomotion.

Quiz Yourself

- What are organelles?
- What is the composition of the plasma membrane?
- What are the functions of the nucleus?
- What are the functions of mitochondria? Of lysosomes?

MATERIALS MOVE THROUGH THE PLASMA MEMBRANE BY BOTH PASSIVE AND ACTIVE PROCESSES

LEARNING OBJECTIVES

5. **Explain how materials pass through cell membranes, distinguishing between passive and active processes.**
6. **Predict whether cells will swell or shrink under various osmotic conditions.**

The plasma membrane is **selectively permeable.** This means that it allows certain materials to enter or leave the cell while preventing the passage of other materials.

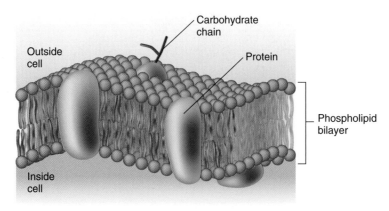

(A) The plasma membrane is a fluid bilayer of lipids in which proteins are embedded. Carbohydrate chains attached to proteins help cells recognize one another, and some are important in cells adhering to one another to form tissues.

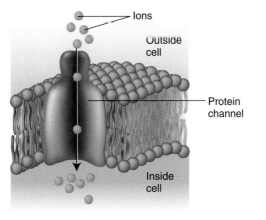

(B) Passive transport through the plasma membrane. Some plasma proteins form channels that allow certain ions or molecules to pass into (or out of) the cell.

FIGURE 2-3 • The plasma membrane.

Passive Transport Does Not Require the Cell to Expend Metabolic Energy

Some materials move through cell membranes passively by physical processes such as diffusion, osmosis, and filtration. These processes do not require the cell to expend metabolic energy.

Diffusion is the net movement of molecules or ions from a region of higher concentration to a region of lower concentration brought about by the energy of the molecules. Diffusion depends on the random movement of individual molecules. The molecules are propelled by collision with other molecules or with the sides of the container. Molecules tend to move down a **concentration gradient,** that is, from where they are more concentrated to where they are less concentrated (Figure

2-4). Eventually the molecules are evenly distributed. Gases and many nutrients move in and out of cells by diffusion.

Osmosis (oz-**mow'**-sis) is the diffusion of water molecules through a selectively permeable membrane from a region where water molecules are more concentrated to a region where they are less concentrated. Recall that the plasma membrane is a selectively permeable membrane. The dissolved ions and molecules (solute) in the more concentrated solution "pull" the water molecules across the membrane. This pulling force is known as **osmotic pressure.**

When living cells are placed in a solution that has a solute concentration that is **isotonic** (equal) to that of the cells, the water molecule concentration is also equal and therefore water molecules move in and out of the cells at the same rate. The net movement of the water molecules is zero (Figure 2-5).

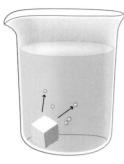 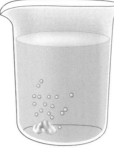 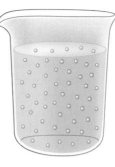

(A) When a lump of sugar is dropped into a beaker of water, its molecules dissolve.

(B) The molecules begin to diffuse through the water.

(C) Eventually, the sugar molecules are evenly distributed throughout the water.

FIGURE 2-4 • Diffusion.

Solute molecules

Water molecules

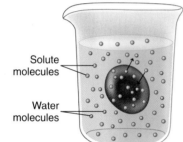 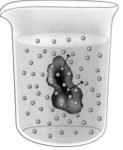 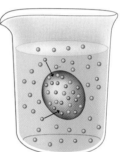

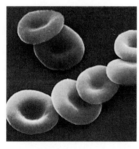 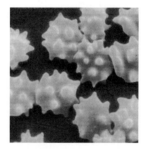 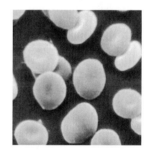

(A) Isotonic solution. When cells are placed in an isotonic solution (one that has the same concentration of solutes as the cells), the net movement of water molecules is zero.

(B) Hypertonic solution. When cells are placed in a hypertonic solution (one with a greater solute concentration than the cells), the solution exerts an osmotic pressure on the cells. This results in a net movement of water molecules out of the cells, causing them to dehydrate, shrink, and perhaps die.

(C) Hypotonic solution. When cells are placed in a hypotonic solution (a solution with a lower solute concentration than the cells), the cell contents exert an osmotic pressure on the solution, drawing water molecules inward. The net diffusion of water molecules into the cells causes them to swell and perhaps even to burst.

FIGURE 2-5 • Osmosis and the living cell. Drawings and photomicrographs show red blood cells. (Micrographs of human red blood cells courtesy Dr. R.F. Baker, University of Southern California Medical School.)

When cells are placed in a solution with a solute concentration that is **hypertonic** (greater compared with that of the cell), water leaves the cells, causing them to dehydrate, shrink, and perhaps die. When cells are placed in a **hypotonic** solution (one of lesser concentration compared with that of the cell), the cell exerts an osmotic pressure on the solution. Water moves into the cells, causing them to swell and perhaps burst.

Filtration is the passage of materials through membranes by mechanical pressure. For example, blood pressure forces some of the liquid part of the blood (plasma) through the capillary wall by filtration. This is how tissue fluid is formed.

Active Transport Requires Metabolic Energy

The cell must actively move some materials from a region of lower concentration to a region of higher concentration, that is, *against* a concentration gradient. Working "uphill" against a concentration gradient requires the cell to expend energy. Thus, in **active transport,** the cell must use some of its stored energy. The cell uses the energy of ATP to drive active transport.

Important examples of active transport are the **sodium-potassium pumps** found in the plasma membrane of virtually all cells in the body. Each pump consists of a group of specific proteins in the plasma membrane. ATP provides energy to pump sodium ions out of the cell. At the same time, potassium ions are moved into the cell.

Phagocytosis (fag'-oh-sigh-**tow**'-sis), which means "cell eating," is a form of active transport. In phagocytosis, the cell ingests large, solid particles such as food or bacteria (Figure 2-6). A small part of the plasma membrane surrounds the particle to be ingested, forming a small vacuole (sac), like a tiny plastic sandwich bag, around it. The vacuole then pinches off from the plasma membrane and floats around in the cytoplasm. White blood cells ingest invading bacteria in this way. Then, lysosomes fuse with the vesicle containing the bacteria. The lysosomes pour their powerful digestive enzymes on the bacteria, destroying them.

⊚ *Quiz Yourself*

- How does active transport differ from diffusion?
- What happens when you place red blood cells in a hypertonic solution? A hypotonic solution?

CELLS COMMUNICATE BY SIGNALING ONE ANOTHER

LEARNING OBJECTIVE

7. **Describe the events that take place in cell signaling.**

Cells of the body must communicate with one another to carry out essential processes. For example, cells must recognize one

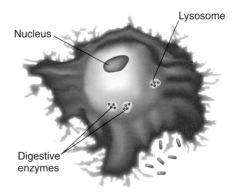

(A) The cell ingests large solid particles such as bacteria. Folds of the plasma membrane surround the particle to be ingested, forming a vacuole around it.

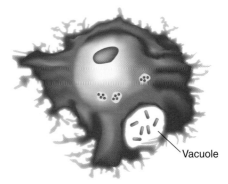

(B) The vacuole then pinches off inside the cell.

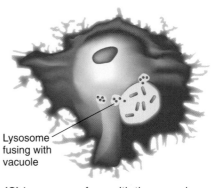

(C) Lysosomes fuse with the vacuole and pour digestive enzymes onto the ingested bacteria.

FIGURE 2-6 • Phagocytosis.

another to form tissues. They signal information about the condition of the body and then send signals to initiate or terminate homeostatic processes. Many types of cells must communicate to protect the body against invading disease organisms.

Cell communication, often referred to as **cell signaling,** takes place through a series of processes (Figure 2-7). First, a cell must send a signal. Cells typically use chemical signals such

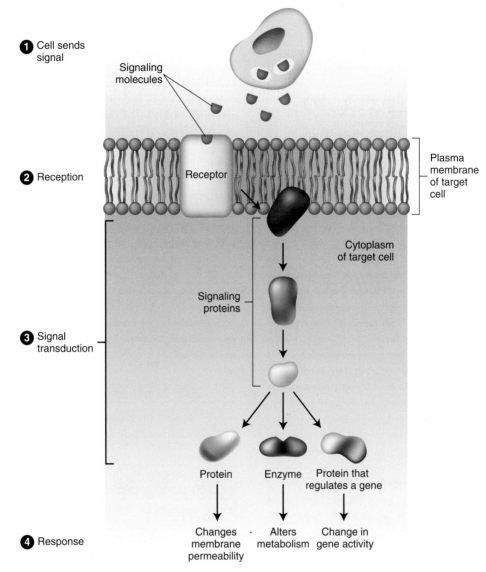

① Cell sends signal

Signaling molecules

② Reception

Receptor

Plasma membrane of target cell

Cytoplasm of target cell

Signaling proteins

③ Signal transduction

Protein   Enzyme   Protein that regulates a gene

④ Response

Changes membrane permeability   Alters metabolism   Change in gene activity

FIGURE 2-7 • Cell signaling. Note that various proteins have different sizes and shapes.

as hormones and other regulatory molecules. Second, **target cells,** the cells that can respond to the particular signal, must receive the signal. This process is called **reception.** In many cases the signal molecules bind to **receptors,** specific molecules on the surface of the target cells that receive chemical messages.

In the third process, the receptor relays information into the cell. Many signal molecules do not enter the cell. Instead, the receptor relays the information through a series of molecules in the plasma membrane and then into the cell. The process by which a receptor converts a signal outside the cell into a signal inside the cell that affects some cellular process is called **signal transduction.**

The final process in cell communication is the **response** by the cell. The cell responds to signals by changing some activity.

Signal molecules may signal the cell to open or close channels in the plasma membrane, affecting the permeability of the membrane. Some signals activate or inhibit specific enzymes. Other signals activate or inhibit specific genes. You will learn more about cell signaling in the discussions of muscle contraction, nerve function, and hormones.

Ⓞ *Quiz Yourself*

• What are the four processes in cell communication? Describe each.

CELLS DIVIDE BY MITOSIS, FORMING GENETICALLY IDENTICAL CELLS

LEARNING OBJECTIVE

8. **Describe the stages of a cell's life cycle and summarize the significance of mitosis with respect to maintaining a constant chromosome number.**

Certain types of cells in the body divide almost continuously. For example, as many as 10 million blood cells are produced every second. Other cells, such as red blood cells, do not divide once they mature.

Before a cell divides to form two cells, the chromosomes are precisely duplicated and the cell undergoes **mitosis** (my-**tow'**-sis). In mitosis, a complete set of chromosomes is distributed to each end of the parent cell. After the parent cell divides, each new cell contains the identical number and types of chromosomes present in the parent cell.

When a fertilized egg divides, each of the new cells receives a complete copy of all its genetic information. During development, hundreds of divisions take place. Most cells in the body contain a complete set of the original chromosomes contributed by the sperm and egg. (Sex cells and mature red blood cells are exceptions. Developing sperm and ova undergo a special process called *meiosis,* which halves their number of chromosomes.)

The life cycle of the cell may be divided into five phases: interphase, prophase, metaphase, anaphase, and telophase (Figure 2-8). The cell spends most of its life in **interphase** (meaning between phases), the period between mitoses. During interphase the cell actively makes new materials and grows. Before mitosis actually begins, the genetic material is duplicated.

During **prophase** (**pro'**-faze), the first stage of mitosis, the chromatin (diffuse strands of genetic material) coils tightly, forming structures that are visible as dark, X-shaped bodies under the light microscope. These are the chromosomes. Each chromosome was duplicated during interphase, but the duplicated chromosome pairs, called **sister chromatids,** remain attached during the first two phases of mitosis.

During prophase, the nucleolus becomes smaller and disappears and the nuclear membrane dissolves. Two pairs of **centrioles,** cylindrical organelles composed of microtubules, function during mitosis. Each pair of centrioles migrates toward an opposite end of the cell. Microtubules in the cytoplasm form a spindle-shaped structure that extends throughout the cell.

During **metaphase** (**met'**-ah-faze), the second phase of mitosis, the chromatids are positioned along the equator of the cell. Each chromatid is now completely coiled so that it appears quite thick. In fact, chromatids can be seen so clearly in metaphase that they can be photographed and studied to determine whether any are abnormal. Threads of the spindle attach to the chromosomes.

During **anaphase** (**an'**-ah-faze) the sister chromatids separate and become independent chromosomes. The duplicated chromosome pairs start to move away from one another. The protein threads of the spindle begin to pull one set of chromosomes to one end of the spindle and the other set to the opposite end.

With the arrival of a complete set of chromosomes at each end of the cell, **telophase** (**tel'**-ah-faze) begins. Each chromosome now begins to uncoil and disperse. The spindle disappears, and a nuclear membrane forms around each set of chromosomes. During telophase, the cell typically constricts around its center and continues to constrict until it has completely divided to form two cells. Each new cell now enters interphase and begins a new cell cycle.

Mitosis ensures that during cell division all the genetic information contained within the chromosomes is precisely duplicated and distributed to each new cell. No genetic information is lost, and no new information is added. Each of the two new cells has the potential to function exactly like the parent cell.

Quiz Yourself

- What are the stages in the life cycle of a cell?
- Why is mitosis important?

TISSUES ARE THE FABRIC OF THE BODY

LEARNING OBJECTIVES

9. **Define the term *tissue* and describe the structure and functions of the principal types of tissues.**
10. **Contrast epithelial tissue with connective tissue.**
11. **Compare the three types of muscle tissue.**

As defined in Chapter 1, a **tissue** is a group of closely associated cells that work together to carry out a specific function or group of functions. Four principal types of tissue make up the body: epithelial tissue, connective tissue, muscle tissue, and nervous tissue. The microscopic study of tissues is called **histology** (his-**tol'**-oh-jee).

Epithelial Tissue Protects the Body

Epithelial tissue, also called **epithelium** (ep'-ih-**theel'**-ee-um), protects the body by covering all its free surfaces and lining its cavities. Some epithelial cells are specialized to *secrete* substances—for example, sweat or mucus. In some parts of the body, epithelial tissue is specialized to *absorb* certain materials. For example, epithelium lining the digestive tract absorbs molecules of digested food.

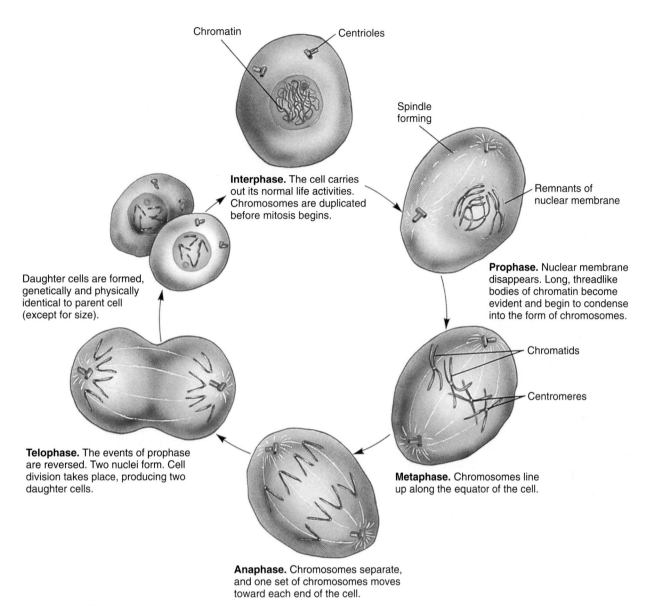

Chromatin

Centrioles

Interphase. The cell carries out its normal life activities. Chromosomes are duplicated before mitosis begins.

Spindle forming

Remnants of nuclear membrane

Prophase. Nuclear membrane disappears. Long, threadlike bodies of chromatin become evident and begin to condense into the form of chromosomes.

Daughter cells are formed, genetically and physically identical to parent cell (except for size).

Chromatids

Centromeres

Telophase. The events of prophase are reversed. Two nuclei form. Cell division takes place, producing two daughter cells.

Metaphase. Chromosomes line up along the equator of the cell.

Anaphase. Chromosomes separate, and one set of chromosomes moves toward each end of the cell.

FIGURE 2-8 • The life cycle of a cell. The generalized cell shown here has a chromosome number of four. A centromere is a constricted region of a chromosome to which spindle cells attach. During prophase and metaphase sister chromatids are attached in the vicinity of their centromeres.

Epithelial cells lining the kidney tubules *excrete* certain materials. In the respiratory passageways, epithelium *transports* mucus containing trapped particles. Such epithelial cells are equipped with cilia that beat a thin sheet of mucus containing trapped dirt particles away from the lungs. The taste buds in the mouth and olfactory (smelling) structures in the nose consist of epithelium specialized to receive *sensory* information.

Epithelial tissue consists of cells that fit tightly together to form a continuous layer, or sheet, of cells. One surface of the sheet is typically exposed because it lines a cavity, such as the lumen (cavity) of the intestine, or covers the body (outer layer of the skin). The other surface of an epithelial layer is attached to the underlying tissue by a noncellular **basement membrane** produced by the epithelial cells. Very little intercellular substance (material between the cells) is present.

Three types of epithelial tissue can be distinguished on the basis of the shape of the cells (Figure 2-9). **Squamous** epithelial cells are thin, flattened cells shaped like pancakes or flagstones. **Cuboidal** epithelial cells are short cylinders that from the side appear cube-shaped, resembling dice. **Columnar** epithelial cells look like columns or cylinders when viewed from the side. The nucleus is usually located near the base of the cell. Viewed from above or in cross section, these cells often appear hexagonal. On its free surface, a columnar epithelial cell may have cilia that beat in a coordinated way, moving materials over the tissue surface. Most of the upper respiratory tract is lined with ciliated columnar epithelium that moves particles of dust and other foreign material away from the lungs.

Epithelial tissue may be **simple** (that is, composed of one layer of cells), **stratified** (composed of two or more layers),

Nuclei

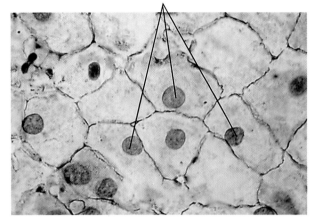

(A) Simple squamous epithelium is found in the air sacs of the lungs and lining the blood vessels (magnified approximately 800x).

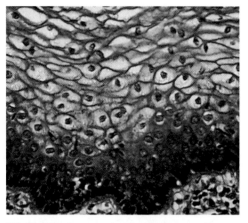

(B) Stratified squamous epithelium makes up the outer layer of the skin (magnified approximately 500x).

Nuclei of cuboidal epithelial cells   Lumen of tubule

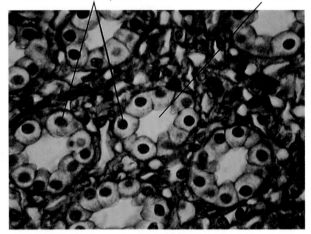

(C) Simple cuboidal epithelium lines the kidney tubules and the ducts of glands (magnified approximately 600x).

Goblet cell   Nuclei of columnar cells

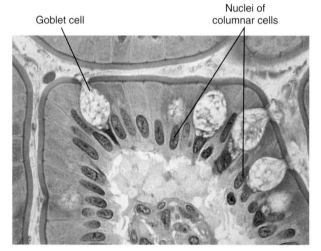

(D) Simple columnar epithelium lines much of the digestive tract (magnified approximately 600x).

Cilia

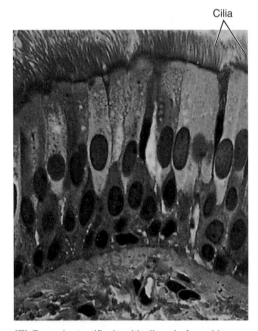

(E) Pseudostratified epithelium is found in some respiratory passages (magnified approximately 500x).

FIGURE 2-9 • Epithelial tissues.

or **pseudostratified** (epithelium that appears to be layered but is not). The pseudostratified impression occurs because the cells are of different heights and their nuclei are at different levels in the tissue. Not every cell extends to the exposed surface of the tissue. This arrangement gives the impression of two or more cell layers. Some of the respiratory passageways are lined with pseudostratified epithelium equipped with cilia.

Simple epithelium is typically present in areas where materials must diffuse through the tissue or where substances are secreted, excreted, or absorbed. Stratified epithelial tissue is located in regions such as the skin, where protection is required. Skin and the lining of the digestive tract are examples of epithelial tissues that are subjected to continuous wear and tear. As outer cells are shed, they must be replaced by new ones from below. Some epithelial tissues have a rapid rate of mitosis, so new cells are continuously produced to take the place of those lost.

A **gland** consists of one or more epithelial cells specialized to produce and secrete a product such as mucus, sweat, saliva, milk, enzymes, or hormones. For example, goblet cells in the lining of the intestine secrete **mucus**—a slippery protective substance (Figure 2-10, *A*). Some epithelial cells form multicellular glands.

Two main types of glands are exocrine and endocrine glands. **Exocrine glands** have ducts (tubes that also consist of epithelial cells) through which the secretion is discharged to some body surface. For example, sweat passes from sweat glands through ducts to the surface of the skin, and salivary gland ducts conduct saliva to the mouth (Figure 2-10, *B* and *C*). Exocrine glands may be unicellular (composed of one cell), such as goblet cells, but most are multicellular (composed of many cells). Compound multicellular glands have branched ducts.

Endocrine glands do not have ducts. They release their products, called *hormones,* into the surrounding tissue fluid. The hormone molecules usually diffuse into the blood, which transports them to their destination. The thyroid gland and the adrenal glands are examples of endocrine glands.

Connective Tissue Joins Body Structures

Connective tissues *join together* the other tissues of the body. Almost every organ in the body has a framework of connective tissue that *supports* and *protects* it. Cartilage and bone are examples of connective tissues that support the body and protect vital organs such as the heart and lungs. Some of the main types of connective tissue are (1) loose connective tissue, (2) adipose (fat) tissue, (3) cartilage, (4) bone, and (5) blood, lymph, and tissues that produce blood cells. Cartilage and bone are discussed in Chapter 4, blood in Chapter 10, and lymph in Chapter 12.

Unlike the closely fitting cells of epithelial tissues, the cells of connective tissue are typically separated by large amounts of **intercellular substance**—nonliving materials produced by the tissue (Figure 2-11). The intercellular substance usually

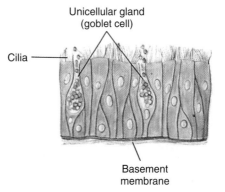

Unicellular gland
(goblet cell)

Cilia

Basement
membrane

(A) A goblet cell is a unicellular gland that secretes mucus. Goblet cells are found in the epithelial lining of the intestine.

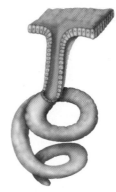

(B) Sweat glands are multicellular, tubular glands.

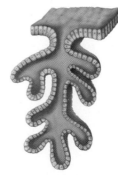

(C) Compound glands have branched ducts. Two types of salivary glands have saclike units that secrete saliva into a duct.

FIGURE 2-10 • Exocrine glands.

consists of threadlike, microscopic fibers scattered throughout a thick gel, or matrix. If the body were composed only of cells, it would be somewhat like a blob of jelly. The intercellular substances give the body strength and help maintain its shape.

Three types of connective tissue fibers are collagen fibers, reticular fibers, and elastic fibers. **Collagen fibers** are the most numerous. These fibers contain the protein **collagen,** the most

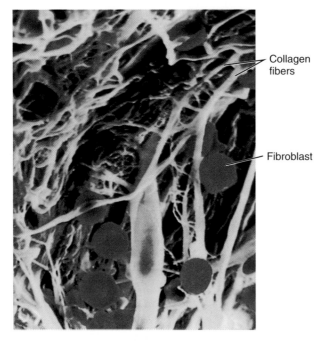

Collagen fibers

Fibroblast

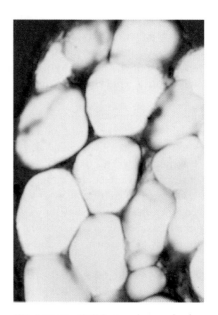

(A) Scanning electron micrograph of loose connective tissue (magnified approximately 440x). Collagen fibers appear as an irregular mass of yellow strands. Fibroblasts are visible between the fibers.

(B) Adipose (fat) tissue (magnified approximately 200x).

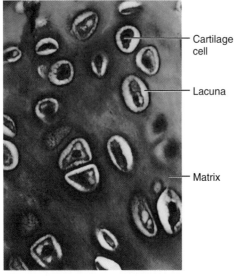

Cartilage cell

Lacuna

Matrix

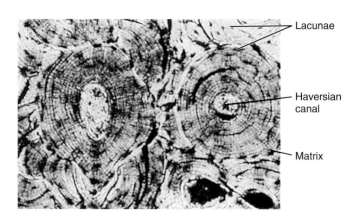

Lacunae

Haversian canal

Matrix

(D) Bone cells are arranged in concentric circles. They are separated by a hard matrix (magnified approximately 100x).

(C) Cartilage cells are separated by a tough matrix (magnified approximately 500x).

FIGURE 2-11 • Connective tissues.

abundant protein in the body. Collagen is a very tough substance, and collagen fibers give great strength to body structures.

Reticular fibers are very fine, branched fibers. They form a network that supports many tissues and organs. **Elastic fibers** stretch easily and are an important component of structures that must stretch. For example, elastic fibers in the walls of the air sacs in the lungs permit these tiny sacs to stretch as they fill with air and then snap back to force air out of the lungs during expiration.

Two types of cells that are common in connective tissues are **fibroblasts** and **macrophages** (**mak′**-row-fajes). Fibroblasts produce the fibers of connective tissues. Macrophages are large scavenger cells that wander through connective tissues phagocytizing cellular debris and foreign matter, including bacteria.

Loose connective tissue (also called *areolar tissue*) joins body structures. It is found as a thin filling between body parts and serves as a reservoir for water and salts. Together with adipose tissue, loose connective tissue forms the subcutaneous (under the skin) tissue layer that attaches the skin to the tissues and organs beneath.

Adipose (fat) tissue stores fat and releases it when the body needs energy. Adipose tissue helps to shape and protect the body and provides insulation.

Muscle Tissue Is Specialized to Contract

Muscle tissue is composed of cells specialized to contract. Because they are long and narrow, muscle cells are referred to as **muscle fibers.** When muscle fibers contract, they become shorter and thicker. As they shorten, they move body parts attached to them. Muscle fibers are usually arranged in bundles or layers surrounded by connective tissue. Three types of muscle tissue are skeletal muscle, cardiac muscle, and smooth muscle (Table 2-1).

When we think of muscles, we normally think of the voluntary muscles that enable us to walk, run, or move the body in some other way. Such movements are the job of the **skeletal muscles,** which are attached to the bones. Skeletal muscle fibers have a striped, or **striated,** appearance. These fibers contract when they are stimulated by nerves. Skeletal muscles will be described in more detail in Chapter 5.

Cardiac muscle, found in the walls of the heart, is considered involuntary because we do not make a conscious decision to contract it. Cardiac muscle fibers are striated and are also characterized by **intercalated** (in-**ter′**-kuh-lay-ted) **disks**—tight junctions between adjacent muscle fibers that allow the muscle impulse to move rapidly from one fiber to another. **Smooth muscle** occurs in the walls of the digestive tract, uterus, blood vessels, and other internal organs. Its fibers are not striated, and its control is involuntary.

Nervous Tissue Controls Muscles and Glands

Nervous tissue receives and transmits messages, allowing various parts of the body to communicate with one another. Nervous tissue consists of **neurons** (**new′**-rons), cells specialized for transmitting nerve impulses, and **glial** (**glee′**-ul) cells (also known as neuroglial cells) that support and nourish the neurons. Typically, a neuron has a large **cell body** that con-

TABLE 2-1	THE TYPES OF MUSCLE TISSUES		
	Skeletal	**Cardiac**	**Smooth**
Location	Attached to skeleton	Wall of heart	Wall of stomach, intestines, etc.
Type of control	Voluntary	Involuntary	Involuntary
Striations	Present	Present	Absent
Number of nuclei per fiber	Many	One or two	One
Speed of contraction	Most rapid	Intermediate	Slowest
Resistance to fatigue (with repeated contraction)	Least	Intermediate	Greatest

Skeletal muscle fibers — Nuclei, Cross striations

Cardiac muscle fibers — Nuclei, Intercalated disks

Smooth muscle fibers — Nuclei

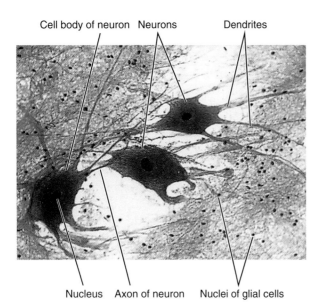

Cell body of neuron   Neurons   Dendrites

Nucleus   Axon of neuron   Nuclei of glial cells

FIGURE 2-12 • Nervous tissue consists of neurons and glial cells (magnified approximately 500×).

tains the nucleus and from which two types of extensions project.

Dendrites are specialized for receiving impulses, whereas the single axon transmits information away from the cell body (Figure 2-12). Neurons receive information from **sensory receptors**—structures that detect information about changes in the internal or external environment (e.g., touch receptors in the skin and photoreceptors in the retina of the eye). Neurons also receive information from other neurons. They transmit information to other neurons and muscles and glands.

Quiz Yourself

- What is a tissue?
- How is connective tissue different from epithelial tissue?
- How is skeletal muscle different from smooth muscle?

MEMBRANES COVER OR LINE BODY SURFACES

LEARNING OBJECTIVE

12. **Identify the main types of membranes and contrast the main types of epithelial membranes.**

Membranes are sheets of tissue that cover or line body surfaces. **Epithelial membranes** consist of epithelial tissue and a layer of underlying connective tissue. The main types of epithelial membranes are mucous membranes, serous membranes, and the skin, which is a cutaneous membrane (discussed in Chapter 3).

A **mucous membrane,** or **mucosa,** lines body cavities that open to the outside of the body. Thus, mucous membranes line the digestive, respiratory, urinary, and reproductive tracts. The epithelial layer of a mucous membrane secretes mucus, which lubricates the tissue and prevents drying.

A **serous membrane,** or **serosa,** lines a body cavity that does not open to the outside of the body. The cavity contains fluid secreted by the serous membrane. A serous membrane consists of a thin layer of loose connective tissue covered by a layer of simple epithelium. A serous membrane folds, forming a double-walled sheet of tissue. The portion of the membrane attached to the wall of the cavity is the **parietal membrane,** whereas the part of the membrane that covers the organs inside the cavity is the **visceral membrane.** Thus the serous membrane lining the thoracic cavity is the parietal pleura, whereas the portion of that membrane covering the lungs is the visceral pleura. Similarly, the serous membrane lining the abdominal cavity is the parietal peritoneum; the portion of the membrane that covers the abdominal and some pelvic organs is the visceral peritoneum.

The membranes that cover bone and cartilage are examples of **connective tissue membranes.** The **synovial membrane** is a connective tissue membrane that lines the joint cavities.

Quiz Yourself

- How does a serous membrane differ from an epithelial membrane?

SUMMARY

LO 1. Describe the general characteristics of cells.
- **Cells,** the building blocks of the body, have specialized **organelles** that carry out specific functions. Most organelles are dispersed within the **cytoplasm**—the jellylike material of the cell.
- Most cells are very small and must be studied with microscopes. Photographs taken with the light microscope are referred to as **light micrographs (LMs);** photographs taken with the electron microscope are **electron micrographs (EMs).**

LO 2. State three functions of cell membranes and describe the structure of the plasma membrane.
- Many organelles are surrounded by membranes that form compartments. Compartments allow the cell to separate various processes.
- Most cells are bounded by a thin **plasma membrane** that protects the cell and regulates the passage of materials into and out of the cell.
- The plasma membrane consists of a double layer of lipids in which proteins are embedded.

LO 3. Describe the structure and functions of the cell nucleus.
- The **nucleus,** the control center of the cell, contains the **chromosomes.** The chromosomes contain the **genes,** units of hereditary information. The genes are composed of DNA.
- The nucleus also contains the **nucleolus**—the site of ribosome assembly.

LO 4. Describe, locate, and list the functions of the principal cytoplasmic organelles and label them on a diagram.
- The **endoplasmic reticulum (ER)** is a system of internal membranes that help transport materials within the cell. The **rough ER** is studded along its outer walls with **ribosomes**—granular organelles that manufacture proteins. The **smooth ER** is an important site of lipid synthesis.
- The **Golgi complex** processes and packages proteins and produces lysosomes. **Lysosomes** contain enzymes that destroy bacteria and other foreign matter.

- **Mitochondria,** the power plants of the cell, are the sites of most of the reactions of **cellular respiration,** a process that captures energy for the cell. During cellular respiration, some of the energy is stored as ATP.
- **Vesicles** and **vacuoles** are membrane-enclosed sacs that contain various materials.
- The **cytoskeleton** provides structural support and plays a role in cell movement. It is composed of **microtubules,** microfilaments, and intermediate filaments. **Cilia** and **flagella,** both composed of microtubules, are important in cell movement.

LO 5. Explain how materials pass through cell membranes, distinguishing between passive and active processes.
- Materials move through the plasma membrane passively by physical processes such as diffusion or osmosis, or they can be actively transported by physiological processes such as active transport and phagocytosis. Passive processes do not require the cell to expend energy, whereas active processes require energy input by the cell.
- **Diffusion** is the movement of molecules or ions from one region to another because of their random molecular motion. The net movement of molecules in diffusion is from a region of greater concentration to a region of lower concentration, that is, down a **concentration gradient.**
- **Osmosis** is a kind of diffusion in which molecules of water diffuse through a selectively permeable membrane.
- In **active transport,** cells expend energy to transport materials across membranes from a region of lower to a region of higher concentration.
- In **phagocytosis,** the cell ingests large, solid particles by enclosing them in a vacuole pinched off from the plasma membrane.

LO 6. Predict whether cells will swell or shrink under various osmotic conditions.
- An **isotonic** solution has a solute concentration equal to that of cells. When cells are placed in an isotonic solution, there is no net movement of water molecules.
- When cells are placed in a **hypertonic** solution, one with a higher solute concentration than that of the cells, water molecules leave the cells, causing them to shrink.

LO = Learning Objective

- When cells are placed in a **hypotonic** solution, one with a lower solute concentration than that of the cells, water molecules move into the cells, causing them to swell.

LO 7. **Describe the events that take place in cell signaling.**
- The following sequence of events takes place in **cell signaling:** (1) a cell must send a signal, for example, a chemical compound such as a hormone; (2) **reception—receptors,** specific proteins on **target cells,** cells that can respond to a specific signal, bind with the signal; (3) **signal transduction,** a process by which a receptor converts a signal outside the cell into a signal inside the cell that affects some cellular process; and (4) **response** by the cell. Some cell activity is altered.

LO 8. **Describe the stages of a cell's life cycle and summarize the significance of mitosis with respect to maintaining a constant chromosome number.**
- **Interphase** is the period of growth and activity between mitoses. A cell reproduces itself by undergoing **mitosis** and then dividing to form two new cells.
- During **prophase,** the first stage of mitosis, the chromatin coils so that the chromosomes are visible; the nuclear membrane dissolves, centrioles migrate toward opposite ends of the cell, and a spindle made of microtubules forms.
- During **metaphase,** the chromosomes position themselves along the equator of the cell.
- During **anaphase,** sister chromatids separate and the two sets of chromosomes move toward opposite ends of the cell.
- During **telophase,** chromosomes begin to uncoil and a nuclear membrane forms around each   set of chromosomes. Cell division occurs during telophase.
- Mitosis ensures that the chromosomes are duplicated and distributed to each new cell.

LO 9. **Define the term *tissue* and describe the structure and functions of the principal types of tissues.**
- A **tissue** is a group of closely associated cells that work together to carry out a specific function or group of functions.
- The major function of **epithelial tissue** is protection. It covers the body and lines the body cavities. Some epithelial tissue is specialized for secretion and forms **glands.** On the basis of shape, epithelial cells may be **squamous, cuboidal,** or **columnar.** Epithelial cells may be

arranged to form **simple, stratified,** or **pseudostratified epithelial tissue.**
- **Connective tissue** joins other tissues of the body, supports the body, and protects underlying organs. Some main types of connective tissue are **loose connective tissue, adipose tissue, cartilage, bone, blood, lymph,** and tissues that produce blood cells. Two types of cells commonly found in connective tissues are **fibroblasts,** which produce fibers, and **macrophages,** which are large scavenger cells. Three types of connective tissue fibers are **collagen fibers, reticular fibers,** and **elastic fibers.**
- **Muscle tissue,** which consists of elongated cells called **muscle fibers,** is specialized to contract.
- **Nervous tissue** is specialized to transmit information. It consists of **neurons** and **glial cells,** which support the neurons. A neuron has a large **cell body** that contains the nucleus. **Dendrites,** which extend from the cell body, are specialized for receiving impulses. The **axon** transmits information away from the cell body.

LO 10. **Contrast epithelial tissue with connective tissue.**
- Epithelial cells fit closely together. In contrast, the cells of connective tissue are separated by **intercellular substance,** which consists of threadlike fibers scattered through a thick gel.

LO 11. **Compare the three types of muscle tissue.**
- **Skeletal muscle** and **cardiac muscle** fibers are **striated,** or striped. Skeletal muscle is attached to bones and is voluntary. Cardiac muscle has **intercalated disks,** tight junctions between adjacent muscle fibers that allow rapid transmission of information. **Smooth muscle** and cardiac muscle are involuntary. Smooth muscle functions in movement of internal organs.

LO 12. **Identify the main types of membranes and contrast the main types of epithelial membranes.**
- **Membranes** are sheets of tissue that cover or line body surfaces.
- Three main types of **epithelial membranes** are **mucous membranes,** which line body cavities that open to the outside of the body; **serous membranes,** which line body cavities that do not open to the outside of the body; and the skin, which is referred to as a cutaneous membrane.
- **Connective tissue membranes** include the membranes that cover bone and cartilage and **synovial membranes** that line joint cavities.

CHAPTER QUIZ

Matching

Select the most appropriate match in column B for each item in column A.

Column A	Column B
1. Regulates passage of materials into the cell	**a.** ribosomes
2. Network of internal membranes that extends throughout cytoplasm	**b.** endoplasmic reticulum (ER)
3. Site of energy capture from fuel molecules	**c.** mitochondria
4. Membranous sacs containing digestive enzymes	**d.** plasma membrane
5. Chromosomes located here	**e.** nucleus
6. Propels sperm	**f.** lysosomes
7. Packages secretions	**g.** Golgi complex
8. Granules that manufacture protein	**h.** flagellum

Fill in the Blank

9. If a cell is placed in a very salty (hypertonic) solution, the net passage of water molecules will be from _____ to _____.

10. A cell engulfs a bacterium; this is an example of _____.

11. Active transport requires the expenditure of _____ by the cell.

12. A complete set of chromosomes is distributed to each end of the cell during the phase of mitosis known as _____.

13. Tiny hairlike structures that project from the surface of some cells and function in movement of materials outside the cell are called _____.

14. Endocrine glands do not have _____.

15. Bone and cartilage are examples of _____ tissue.

Multiple Choice

16. Muscle tissue: a. covers body surfaces; b. is specialized to contract; c. contains collagen fibers; d. supports and protects major organs.

17. Nervous tissue: a. covers body surfaces; b. is specialized to contract; c. contains collagen fibers; d. contains glial cells.

18. Connective tissue: a. secretes hormones; b. is specialized to contract; c. contains collagen fibers; d. forms glands.

19. Mucous membranes: a. are composed of connective tissue; b. line body cavities that open to the outside of the body; c. contain large numbers of collagen fibers; d. line joint cavities.

20. Fibroblasts are most likely to be found in: a. connective tissue; b. epithelial tissue; c. muscle tissue; d. fibrous nervous tissue.

REVIEW QUESTIONS

1. What are the functions of the plasma membrane?

2. What is the function of mitochondria?

3. Draw a diagram of a cell and label at least eight organelles. Give the function of each organelle you label.

4. Explain why the nucleus is considered the control center of the cell.

5. Compare diffusion with active transport.

6. If red blood cells are accidentally placed in a hypotonic solution (one containing less solute than the cells), what happens to them? What would happen if red blood cells were placed in a hypertonic solution (one containing more solute than the cell)? An isotonic solution?

7. Why is mitosis important? Draw a series of diagrams illustrating mitosis in a cell with two chromosomes.

8. What are some of the differences between epithelial and connective tissue?

9. The heart (like most organs) contains epithelial, connective, muscle, and nervous tissue. What function might each of these tissues perform in the heart?

10. What are the functions of epithelial tissue?

11. Where would you expect to find a mucous membrane? A serous membrane? A connective tissue membrane?

12. Label the diagram. (See Figure 2-2 to check your answers.)

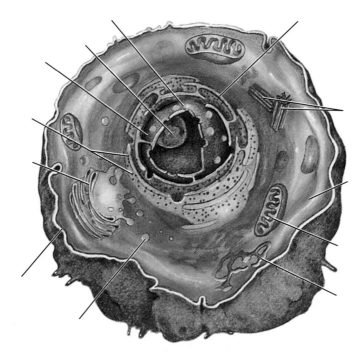

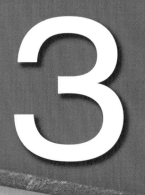

3

The Integumentary System

Chapter Outline

The skin is the body's outer protective covering. Together with its hair, nails, and glands, the skin makes up the **integumentary** (in-teg'-u-men'-tar-y) **system.** Because it is at least partly exposed to view, we give this organ system a lot of attention. We scrub our skin, cream it, and coat it with makeup. We cut, shave, and curl our hair, and we manicure our nails.

The skin is important in communication. It has sensory receptors that permit us to feel a handshake, kiss, stroke, squeeze, or slap. Involuntary changes in the skin reflect emotional states. For example, you may blush with embarrassment, blanch with fear or rage, redden with exertion, or sweat excessively when anxious. In addition, the appearance, coloration, temperature, and feel of the skin are important indicators of general health and of many disease states.

THE INTEGUMENTARY SYSTEM PROTECTS THE BODY

LEARNING OBJECTIVE

1. **List six functions of the integumentary system and explain how each is important in maintaining homeostasis.**

The integumentary system is the outer boundary of the body—the part in direct contact with the external environment. The 20 or so square feet of skin that cover the body must resist continuous wear and tear, drying, and exposure to cold, heat, and toxic substances. This outer covering is frequently cut, bruised, scraped, and burned and must heal such wounds. The skin is important in maintaining **homeostasis**—the balanced internal environment. The skin performs the following functions:

1. Protects the body against injury and is the body's first line of defense against harmful bacteria and other agents of disease.
2. Receives and communicates information about the outside world. Located within the skin are sensory receptors that detect touch, pressure, heat, cold, and pain.
3. Prevents drying out. The cells of the body are bathed in an internal sea—a carefully regulated, dilute salt solution essential to life. As we move about in the air, a relatively dry environment, the skin prevents loss of fluid so that the cells do not dry out.
4. Helps maintain body temperature. Capillary (tiny blood vessels) networks and sweat glands in the skin are an important part of the body's temperature-regulating system.
5. Has sweat glands that excrete excess water and some wastes from the body.
6. Contains a compound that is converted to vitamin D when the skin is exposed to the ultraviolet rays of the sun.

Quiz Yourself

- How does the skin help maintain homeostasis?

THE SKIN CONSISTS OF THE EPIDERMIS AND DERMIS

LEARNING OBJECTIVES

2. **Compare the structure and function of the epidermis with that of the dermis.**
3. **Describe the subcutaneous layer.**

Skin consists of two main layers: an outer **epidermis** (ep′-ih-**der**′-mus) and an inner **dermis** (**der**′-mus). Beneath the skin is an underlying **subcutaneous** (sub′-koo-**tay**′-nee-us) **layer** (Figure 3-1).

The Epidermis Continuously Replaces Itself

The epidermis consists of stratified squamous epithelial tissue. The outer cells of the epidermis continuously wear off and are immediately replaced by new cells. Over most parts of the body, the epidermis is only about as thick as a page of this book, yet it consists of several sublayers, or strata (**stray**′-tah).

New epidermal cells are constantly produced in the deepest sublayer of the epidermis, the **stratum basale** (ba-**say**′-lee). These cells mature as they are pushed toward the outer surface by newer cells beneath.

As they move toward the body surface, epidermal cells manufacture **keratin** (**ker**′-ah-tin)—a tough waterproofing protein that gives the skin mechanical strength and flexibility. As epidermal cells move through the outer sublayer of epidermis, they die. The cells at the surface of the skin resemble dead scales. They are closely packed together and serve as a waterproof protective covering for the body. The outer sublayer of the skin is **stratum corneum (kor**′-nee-um). It takes about 2 weeks for a new epidermal cell to be pushed up from the stratum basale into the stratum corneum.

The Dermis Provides Strength and Elasticity

The dermis is the thick layer of skin beneath the epidermis (see Figure 3-1). Dermis consists of dense connective tissue composed mainly of collagen fibers. Collagen is largely responsible for the mechanical strength of the skin. It also permits the skin to stretch and then return to its normal form again. Blood vessels and nerves, which are generally absent in the epidermis, are found throughout the dermis. Specialized skin structures such as hair follicles and glands are found in the dermis. They develop from cells of the epidermis that push down into the dermis.

The upper portion of the dermis has many small, fingerlike extensions, called **dermal papillae** (pah-**pil**′-ee), that project into the epidermal tissue. Extensive networks of capillaries in the papillae deliver oxygen and nutrients to the cells of the epidermis and also function in temperature regulation. The patterns of ridges and grooves visible on the skin of the soles and palms (including the fingertips) reflect the arrangement of the dermal elevations beneath. Unique to each individual, these patterns provide the fingerprints so useful to law enforcement officials. They also serve as friction ridges that help us hold onto the objects we grasp.

The Subcutaneous Layer Attaches the Skin to Underlying Tissues

The subcutaneous layer beneath the dermis is also known as the **superficial fascia** (**fash**′-ee-ah). This layer consists of loose connective tissue, usually containing a lot of adipose (fat) tissue. The subcutaneous layer attaches the skin to the muscles and other tissues beneath.

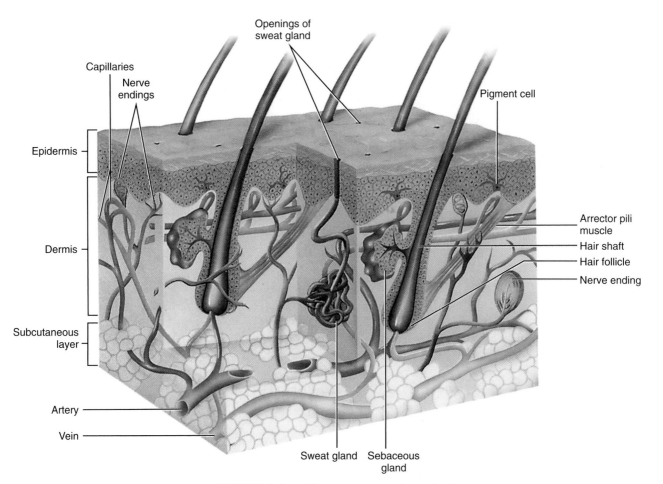

FIGURE 3-1 • Microscopic structure of skin.

The thick fatty subcutaneous layer helps protect underlying organs from mechanical shock. It also insulates the body, which conserves heat. Fat stored within the adipose tissue can be mobilized and used as an energy source when adequate food is not available. Distribution of fat in the subcutaneous layer is largely responsible for characteristic male and female body shapes.

> **Quiz Yourself**
>
> • How does the dermis differ from the epidermis?
> • What is the functional importance of fat in the subcutaneous layer?

THE SKIN HAS SPECIALIZED STRUCTURES

LEARNING OBJECTIVES

4. **Describe the structure of hair.**
5. **Describe the functions of sebaceous glands.**
6. **Describe the structure and functions of sweat glands.**
7. **Describe the structure and function of nails.**

During embryonic development, thousands of small groups of epidermal cells from the stratum basale push down into the dermis. They multiply and develop into hair follicles and glands.

The Hair Shaft Consists of Dead Cells

Hair, which helps protect the body, is found on all skin surfaces except the palms and the soles. The part of the hair that we see is the **shaft;** the portion below the skin surface is the **root.** The root, together with its epithelial and connective tissue coverings, is called the **hair follicle** (Figure 3-2). At the bottom of the follicle, there is a little mound of connective tissue containing capillaries. These blood vessels deliver nutrients to the cells of the follicle.

Each hair consists of cells that multiply, manufacture keratin as they move outward, and then die. The shaft of the hair consists of dead cells and their products. That is why we can cut hair without any sensation of pain. As long as the follicle remains intact, new hair will continue to grow. If the follicle is destroyed, as by laser treatment, no new hair can form.

Tiny bundles of smooth muscle are associated with hair follicles. These arrector pili muscles contract in response to

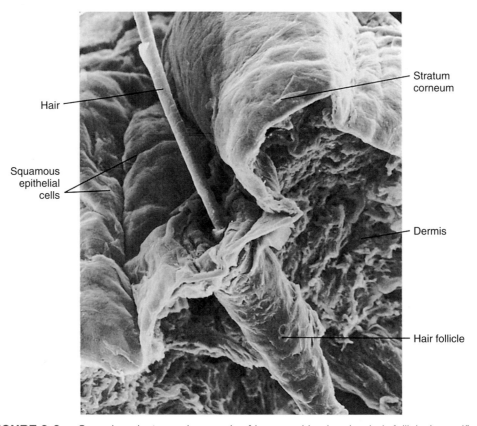

FIGURE 3-2 • Scanning electron micrograph of human skin showing hair follicle (magnified approximately ×250). (Courtesy Dr. Karen A. Holbrook.)

cold or fear, making the hairs stand up straight. Skin around the hair shaft is pulled up into "gooseflesh."

Sebaceous Glands Lubricate the Hair and Skin

Sebaceous glands (see-**bay′**-shus), also known as *oil glands,* are generally attached to hair follicles by little ducts through which they release their secretions. These glands are most numerous on the face and scalp. Sebaceous glands secrete an oily substance called **sebum** (**see′**-bum) that oils the hair, lubricates the surface of the skin, and helps prevent water loss. Sebum inhibits the growth of certain bacteria and may also have antifungal action.

Sometimes sebum accumulates in the duct of the sebaceous gland and hair follicle and blocks it, forming a blackhead (comedo). In a blackhead, sebum and dead cells containing the dark pigment *melanin* block the duct. The black color results from melanin, rather than from dirt.

Sometimes the duct of a sebaceous gland ruptures, allowing sebum to spill into the dermis. The skin may become inflamed, and a pimple may form. During childhood, sebaceous glands are relatively inactive. At puberty they are activated by increased secretion of male hormone in both males and females. This stepped-up activity can lead to *acne*—a condition very common during adolescence.

Sweat Glands Help Maintain Body Temperature

Each **sweat gland** is a tiny coiled tube in the dermis or subcutaneous tissue, with a duct that extends up through the skin and opens onto the surface (see Figure 3-1). About three million sweat glands in the skin help maintain body temperature. Muscle movement and metabolic activity generate heat and so raise body temperature. Because heat is required for evaporation, the body becomes cooler as sweat evaporates from the skin.

Sweat glands excrete excess water, salts, and small amounts of nitrogen wastes. About 1 quart of water is excreted in sweat each day. Normally, sweat, also called perspiration, is not noticed. Only when it is produced more quickly than it can evaporate does it accumulate on the skin and become annoying. This is most apt to happen on a humid day, when the air already contains a great deal of water vapor. When profuse sweating occurs, proportionately more salt is lost in the sweat. This is why people engaged in strenuous physical exercise must replace salts lost in sweat.

Certain sweat glands found in association with hairs are concentrated in a few specific areas of the body such as the armpits and genital areas. These glands discharge into hair follicles. Their secretion is thick, sticky, and initially odorless. However, certain bacteria that inhabit the skin surface begin to decompose this secretion, producing a noticeable odor. Deodorants kill these bacteria and replace the odor with a more perfumed scent; antiperspirants reduce moisture and so inhibit the growth of bacteria. Emotional stress or sexual stimulation promotes secretion of these glands.

Nails Protect the Ends of the Fingers and Toes

Nails develop from horny epidermal cells and consist mainly of a closely compressed, tough keratin. The nail bed beneath the body (the visible part) of the nail lacks a stratum corneum. Nails appear pink because of underlying capillaries. The actively growing area is the white crescent (lunula) at the base of the nail. Nails lost as a result of injury are regenerated, but the process requires several months.

Quiz Yourself

- Why doesn't it hurt when you cut your hair?
- What is the function of sebaceous glands?
- How do sweat glands help maintain homeostasis?

MELANIN HELPS DETERMINE SKIN COLOR

LEARNING OBJECTIVE

8. Explain the function of melanin.

Scattered throughout the lowest layer of the epidermis are cells that produce granules containing pigment. These granules are composed of a type of protein called **melanin** (**mel′**-ah-nin), which gives color to hair and skin. Skin color is inherited. In dark-skinned individuals, the pigment cells are more active and produce more melanin. Asians have the yellowish pigment **carotene** in their skin as well as melanin. The pinkish hue of light skin is caused by the color of blood in the vessels of the dermis. In **albinism** (**al′**-bih-nizm), an inherited condition that can occur in a person of any race, the cells are not able to produce melanin. An albino typically has very light skin and white hair.

Melanin is an important protective screen against the sun because it absorbs harmful ultraviolet rays. Exposure to the sun stimulates an increase in the amount of melanin produced and causes the skin to become darker. The tan so prized by sun worshipers is actually a protective response—a sign that the skin has been exposed to too much ultraviolet radiation. When the melanin is not able to absorb all the ultraviolet rays, the skin becomes inflamed, or sunburned. Excessive exposure to sun over a period of years, especially in fair-skinned individuals, eventually results in wrinkling of the skin and sometimes in skin cancer. In fact, most cases of skin cancer are caused by excessive, frequent exposure to ultraviolet radiation. Because dark-skinned people have more melanin, they have less sunburn, less wrinkling, and a lower incidence of skin cancer.

SUMMARY

LO 1. **List six functions of the integumentary system and explain how each is important in maintaining homeostasis.**

- The **integumentary system** consists of the **skin** and its hair, nails, and glands. This system protects the body against injury and disease organisms; has sensory receptors that receive and transmit information about the outside world; prevents drying; helps maintain constant body temperature; helps excrete water and some wastes; and produces vitamin D.

LO 2. **Compare the structure and function of the epidermis with that of the dermis.**

- The skin consists of an outer **epidermis** and an inner **dermis.** The epidermis consists of stratified squamous epithelial tissue. New epidermal cells are produced in the **stratum basale,** the deepest sublayer of the epidermis. As a cell moves outward through the layers of the epidermis, it produces **keratin,** a tough waterproofing protein. Epidermal cells die as they move through the **stratum corneum,** the outer sublayer of the epidermis.
- The dermis consists of connective tissue containing large amounts of collagen. It gives strength to the skin and holds the blood vessels that nourish the epidermal cells. Capillaries extend into **dermal papillae,** projections in the upper region of the dermis that extend into the epidermis. The dermis is rich in capillaries and contains hair follicles and glands.

LO 3. **Describe the subcutaneous layer.**

- The **subcutaneous layer** consists of connective tissue, including fat. This tissue cushions underlying structures against mechanical injury, connects skin with tissues beneath, and stores energy in the form of fat.

LO 4. **Describe the structure of hair.**

- Hair helps protect the body. The part of a hair that we see is its **shaft;** the part below the skin is the **root.** The root plus its epithelial and connective tissue coverings is the **hair follicle.**

LO 5. **Describe the functions of sebaceous glands.**

- **Sebaceous glands** produce **sebum,** an oily substance that lubricates the surface of the skin and helps prevent water loss. It also inhibits growth of bacteria.

LO 6. **Describe the structure and functions of sweat glands.**

- Most **sweat glands** are coiled tubes that excrete a dilute salt water through a pore onto the skin surface. When body temperature increases, more sweat is produced. As sweat evaporates, the body is cooled.

LO 7. **Describe the structure and function of nails.**

- Nails consist mainly of keratin. The actively growing area is the white crescent at the base of the nail. The nails protect the fingers and toes.

LO 8. **Explain the function of melanin.**

- Pigment cells in the epidermis produce **melanin,** which gives color to skin and hair. Melanin absorbs ultraviolet rays from the skin, preventing damage to the dermis and blood vessels. Some individuals have the yellowish pigment **carotene** in their skin as well as melanin. In **albinism,** cells are unable to produce melanin.

LO = Learning Objective

CHAPTER QUIZ

Fill in the Blank

1. The skin, with its glands, hair, nails, and other structures, makes up the _____ system.
2. The two main layers of the skin are the outer _____ and the inner _____.
3. The tough waterproofing protein of the epidermis is _____.
4. The _____ layer beneath the dermis consists of loose connective tissue.
5. _____ glands are attached to each hair follicle by ducts; they secrete an oily substance called _____.
6. Sweat consists mainly of _____ with some _____ and small amounts of nitrogen wastes.
7. The root of a hair together with its coverings is called a _____ _____.
8. Nails consist mainly of tough, compressed _____.
9. Pigment granules in the skin produce the dark pigment _____.
10. Melanin protects against the sun by absorbing _____ rays.

REVIEW QUESTIONS

1. In what ways does the skin help maintain homeostasis?
2. How is the structure of the epidermis different from that of the dermis?
3. Which cells of the epidermis actively divide? Which are dead?
4. What are the functions of the dermis? The subcutaneous layer?
5. What is the function of the sebaceous glands? What happens when they malfunction?
6. Why is melanin important?
7. Label the diagram. (See Figure 3-1 to check your answers.)

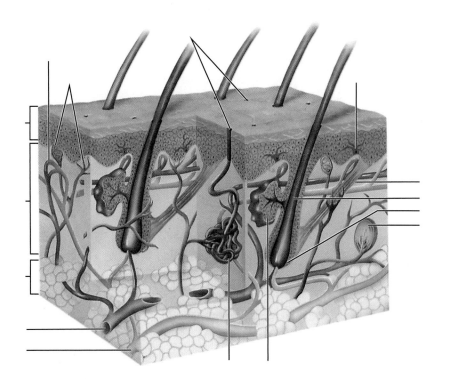

4 The Skeletal System

Chapter Outline

I. The skeletal system supports and protects the body

II. A bone consists of compact and spongy bone tissue

III. Bone develops by replacing existing connective tissue

IV. The bones of the skeleton are grouped in two divisions

V. The axial skeleton consists of 80 bones

    A. The skull is the bony framework of the head
    B. The vertebral column supports the body
    C. The thoracic cage protects the organs of the chest

VI. The appendicular skeleton consists of 126 bones

    A. The pectoral girdle attaches the upper extremities to the axial skeleton
    B. The bones of the upper extremity are located in the arm, forearm, wrist, and hand
    C. The pelvic girdle supports the lower extremities
    D. The bones of the lower extremity are located in the thigh, knee, leg, ankle, and foot

VII. Joints are junctions between bones

    A. Joints can be classified according to the degree of movement they permit
    B. A diarthrosis is surrounded by a joint capsule

The skeleton found in science laboratories consists of dry, dead bones. In contrast, the **skeletal system** in a living body is made up of active, living tissues, including bone, cartilage, and other connective tissues. The cells of skeletal tissues must have nutrients, oxygen, and energy to carry on metabolism. These tissues produce waste products and some aspects of their metabolism are regulated by hormones. The skeletal system functions closely with the muscular system.

THE SKELETAL SYSTEM SUPPORTS AND PROTECTS THE BODY

LEARNING OBJECTIVE

1. List five functions of the skeletal system.

The skeletal system serves several important functions:

1. It *supports* the body by serving as a bony framework for the other tissues and organs.
2. It *protects* delicate vital organs. For example, the bones of the skull surround and protect the brain; the sternum (breastbone) and ribs protect the heart and lungs. For their weight, bones are nearly as strong as steel.
3. Bones serve as levers that *transmit muscular forces.* Muscles are attached to bones by bands of connective tissue called **tendons.** When muscles contract, they pull on bones and in this way they move parts of the body. Bones are held together at joints by bands of connective tissue called **ligaments.** Most joints are movable. The interaction of bones and muscles also makes breathing possible.
4. The marrow within some bones *produces blood cells.*
5. Bones serve as banks for the *storage and release of minerals* such as calcium and phosphorus. When the concentration of calcium in the blood increases above normal, calcium is

deposited in the bones. When the concentration of calcium decreases, calcium is withdrawn from the bones and enters the blood. These actions, which are regulated by hormones, help maintain homeostasis.

Quiz Yourself

* What are five functions of the skeletal system?

A BONE CONSISTS OF COMPACT AND SPONGY BONE TISSUE

LEARNING OBJECTIVE

2. Describe the gross and microscopic structure of a typical bone.

The main shaft of a long bone is known as its **diaphysis** (dye′-af′-ih-sis) (Figure 4-1). The expanded ends of the bone are called **epiphyses** (eh-**pif′**-ih-sees). In children, a disk of cartilage, the **metaphysis** (meh-**taf′**-ih-sis), is found between the epiphyses and the diaphysis. The metaphyses are growth centers that disappear at maturity, becoming vague epiphyseal lines. At its joint surfaces, the outer layer of a bone consists of a thin layer of hyaline cartilage—the **articular cartilage.** Some important types of bone markings are described in Table 4-1.

TABLE 4-1	BONE MARKINGS

PROCESS: ANY PROMINENT BONY PROJECTION

Processes That Help form Joints

Condyle (**kon′**-dil)	Rounded projection
Head	Rounded projection supported by narrow neck (constricted region); usually the upper or proximal extremity of a bone; often bears the ball of ball-and-socket joint
Facet	Smooth, flat surface; found on vertebrae for articulation with ribs

Processes That Are Sites of Attachment for Tendons and Ligaments

Crest	Projecting line or ridge, often on long border of bone
Epicondyle	Bony bulge adjacent to condyle
Spine	Sharp projection; sometimes a long, strongly raised ridge
Trochanter (tro-**kan′**-ter)	Pulley-like process found only on femur
Tubercle (**too′**-ber-kul)	Small, rounded process
Tuberosity	Large, rounded, often roughened process

DEPRESSIONS AND OPENINGS

Fissure (**fish′**-er)	Narrow cleft or groove between adjacent bones through which blood vessels and nerves pass
Foramen (foe-**ray′**-men)	Natural opening or passage into or through bony structure, often round; term means "hole"
Fossa	Trench or shallow depression on surface of bone; term means "basin-like depression"
Sulcus	Elongated groove through which blood vessel or nerve may pass
Meatus (me-**a′**-tus)	Opening into some passageway in body, not necessarily bony; usually lengthy and tunnel-like
Sinus	Air-filled cavity (paranasal sinuses are connected to nasal cavity)

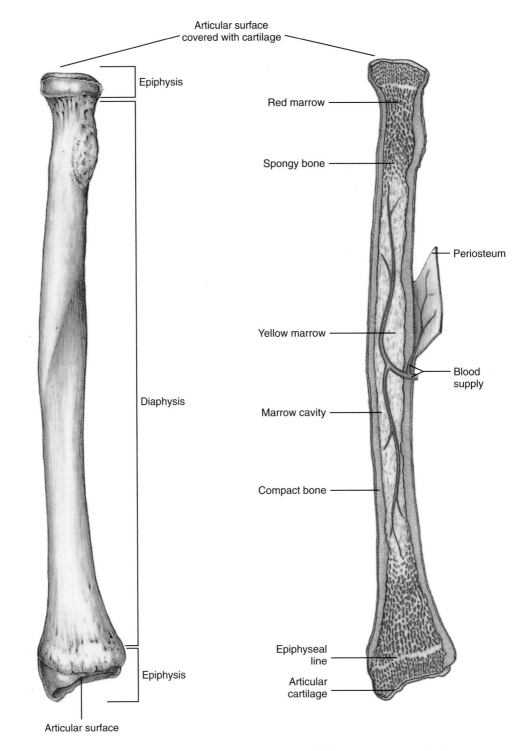

(A) The structure of a typical long bone.   **(B)** Internal structure of a long bone.

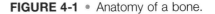

FIGURE 4-1 • Anatomy of a bone.

The bone is covered by a layer of specialized connective tissue—the **periosteum** (per′-ee-**os**′-tee-um). The inner layer of the periosteum contains cells that produce bone. A long bone has a central marrow cavity filled with a fatty connective tissue known as *yellow bone marrow*. The marrow cavity is lined with a thin layer of cells—the **endosteum** (en-**dos**′-tee-um).

Two types of bone tissue are compact and spongy bone. **Compact bone** is very dense and hard. It is found near the surfaces of the bone, where great strength is needed. Compact bone consists of interlocking, spindle-shaped units called **osteons** (**os**′-tee-ons), or **haversian systems** (Figure 4-2, also see Figure 2-9, *D*). Within an osteon, **osteocytes** (**os**′-tee-oh-

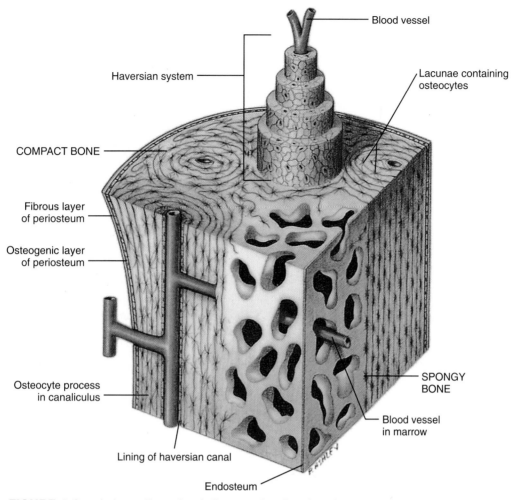

Blood vessel

Haversian system

Lacunae containing osteocytes

COMPACT BONE

Fibrous layer of periosteum

Osteogenic layer of periosteum

Osteocyte process in canaliculus

SPONGY BONE

Blood vessel in marrow

Lining of haversian canal

Endosteum

FIGURE 4-2 • A three-dimensional diagram showing the microscopic structure of bone. A cross section and longitudinal section of compact bone are shown.

sites'), the mature bone cells, are found in small cavities called **lacunae** (la-**koo′**-nee). The lacunae are arranged in concentric circles around central **haversian canals.** Blood vessels that nourish the bone tissue pass through the haversian canals. Threadlike extensions of the osteocyte cytoplasm extend through narrow channels (called *canaliculi*). These cellular extensions connect the osteocytes.

Spongy bone, also called **cancellous bone,** is found within the epiphyses and makes up the inner part of the wall of the diaphysis. Spongy bone consists of a network of thin strands of bone. The spaces within the spongy bone are filled with **bone marrow.** In an infant, **red marrow** fills the cavities of most bones. With age, red marrow is replaced by **yellow marrow** in most bones. In the adult, red marrow is found mainly in the bones of the skull, the vertebrae, ribs, sternum, clavicles, and pelvis. Blood cells are manufactured in red bone marrow, and this marrow is also an important site of antibody production. Yellow marrow contains numerous fat cells, which store fat.

Quiz Yourself

• What is a diaphysis? What are epiphyses?
• How does spongy bone differ from compact bone?

BONE DEVELOPS BY REPLACING EXISTING CONNECTIVE TISSUE

LEARNING OBJECTIVES

3. **Contrast endochondral with intramembranous bone development.**
4. **Describe the functions of osteoblasts and osteoclasts in bone production and remodeling.**

Bone formation is called **ossification** (os′-ih-fih-**kay**′-shun). During fetal development, bones form in two ways. Long bones such as the radius develop from cartilage templates—a process called endochondral (en´-doe-**kon**´-dral) bone development. A bone begins to ossify in its diaphysis. Secondary sites of bone production develop in the epiphyses. The part of the bone between the ossified regions grow and eventually fuse. In contrast, the flat bones of the skull, the irregular vertebrae, and some other bones develop from a noncartilage connective tissue scaffold. This process is called **intramembranous** (in´-trah-**mem**´-brah-nus) bone development.

Osteoblasts (**os**´-tee-oh-blasts´) are cells that produce bone. They secrete the protein *collagen* that forms the strong, elastic fibers of bone. The compound *hydroxyapatite* is present in the tissue fluid. This compound, composed mainly of calcium phosphate, automatically crystallizes around collagen fibers, forming the hard matrix of bone. As the matrix forms around the osteoblasts, they become isolated within lacunae. When osteoblasts become embedded in the bone matrix, they are referred to as **osteocytes**.

Bones are modeled during growth and remodeled continuously throughout life in response to physical stresses on the body. **Osteoclasts** (**os**´-tee-oh-klasts´) are very large cells that **resorb** (break down) bone. Osteoclasts move about secreting enzymes that digest collagen and hydrogen ions that dissolve the crystals. Osteoclasts and osteoblasts work side by side to shape bones and to form the precise grain needed in the finished bone.

As muscles develop in response to physical activity, the bones to which they are attached thicken and become stronger. As bones grow, bone tissue is removed from the interior, especially from the walls of the marrow cavity. This process keeps bones from getting too heavy. Bone remodeling is extensive—the adult skeleton is replaced every 10 years!

Quiz Yourself

- How does intramembranous bone development differ from endochondral bone development?
- What is the function of osteoclasts?

THE BONES OF THE SKELETON ARE GROUPED IN TWO DIVISIONS

LEARNING OBJECTIVES

5. Distinguish between the axial skeleton and the appendicular skeleton.

The human skeleton consists of 206 named bones (Figures 4-3 and 4-4). For convenience, these bones are classified as belonging to either (1) the **axial** (**ak**´-se-al) **skeleton,** which forms the central axis of the body, or (2) the **appendicular** (ap-en-**dik**´-u-lar) **skeleton,** which consists of the bones of the upper and lower extremities (arms and legs) plus the bones that attach them to the axial skeleton.

Quiz Yourself

- In general terms, compare the axial and appendicular skeletons.

THE AXIAL SKELETON CONSISTS OF 80 BONES

LEARNING OBJECTIVES

6. Identify the bones of the axial skeleton and locate each on a diagram or skeleton.
7. Describe and give the function of each of the cranial and facial bones.
8. Describe and give the function of each of the bones of the vertebral column and of the thoracic cage.

The axial skeleton consists of the skull, vertebral column, ribs, and breast bone (sternum). These bones are described in Table 4-2.

The Skull Is the Bony Framework of the Head

The **skull,** the bony framework of the head, consists of 22 bones grouped in two sets: the eight bones of the **cranium** (those that enclose the brain) and the 14 bones that make up the face (the anterior part of the skull). Also within the head are six very small bones (auditory ossicles) in the middle ears. Functions and descriptions of the bones of the head are given in Table 4-2 and are illustrated in Figures 4-5 through 4-8.

Most of the bones of the skull are joined by immovable joints (points of contact) called **sutures** (see Figure 4-14, *A*). The two parietal bones are joined in the midline by the **sagittal suture.** The **coronal suture** joins the parietal bones to the frontal bone. The **lambdoid suture** is the joint between the parietal bones and the occipital bone.

At birth, ossification at the skull joints is not complete. Many of these bones are loosely joined by fibrous connective tissue or cartilage. Six such joints, called **fontanelles** (fon-tah-**nells**´), occur at the angles of the parietal bone. The largest fontanelle is the anterior fontanelle at the junction of the sagittal and coronal sutures (located between the unfused halves of the frontal bones at birth). The fontanelles, popularly referred to as *soft spots,* permit the baby's head to be compressed slightly as it passes through the bony pelvis during birth. They also allow the infant's brain to grow during the latter weeks of prenatal development and permit growth of the skull bones.

Certain cranial bones contain **sinuses,** air-filled spaces lined with mucous membranes. Four pairs of sinuses, the *paranasal sinuses* (located in the frontal, maxillary, sphenoid, and ethmoid bones), are continuous with the nose and throat. Sometimes the mucous membranes of the sinuses become swollen and inflamed—the condition we know as *sinusitis.*

Text continues on p. 62.

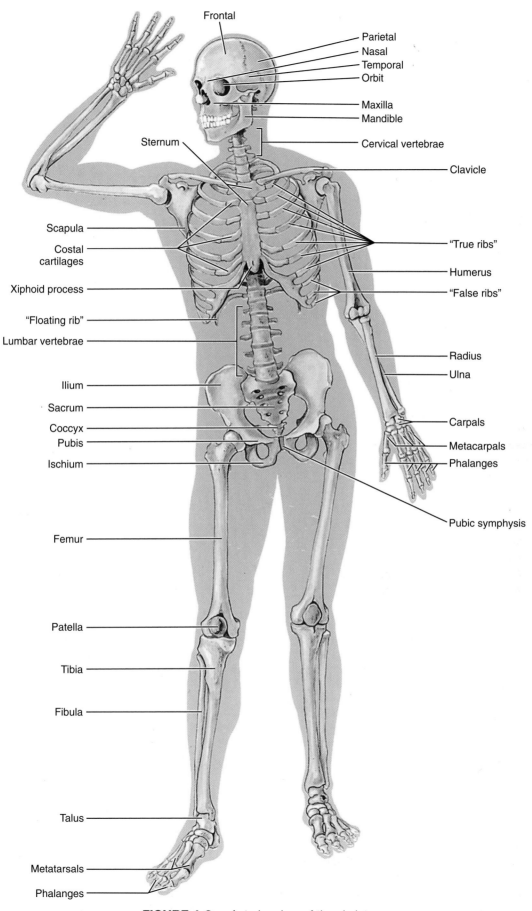

Frontal

Parietal
Nasal
Temporal
Orbit

Maxilla
Mandible

Cervical vertebrae

Sternum

Clavicle

Scapula

Costal
cartilages

"True ribs"

Humerus

Xiphoid process

"False ribs"

"Floating rib"

Lumbar vertebrae

Radius
Ulna

Ilium

Sacrum

Coccyx

Carpals

Pubis

Metacarpals

Ischium

Phalanges

Pubic symphysis

Femur

Patella

Tibia

Fibula

Talus

Metatarsals

Phalanges

FIGURE 4-3 • Anterior view of the skeleton.

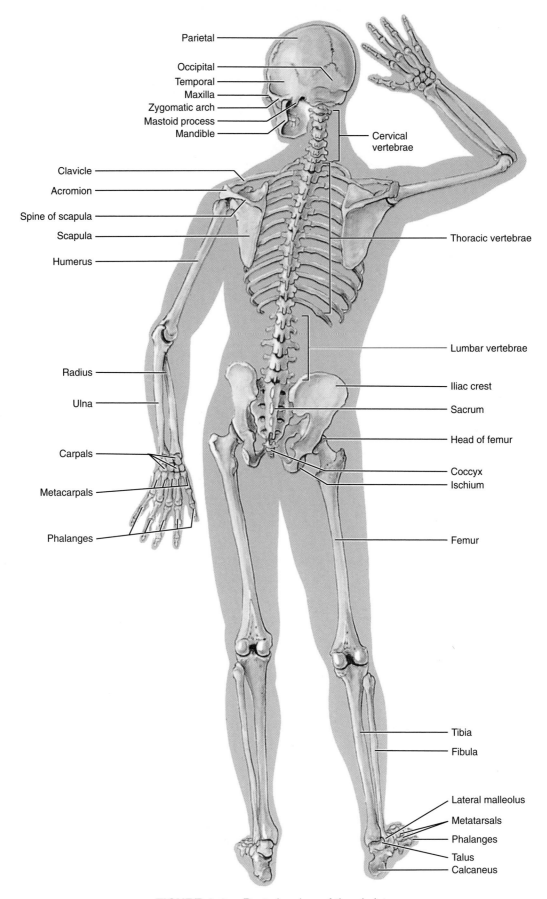

FIGURE 4-4 • Posterior view of the skeleton.

TABLE 4-2	BONES THAT MAKE UP THE AXIAL SKELETON	
Name of Bone (Number)	**Function**	**Description**
CRANIAL BONES		
Frontal (1)	Forms forehead and front part of cranium floor; forms part of roof over eyes and nasal cavity	Large, curved bone
		Frontal sinuses: air-filled cavities lined with mucous membrane
		Supraorbital ridge: just below eyebrows
Parietal (2) (pah-**rye'**-eh-tal)	Form much of walls and roof of cranium	Curved, flattened bones that meet at midline of cranium just behind frontal bone
Temporal (2)	Helps form floor and lateral wall of cranial cavity; contains ear canal, middle ear bones, and sensory portions of ear; bears temporomandibular joint (see "Mandible" below)	Pointed **styloid process** serves as point of attachment for certain neck muscles; **mastoid process** contains air-filled sinuses that may become infected when a middle ear infection spreads; **zygomatic process** helps form cheek
Occipital (1)	Forms most of floor and posterior part of skull; articulates with neck	Contains **foramen magnum** through which spinal cord passes; **occipital condyles** articulate with first vertebra of spinal column
Sphenoid (1) (**sfee'**-noyd)	Forms floor of cranium; helps form eye orbits	Shaped like butterfly
		Sella turcica (**sell'**-ah **tur'**-si-kah): saddle-shaped depression on superior surface holds pituitary gland; also called *Turkish saddle*
		Sphenoid sinus: air-filled spaces lined with mucous membrane
Ethmoid (1) (**eth'**-moyd)	Forms roof of nasal cavity and part of medial walls of eye orbits	Has irregular shape
		Crista galli: beak-shaped process to which an extension (falx cerebri) of outermost membrane surrounding brain attaches
		Cribiform plate: area of ethmoid perforated by tiny holes through which fibers of olfactory nerves pass from nose to brain
		Superior and middle turbinates (conchae): projections that form ledges along lateral walls of nasal cavity
		Ethmoid sinuses: air-filled spaces lined with mucous membrane
FACIAL BONES		
Mandible (1) (**man'**-dih-bal)	Lower jawbone; joins with temporal bone on each side forming **temporomandibular joints** (only freely movable joints in the skull); used in many mouth movements, especially chewing	U-shaped bone; its body (horizontal part) forms chin; its rami (vertical parts) have condyles (heads) that articulate with temporal bones
		Alveolar process: bony ridge in which lower teeth are rooted
Maxilla (2) (mak-**sil'**-ah)	Fuse to form upper jaw bone; form lateral walls of nose, floor of orbits, anterior part of hard palate (roof of mouth)	Very irregular shape; all facial bones except mandible touch maxilla

Continued

TABLE 4-2	BONES THAT MAKE UP THE AXIAL SKELETON—cont'd	
Name of Bone (Number)	**Function**	**Description**
		Palatine processes: form anterior part of hard palate
		Alveolar process: bony ridge in which upper teeth are rooted
		Maxillary sinuses: largest sinuses; drain into nasal passages and throat
Palatine (2)	Forms posterior part of hard palate	Irregular shape; cleft palate occurs when these bones (or palatine processes) do not fuse
Malar (zygomatic) (2)	Cheekbones; form walls and floors of orbits	Curved, irregular shape
Nasal (2)	Form upper part of bridge of nose	Small, thin, triangular shape
Lacrimal (2) (**lak'**-rih-mal)	Help form medial wall of orbit; contain a groove through which tears pass into nasal cavity	About size and shape of fingernail
Vomer (1) (**voe'**-mar)	Forms inferior, back part of nasal septum	Trapezoid shaped
Inferior turbinate (2)	Forms ledge along lateral walls of nose; increases surface area of nasal cavity	Scroll shaped
EAR BONES AND HYOID A chain of three tiny bones, or ossicles, in each middle ear cavity		
Malleus (2)	Transmits vibration from eardrum	Attached to eardrum; shaped somewhat like hammer
Incus (2)	Transmits vibration in middle ear	Shaped somewhat like anvil
Stapes (2)	Transmits vibration to oval window	Shaped like stirrup
Hyoid (1)	Important during swallowing	U-shaped, located in neck between mandible and larynx; does not articulate directly with any other bone
VERTEBRAL COLUMN Cervical vertebrae (7)		
Atlas (C1)	First cervical vertebra; forms joints with occipital condyles that allow head to nod "yes"	Has no centrum; no neural spine
Axis (C2)	Second cervical vertebra; its odontoid process serves as pivot for rotation of atlas and skull; permits you to shake your head "no"	**Odontoid process** (dens) projects upward from centrum
Inferior cervical vertebrae	**Spines** serve as points of attachment for neck and back muscles	Can be identified by **transverse foramina** through which vertebral arteries and veins pass
Thoracic vertebrae (12)	Ribs attach to these vertebrae; part of thoracic cage	Have facets for articulation with ribs
Lumbar vertebrae (5)	Make up part of vertebral column in small of back; support most of body weight; responsible for much of flexibility of trunk; many back muscles attach to them	Large, heavy vertebrae
Sacrum (1) (**say'**-krum)	Part of pelvic girdle	5 separate vertebrae in child; fuse to form a single bone in adult
Coccyx (1) (**kok'**-six)	Several pelvic and hip muscles originate on coccyx	3-5 separate vertebrae in child; fuse in adult

TABLE 4-2	BONES THAT MAKE UP THE AXIAL SKELETON—cont'd	
Name of Bone (Number)	Function	Description
THORACIC CAGE		
Ribs (24)	Protect organs of thoracic cavity; form part of thoracic cage	Long, curved bones
		True ribs: upper 7 pairs; attach directly to sternum by way of costal cartilages
		False ribs: pairs 8, 9, and 10; attach to sternum by way of common bar of cartilage that joins costal cartilage of seventh ribs
		Floating ribs: pairs 11 and 12; not connected to sternum
Sternum (1)	Breastbone; protects heart and anchors anterior ends of ribs; produces red blood cells in its marrow cavity	Consists of 3 parts: thick, superior **manubrium;** long **body;** inferior **xiphoid process** composed of cartilage (xiphoid process important landmark for cardiopulmonary resuscitation)

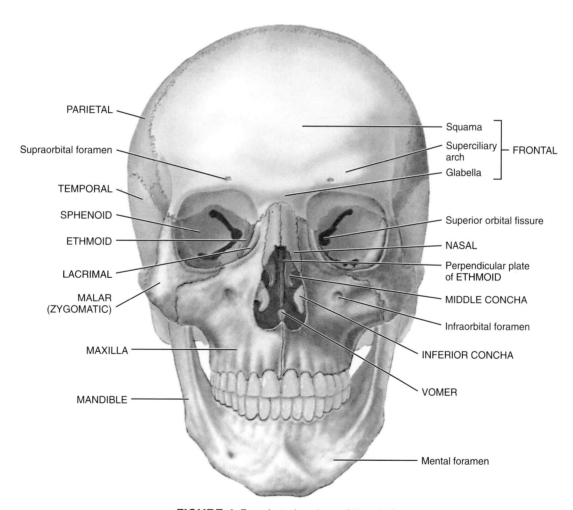

FIGURE 4-5 • Anterior view of the skull.

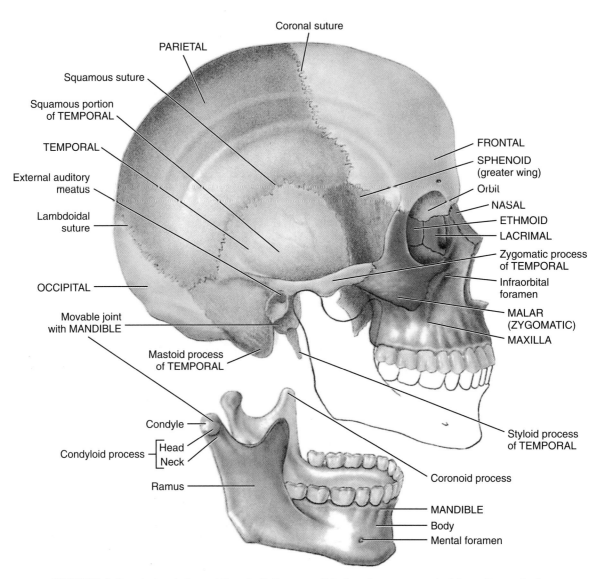

Coronal suture

PARIETAL

Squamous suture

Squamous portion
of TEMPORAL

TEMPORAL

External auditory
meatus

Lambdoidal
suture

OCCIPITAL

Movable joint
with MANDIBLE

Mastoid process
of TEMPORAL

Condyle

Condyloid process ⎡Head
                  ⎣Neck

Ramus

FRONTAL

SPHENOID
(greater wing)

Orbit

NASAL

ETHMOID

LACRIMAL

Zygomatic process
of TEMPORAL

Infraorbital
foramen

MALAR
(ZYGOMATIC)

MAXILLA

Styloid process
of TEMPORAL

Coronoid process

MANDIBLE

Body

Mental foramen

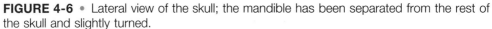

FIGURE 4-6 • Lateral view of the skull; the mandible has been separated from the rest of
the skull and slightly turned.

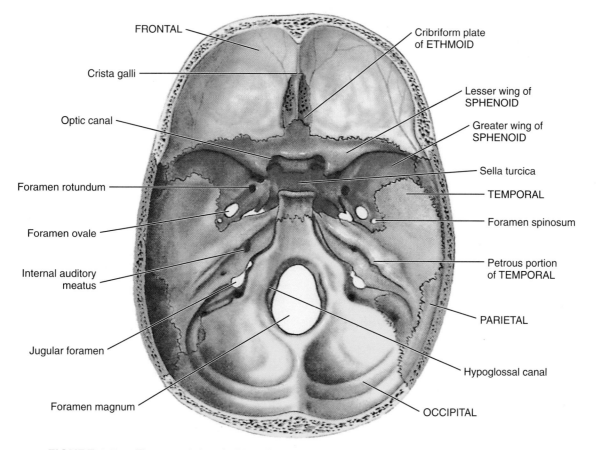

FRONTAL

Crista galli

Optic canal

Foramen rotundum

Foramen ovale

Internal auditory
meatus

Jugular foramen

Foramen magnum

Cribriform plate
of ETHMOID

Lesser wing of
SPHENOID

Greater wing of
SPHENOID

Sella turcica

TEMPORAL

Foramen spinosum

Petrous portion
of TEMPORAL

PARIETAL

Hypoglossal canal

OCCIPITAL

FIGURE 4-7 • The top of the skull has been removed to expose the superior surface of the cranial floor. Superior views of portions of the ethmoid and sphenoid bones can be seen in the floor of the cranial cavity.

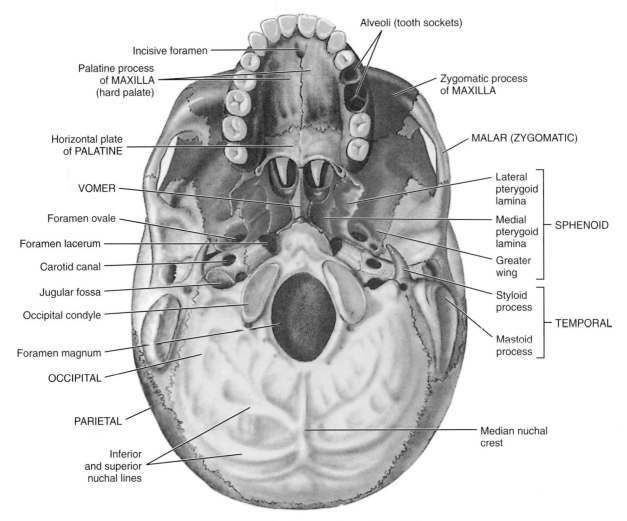

FIGURE 4-8 • Inferior view of the skull.

The Vertebral Column Supports the Body

The **vertebral column,** or spine, supports the body and bears its weight. It consists of 24 vertebrae and two fused bones—the **sacrum** (**say′**-krum) and **coccyx** (**kok′**-six) (Figure 4-9). The regions of the vertebral column are the **cervical** (neck), composed of seven vertebrae; the **thoracic** (chest), which consists of 12 vertebrae; the **lumbar** (back), composed of five vertebrae; the **sacral** (pelvic), which is a single bone (sacrum) composed of five fused vertebrae; and the **coccygeal,** made up of three to five fused vertebrae (see Table 4-2.). The vertebral column is S-shaped because of four curves that develop before birth and during childhood. These curves provide strength and flexibility for the vertebral column.

Vertebrae articulate with each other by means of synovial joints and by means of **intervertebral disks** composed of cartilage. The intervertebral disks are tiny pads that act as shock absorbers. Occasionally an intervertebral disk herniates (ruptures); the soft, central part of the disk bulges out and puts pressure on the root of a spinal nerve. This condition, popularly known as a *slipped disk,* can be extremely painful.

A "typical" vertebra consists of two main parts. The anterior region is the **body,** or **centrum.** The posterior, curved region of the vertebra is the **neural arch** (also called *vertebral arch*). The body and neural arch enclose a large opening called the **vertebral foramen.** The adjacent vertebral foramina form the **vertebral canal,** which contains the spinal cord. Vertebrae also have projections for the attachment of ribs and muscles and for joining with other vertebrae. Some structural features of vertebrae are shown in Figures 4-9 and 4-10 and are described in Table 4-3.

The Thoracic Cage Protects the Organs of the Chest

The **thoracic cage,** or rib cage, protects the internal organs of the chest, including the heart and lungs. This bony cage is formed by the **sternum,** or breast bone, the thoracic vertebrae, and 12 pairs of **ribs.** The thoracic cage protects the heart and lungs, provides support for the bones of the pectoral girdle and upper **extremities** (the limbs), and is important in breathing.

Text continues on p. 65.

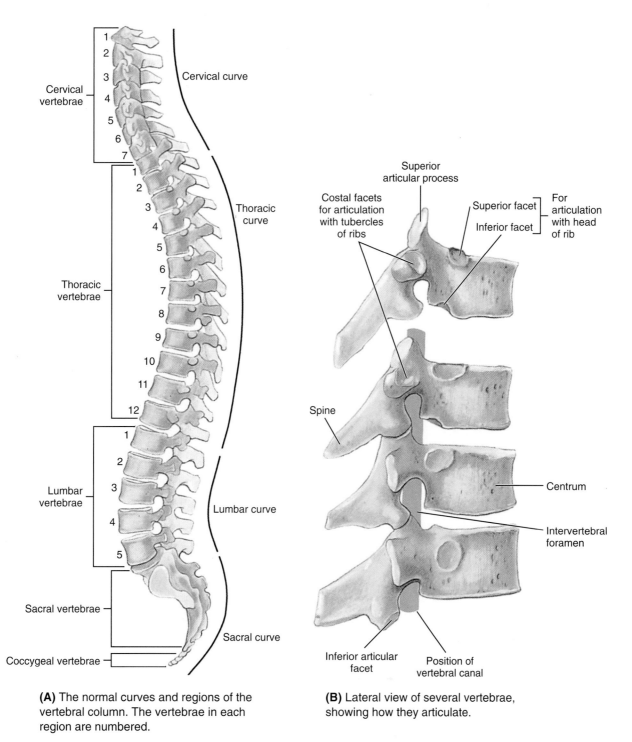

Cervical vertebrae
1
2
3
4
5
6
7

Cervical curve

Thoracic vertebrae
1
2
3
4
5
6
7
8
9
10
11
12

Thoracic curve

Lumbar vertebrae
1
2
3
4
5

Lumbar curve

Sacral vertebrae

Coccygeal vertebrae

Sacral curve

Superior articular process

Costal facets for articulation with tubercles of ribs

Superior facet
Inferior facet

For articulation with head of rib

Spine

Centrum

Intervertebral foramen

Inferior articular facet

Position of vertebral canal

(A) The normal curves and regions of the vertebral column. The vertebrae in each region are numbered.

(B) Lateral view of several vertebrae, showing how they articulate.

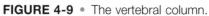

FIGURE 4-9 • The vertebral column.

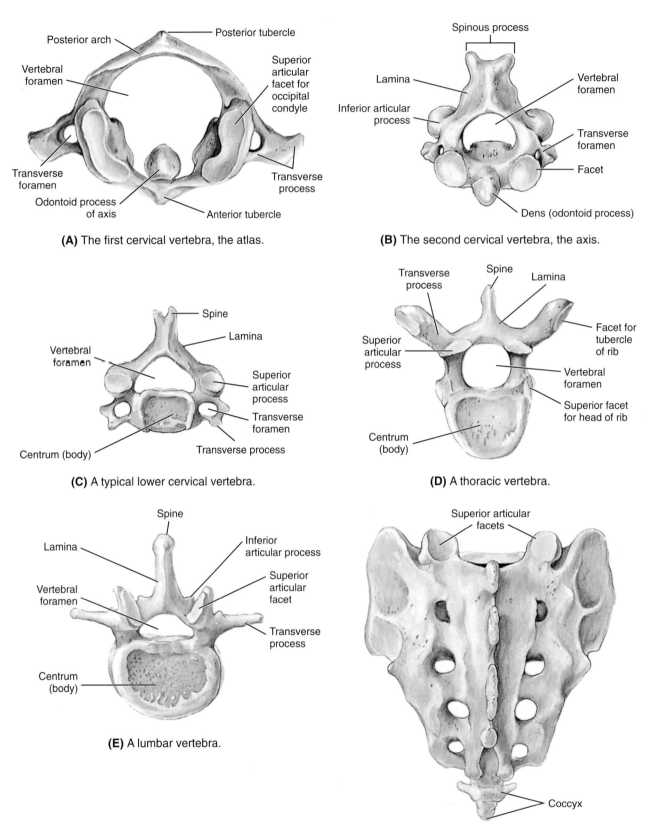

(A) The first cervical vertebra, the atlas.

(B) The second cervical vertebra, the axis.

(C) A typical lower cervical vertebra.

(D) A thoracic vertebra.

(E) A lumbar vertebra.

(F) The sacrum and coccyx.

FIGURE 4-10 • Vertebrae from different regions of the vertebral column have distinctive features.

TABLE 4-3	VERTEBRAE STRUCTURE
Structural Feature	**Definition**
Centrum (or body)	The bony central part of the vertebra that bears most of the body weight
Lamina	Posterolateral sides of the neural arch
Vertebral foramen	Passageway through which the spinal cord passes
Spinous process	Posterior projection from the lamina; back muscles attach to this process
Transverse processes	Lateral projections from the centrum; provided with articular surfaces for joining with other vertebrae and ribs
Superior and inferior articular processes	Projections lateral to the vertebral foramen; where vertebra forms joints with adjacent vertebrae

Quiz Yourself

- What are the eight bones of the cranium?
- What are the regions of the vertebral column?
- Which bones form the thoracic cage?

THE APPENDICULAR SKELETON CONSISTS OF 126 BONES

LEARNING OBJECTIVES

9. **Identify the bones of the appendicular skeleton and locate each on a diagram or skeleton.**
10. **Describe and give the function of each of the bones of the pectoral girdle, upper extremity, pelvic girdle, and lower extremity.**

The **appendicular** (ap-en-**dik′**-u-lar) **skeleton** consists of the bones of the upper and lower extremities (limbs) plus the bones making up the pectoral (shoulder) girdle and the pelvic girdle (with the exception of the sacrum). Descriptions and functions of these bones are given in Table 4-4.

The Pectoral Girdle Attaches the Upper Extremities to the Axial Skeleton

Each half of the **pectoral girdle** consists of a **scapula** (shoulder blade) and a **clavicle** (collarbone). The pectoral girdle articulates with the sternum but not with the vertebral column.

The Bones of the Upper Extremity Are Located in the Arm, Forearm, Wrist, and Hand

Each upper extremity consists of 30 bones—the **humerus** (**hu′**-mer-us) in the upper limb, the **ulna** (**ul′**-nuh) and radius (**ray′**-dee-us) in the forearm, eight small **carpal** (**kar′**-pal) **bones** in the wrist, five **metacarpal** bones in the palm of the

hand, and 14 **phalanges** (fay-**lan′**-jeez) in the fingers (Figure 4-11, p. 68).

The Pelvic Girdle Supports the Lower Extremities

The **pelvic girdle** is a broad basin of bone that encloses the pelvic cavity. The pelvic girdle supports the lower extremities and is the site of attachment of major muscles of the trunk and lower limbs. It supports the weight of the upper body and protects the organs that lie within the pelvic cavity—the reproductive organs, urinary bladder, and part of the large intestine. The hip bones are called **coxal bones** (also called *os coxae* or *innominate bones*). The coxal bones, together with the sacrum and coccyx, form the pelvic girdle (Figure 4-12, p. 68).

Each coxal bone is formed from the fusion of three bones during development. The largest of the three, the **ilium,** lies on top of the other two bones. The most posterior bone is the **ischium** (**is′**-kee-um). The anterior bone is the **pubis.** In the adult, the ilium, ischium, and pubis are not separate bones; they form the parts of the coxal bone. The joint where the coxal bones come together anteriorly is called the **pubic symphysis** (**sim′**-fih-sis).

The female pelvis is adapted for holding a developing baby and permitting its passage to the outside world at birth. Accordingly, it is broader and shallower than the male pelvis (see Figure 4-12). The pelvic inlet in the female is larger and more circular. The ischial spines of the female are shorter, so there is a greater relative distance between them. The female pelvis also has a greater angle between the pubic bones.

The Bones of the Lower Extremity Are Located in the Thigh, Knee, Leg, Ankle, and Foot

The lower extremity consists of 30 bones—the **femur** (**fee′**-mer) in the upper limb, or thigh; the **patella** (pah-**tel′**-uh), or kneecap; the **tibia** (**tib′**-ee-ah) and **fibula** (**fib′**-u-lah) in the lower leg, or shin; the 7 **tarsal bones** in the back part of the

TABLE 4-4	BONES THAT MAKE UP THE APPENDICULAR SKELETON	
Name of Bone (Number)	**Function**	**Description**
PECTORAL GIRDLE		
Scapula (2) (**skap'**-u-lah)	Shoulder blade	Somewhat flat, triangular bone **Spine:** sharp ridge that runs diagonally across posterior surface of shoulder blade **Acromion process:** helps hold head of humerus in place **Glenoid fossa:** socket that receives head of humerus
Clavicle (2) (**klav'**-ih-kle)	Collarbone; connects scapula with sternum; helps form shoulder joint	Small, curved bone
UPPER LIMB		
Humerus (2) (**hu'**-mer-us)	Upper arm bone; forms joint with scapula above and with the radius and ulna at the elbow	Longest, largest bone of upper limb **Head:** fits into glenoid process of scapula
Radius (2)	Bone on thumb side of lower arm	Curved with lengthwise ridge
Ulna (2)	Medial bone of forearm; main forearm bone in elbow joint	**Styloid process:** sharp projection at distal end
Carpal bones (16) (**kar'**-pal)	Wrist bones	Irregular bones at proximal end of hand
Metacarpal bones (10)	Form palm of hand	Numbered I through V starting with the thumb; heads of metacarpals are knuckles
Phalanges (28) (fay-**lan'**-jeez)	Bones of fingers; 3 in each finger; 2 in each thumb; serve for attachment of several muscles and ligaments	Each has a proximal base, a shaft, and a distal head
PELVIC GIRDLE		
Coxal (innominate) (2)	Hipbone; supports weight of upper body	Formed by fusion of 3 bones: ilium, ischium, and pubis **Acetabulum:** hip socket; receives head of femur
Ilium (**il'**-ee-um)	Large flaring part of coxal bone; connects posteriorly with sacrum at sacroiliac joint	**Iliac crest:** upper edge of ilium (feels somewhat like a shelf) **Anterior superior spine:** projection at anterior end of iliac crest
Ischium (**iss'**-kee-um)	Lower, posterior portion of coxal bone	**Ischial tuberosity:** large, rough area on which body rests when sitting erect **Ischial spine:** superior to tuberosity; narrows pelvic outlet through which baby passes during delivery
Pubis (**pu'**-bis)	Most anterior part of coxal bone	**Obturator foramen:** largest foramen in body; formed by pubis and ischium **Pubic symphysis:** joint between pubic bones; made of fibrocartilage **Pelvic brim (inlet):** opening within flaring parts of ilia that leads into true pelvis **True (lesser) pelvis:** space inferior to pelvic brim; bounded by muscle and bone; pelvic organs located here; superior opening is **pelvic inlet;** inferior opening is **pelvic outlet** (true pelvis must be large enough in female to permit passage of infant's head during childbirth)

TABLE 4-4	BONES THAT MAKE UP THE APPENDICULAR SKELETON—cont'd	
Name of Bone (Number)	**Function**	**Description**
LOWER LIMB		
Femur (2) (**fee'**-mur)	Thigh bone; largest bone in the body	Slightly curved bone
		Head: ball-like end; fits into acetabulum
		Condyles: rounded projections at distal end; articulate with tibia
		Greater trochanter: prominent projection from upper part of shaft; large muscles (including gluteus maximus) attach here
		Lesser trochanter: smaller projection located inferiorly and medially to greater trochanter
Patella (2) (pah-**tell'**-ah)	Kneecap	Largest sesamoid bone (one that occurs in a tendon or other soft tissue and does not articulate with any other bone)
Tibia (2) (**tib'**-ee-ah)	Larger and more medial of the two shank bones	**Medial and lateral condyles:** articulate with condyles of femur, forming knee joint
		Medial malleolus: medial, rounded process at distal end
Fibula (2) (**fib'**-u-lah)	Smaller bone of shank; foot muscles attach to it	Slender bone. **Lateral malleolus:** lateral, rounded process at distal end; the medial and lateral malleoli are popularly referred to as the *ankle bones*
Tarsals (14)	Ankle and proximal foot bones; 4 (3 cuneiforms and 1 cuboid) articulate with long bones (metatarsals) of each foot; the largest tarsal is the calcaneus (kal-**kay'**-nee-us), or heelbone	2 longitudinal and 1 transverse arch are formed by arrangement of tarsals and metatarsals; these bones are held in arched position by tendons and ligaments; arches permit bones and their ligaments to act as shock absorbers
Metatarsals (10)	Form middle part of foot	Numbered I through V starting with the most medial
Phalanges (28)	Toe bones; 3 in each toe; 2 in each great toe	Each has a proximal base, a shaft, and a distal head

foot and heel; the 5 **metatarsals** in the main part of the foot; and the 14 **phalanges** in the toes (Figure 4-13).

Quiz Yourself

- Which bones are found in the upper extremity?
- Which bones make up the coxal bone?

JOINTS ARE JUNCTIONS BETWEEN BONES

LEARNING OBJECTIVES

11. **Compare the main types of joints.**
12. **Describe the structure and functions of a diarthrosis and describe types of body movements.**

A **joint,** or **articulation,** is the point of contact between two bones. Joints hold bones together, and many of them permit flexibility and movement.

Joints Can Be Classified According to the Degree of Movement They Permit

Joints can be classified into three main groups according to the degree of movement they permit. **Synarthroses** (sin'-ar-**throw'**-sees) do not permit movement. They connect bones by means of a thin layer of fibrous connective tissue that may be replaced by bone in the adult. The sutures that join skull bones are synarthroses (Figure 4-14, *A*, p. 70).

Amphiarthroses (am'-fee-ar-**throw'**-sees) permit slight movement and help absorb shock. In this type of joint, bones are joined by cartilage. The pubic symphysis of the pelvis and

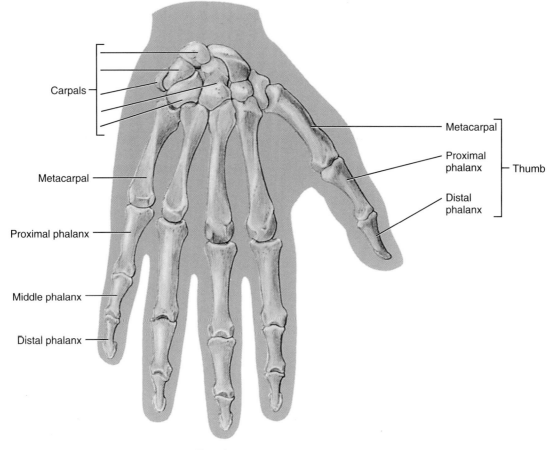

Dorsal

FIGURE 4-11 • The skeleton of the hand.

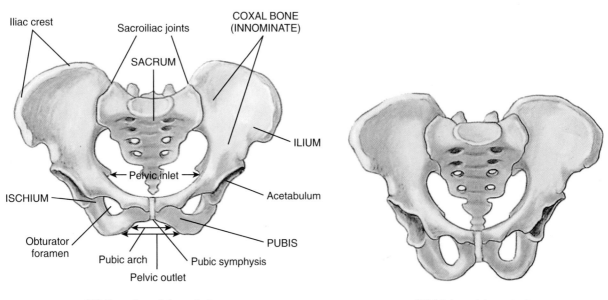

(A) Female pelvis, anterior

(B) Male pelvis, anterior

FIGURE 4-12 • Generally, the male pelvis **(B)** is narrower than the female pelvis **(A)**. However, some pelvises are hard to classify by gender. In this illustration, extreme examples are shown. In the adult, the ilium, ischium, and pubis are fused with one another and should be considered regions of the coxal bone rather than separate bones.

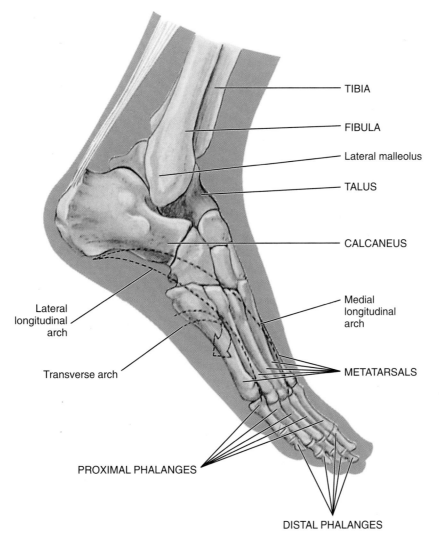

TIBIA

FIBULA

Lateral malleolus

TALUS

CALCANEUS

Medial
longitudinal
arch

METATARSALS

Lateral
longitudinal
arch

Transverse arch

PROXIMAL PHALANGES

DISTAL PHALANGES

FIGURE 4-13 • The bones of the right foot (lateral view). As indicated in the figure, the tarsal and metatarsal bones form several arches that help the foot support the weight of the body.

the intervertebral joints of the vertebral column are examples of amphiarthroses (Figure 4-14, *B*).

Diarthroses (dye′-ar-**throw**′-sees), or **synovial joints,** are referred to as *freely movable joints,* but their flexibility varies. Most of the body's joints are diarthroses. The six types of synovial joints are gliding, condyloid, saddle, pivot, hinge, and ball-and-socket. These are described in Table 4-5 and are shown in Figure 4-14, *C* and *D*. Some of the types of movement at the joints are described and illustrated in Table 4-6, p. 72.

A Diarthrosis Is Surrounded by a Joint Capsule

The ends of the bones forming a diarthrodial joint are covered with hyaline cartilage that lacks any sort of covering membrane. This articular cartilage also lacks nerves and blood vessels. The joint is surrounded by a connective tissue capsule,

the **joint capsule,** made of tough, fibrous connective tissue (Figure 4-15). This tissue is continuous with the periosteum of the bones but does not cover the articular cartilage. The joint capsule is generally reinforced with ligaments—bands of fibrous connective tissue that connect the bones and also limit movement at the joint.

The joint capsule is lined with a membrane that secretes a lubricant called **synovial fluid.** This viscous fluid reduces friction during movement and absorbs shock. In *rheumatoid arthritis,* the synovial membrane thickens and becomes inflamed. Synovial fluid accumulates, causing pressure, stiffness, and pain. The affected joints become deformed, resulting in loss of function.

Fluid-filled sacs called **bursae** (**bur**′-see) (singular—*bursa*) are located between bone and tendons and between bone and some other tissues. Bursae cushion the movement of bone over other tissues. Inflammation of a bursa is a painful condition known as *bursitis.*

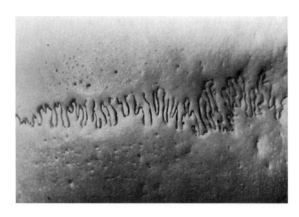

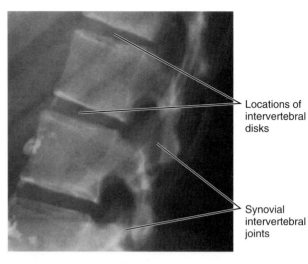

Locations of intervertebral disks

Synovial intervertebral joints

(A) Skull sutures are immovable joints, or synarthroses. This joint looks like an elaborate jigsaw puzzle.

(B) Intervertebral joints are amphiarthroses, or slightly movable joints.

Hinge joints

Epiphyses

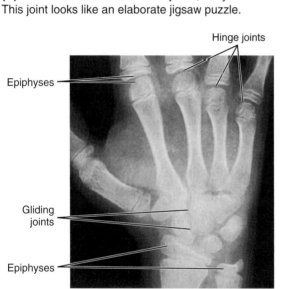

Gliding joints

Epiphyses

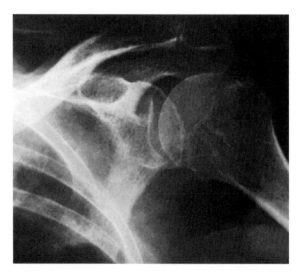

(C) Gliding joints between the wrist bones and hinge joints between the phalanges are synovial joints.

(D) The shoulder joint, also a synovial joint, is a ball-and-socket joint. It is one of the most freely movable joints and also the loosest joint in the body.

FIGURE 4-14 • X-ray images of several types of joints.

Joints wear down with time and use. In the common degenerative joint disorder *osteoarthritis*, cartilage repair does not keep up with degeneration, and the articular cartilage wears out. Inflammation results in joint pain.

Quiz Yourself

- How is an amphiarthrosis different from a synarthrosis?
- What is synovial fluid? Where is it found?

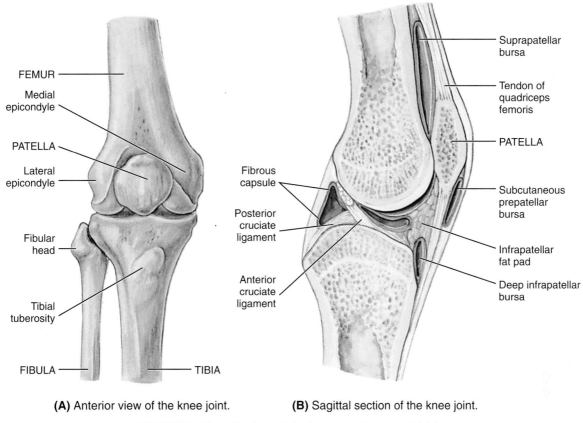

(A) Anterior view of the knee joint.   **(B)** Sagittal section of the knee joint.

FIGURE 4-15 • The knee joint is a complex synovial joint.

TABLE 4-5	SOME TYPES OF SYNOVIAL JOINTS		
Type	**Example**	**Shape of Joint Surface**	**Range of Movement**
Condyloid	Joints between metacarpals and phalanges	Oval-shaped condyle fits into elliptical cavity	Angular movement
Gliding	Carpal joints of wrist; tarsal joints of ankle	Flat or slightly curved	One bone glides over another without circular movement
Saddle	Carpometacarpal joint of thumb	Saddle-shaped	Permits wide range of movement
Pivot	Atlantoaxial joint of first two cervical vertebrae; radioulnar joint of elbow	Small projection of one bone pivots in ring-shaped socket of another bone	Rotation
Hinge	Elbow; knee	Convex surface of one bone fits into concave surface of another bone	Motion in one plane only; permits only flexion and extension
Ball-and-socket	Shoulder; hip joint	Ball-shaped end of one bone fits into cup-shaped socket of another bone	Permits widest range of movement, including rotation

TABLE 4-6   TYPES OF BODY MOVEMENTS

Movement	Description	Illustration
Flexion (**flek'**-shun)	Bending of joint; usually a movement that reduces angle of joint and brings two bones closer together (when you crouch, your knees are flexed; when you touch your shoulder, your elbow is flexed)	(A)
Extension	Opposite of flexion; increases angle of joint, increasing distance between two bones; examples of extension include straightening the knee or the elbow	(B)
Abduction (ab-**duk'**-shun)	Movement of bone or limb away from midline, or median plane of body; abduction in hands and feet is movement of digit away from central axis of limb (one abducts fingers by spreading them apart)	(C)
Adduction	Movement of bone or limb toward the midline of body or, for extremities, movement toward axis of limb; opposite of abduction	(D)
Circumduction (ser'-kum-**duk'**-shun)	Combination of movements that makes body part describe a circle; characteristic of ball-and-socket joints such as shoulder	(E)

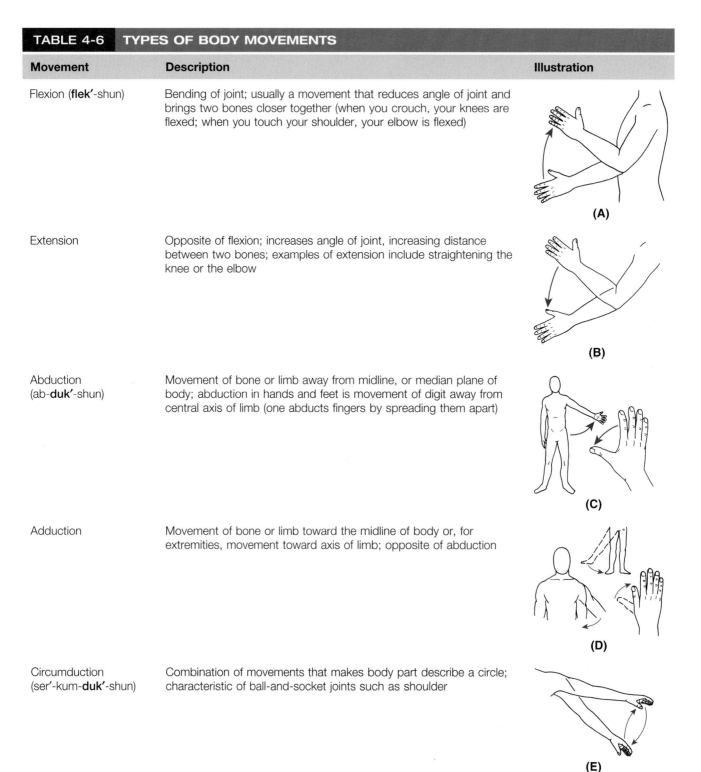

TABLE 4-6	TYPES OF BODY MOVEMENTS—cont'd	
Movement	**Description**	**Illustration**
Rotation	Pivoting of body part around its axis, as in shaking the head "no"; no rotation of any body part is complete (i.e., 360 degrees)	
Pronation	Movement of forearm that in extended position brings palm of hand from upward-facing to downward-facing position; applies only to arm; this action moves distal end of radius across ulna	
Supination	Opposite of pronation; when forearm is in extended position, this movement brings palm of hand facing upward	
Inversion	Ankle movement that turns sole of foot medially; applies only to foot	
Eversion	Opposite of inversion; turns sole of foot laterally	

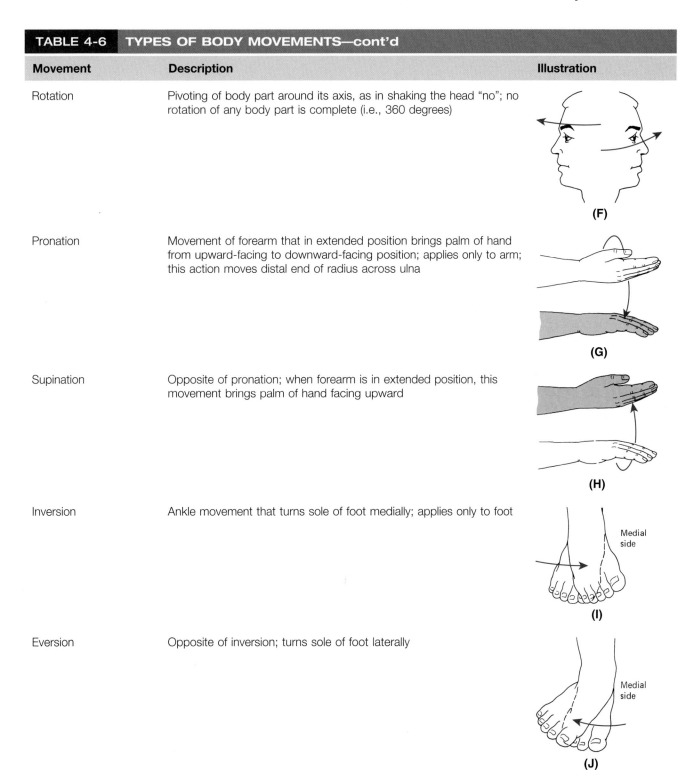

(F)

(G)

(H)

Medial side

(I)

Medial side

(J)

SUMMARY

LO 1. **List five functions of the skeletal system.**
- The **skeletal system** supports and protects the body, produces blood cells, and stores and releases minerals such as calcium and phosphorus.
- Bones serve as levers that transmit muscular forces. Muscles are attached to bones by bands of connective tissue called **tendons.** When muscles contract, they pull on bones, thereby moving parts of the body.

LO 2. **Describe the gross and microscopic structure of a typical bone.**
- A long bone consists of a **diaphysis** (shaft) with flared ends called **epiphyses.**
- It has growth centers called **metaphyses** that disappear at maturity. The bone has a central marrow cavity filled with yellow marrow and lined with an **endosteum.**
- The bone is covered by a **periosteum** that contains **osteoblasts.**
- **Compact** bone consists of **osteons,** or **haversian systems. Osteocytes,** the mature bone cells, are found in small cavities called **lacunae,** which are arranged in concentric circles around central **haversian canals.**
- **Spongy bone** consists of thin strands of bone. The spaces within spongy bone are filled with **bone marrow.** Blood cells are manufactured in **red bone marrow.**

LO 3. **Contrast endochondral with intramembranous bone development.**
- **Endochondral bones** develop from a cartilage model; **intramembranous bones** develop from a noncartilage connective tissue model.

LO 4. **Describe the functions of osteoblasts and osteoclasts in bone production and remodeling.**
- Osteoblasts are cells that produce bone; **osteoclasts** break down bone.

LO 5. **Distinguish between the axial skeleton and the appendicular skeleton.**
- The **axial skeleton** forms the vertical axis of the body; it consists of the skull, vertebral column, ribs, and sternum. The **appendicular skeleton** consists of the upper and lower extremities, the pectoral girdle, and the pelvic girdle.

LO = Learning Objective

LO 6. **Identify the bones of the axial skeleton, and locate each on a diagram or skeleton.**
- The axial skeleton consists of the skull, vertebral column, ribs, and **sternum** (breast bone). The **thoracic cage** (rib cage) is formed by the sternum, thoracic vertebrae, and 12 pairs of **ribs.**

LO 7. **Describe and give the function of each of the cranial and facial bones.**
- The **skull** is formed by the **cranium** and facial bones. The cranial bones include the **frontal bone, occipital bone, ethmoid bone, sphenoid bone,** and the paired **parietal bones** and **temporal bones.** The facial bones include the **maxilla, mandible, vomer,** and the paired **malars, palatines, nasals, lacrimals,** and **inferior turbinates.** See Table 4-2 for descriptions and functions of each of these bones.
- Most bones of the skull are joined by immovable joints called **sutures.** The **sagittal suture** joins the parietal bones in the midline. **Fontanelles** are joints that are present in the skull at birth before ossification is complete. They consist of fibrous connective tissue or cartilage.

LO 8. **Describe and give the function of each of the bones of the vertebral column and of the thoracic cage.**
- The vertebral column consists of seven cervical vertebrae, 12 thoracic vertebrae, five lumbar vertebrae, the sacrum, and the coccyx. The first cervical vertebra is the atlas; the second is the axis.
- A typical vertebra consists of a body, or centrum, and a neural arch that enclose the vertebral foramen. Adjacent vertebral foramina form the vertebral canal that holds the spinal cord. The posterolateral sides of the neural arch are the laminae. The transverse processes are lateral projections from the centrum that provide surfaces for joining with other vertebrae and ribs. The superior articular processes and inferior articular processes are projections where a vertebra forms joints with other vertebrae.

LO 9. **Identify the bones of the appendicular skeleton and locate each on a diagram or skeleton.**
- The **appendicular skeleton** consists of the upper and lower extremities, the pectoral girdle, and the pelvic girdle (see Table 4-4, pp. 66-67).

LO 10. **Describe and give the function of each of the bones of the pectoral girdle, upper extremity, pelvic girdle, and lower extremity.**
- The **pectoral girdle** attaches the upper extremities to the axial skeleton; it consists of the **scapulae** and **clavicles.**
- Each upper extremity consists of a **humerus, ulna, radius,** 8 **carpal bones,** 5 **metacarpals,** and 14 **phalanges.**
- The **pelvic girdle** consists of the **coxal bones** together with the **sacrum** and **coccyx.**
- Each coxal bone consists of three fused bones: an **ilium, ischium,** and **pubis.** The female pelvis is broader and shallower than the male pelvis; the pelvic inlet is larger and more circular.
- Each lower extremity consists of a **femur, tibia, fibula,** 7 **tarsal bones,** 5 **metatarsals,** and 14 **phalanges.**

LO 11. **Compare the main types of joints.**
- An **articulation,** or **joint,** is the junction between two or more bones. **Synarthroses** are immovable joints such as sutures in the skull. **Amphiarthroses** are slightly movable joints such as the pubic symphysis. **Diarthroses,** also called **synovial joints,** are movable joints. The body has several types of diarthroses. The ball-and-socket joint permits the greatest freedom of movement.

LO 12. **Describe the structure and functions of a diarthrosis and describe types of body movements.**
- In diarthroses, the articulating bone surfaces are covered with hyaline cartilage and are enclosed in a **joint capsule. Ligaments** are bands of fibrous connective tissue that bind bones together at joints.
- Types of body movements are described in Table 4-6, pp. 72-73.

CHAPTER QUIZ

Fill in the Blank

1. The _____ _____ within some bones produces blood cells.

2. Bone is covered by a connective tissue membrane, the _____.

3. The main shaft of a long bone is its _____.

4. Compact bone consists of spindle-shaped units called _____.

5. Osteocytes are found in small cavities called _____.

6. Osteoclasts are cells that _____.

7. The skull and ribs are part of the _____ skeleton.

8. The skull consists of the _____ and _____ bones.

9. The _____ _____ joins the parietal bones at the midline.

10. The vertebral foramen is a passageway for the _____ _____.

11. The scapula is part of the _____ _____.

12. The ribs are attached to the _____ vertebrae.

13. The bony central body of a vertebra is its _____.

14. An example of an immovable joint is a _____.

15. _____ fluid is found in diarthroses.

16. The bending of a joint is known as _____; movement of a limb away from the midline of the body is _____.

17. A joint, like the elbow joint, that moves in one plane only is a _____ joint.

Multiple Choice

18. The lower jaw bone is the: a. atlas; b. mandible; c. calcaneus; d. maxilla.

19. The metacarpals are found in the: a. skull; b. hand; c. foot; d. vertebral column.

20. The most anterior part of the coxal bone is the: a. pubis; b. sacrum; c. ischium; d. ilium.

21. The bone that articulates with occipital condyles is the: a. atlas; b. axis; c. coccyx; d. sphenoid.

22. Blood vessels and nerves would most likely pass through a: a. facet; b. crest; c. fissure; d. sinus.

23. The sella turcica is part of the: a. ethmoid; b. parietal; c. palatine; d. sphenoid.

24. The structure that is *not* characteristic of a thoracic vertebra is the: a. centrum; b. spine; c. styloid process; d. superior articular process.

REVIEW QUESTIONS

1. What are the functions of the skeletal system? How does the skeletal system help maintain homeostasis?

2. Compare spongy bone with compact bone.

3. How does the development of a skull bone differ from the development of a long bone such as the femur?

4. How do osteoblasts and osteoclasts function together in bone remodeling?

5. Describe the structure of the vertebral column. What are the advantages of a curved vertebral column over a straight one?

6. Where is the vertebral foramen? Why is it important?

7. Locate the following and give their functions: (a) sella turcica; (b) cribriform plate; (c) occipital condyles; (d) temporomandibular joint.

8. Locate each of the following: (a) metacarpals; (b) malar; (c) palatine; (d) axis.

9. How do false ribs differ from true ribs? How many pairs of ribs are there in a male? In a female?

10. Contrast the three main types of joints. What are ligaments? What are bursae?

11. What are the functions of: (a) condyles; (b) foramina; (c) facets?

12. Label the diagram below and the diagram on the following page. (See Figures 4-3 and 4-5 to check your answers.)

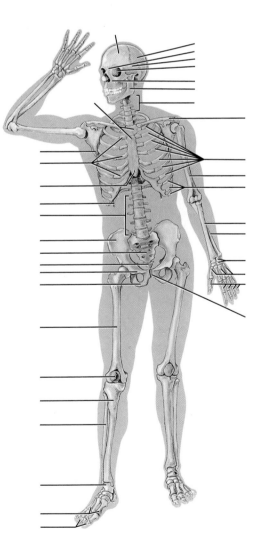

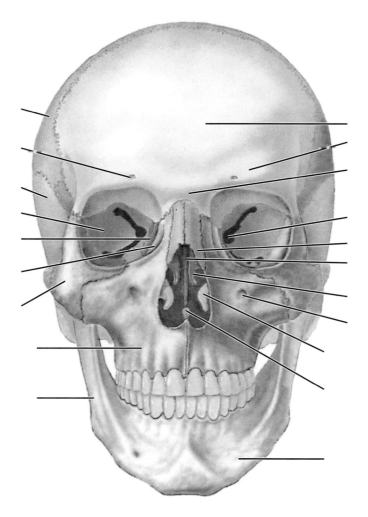

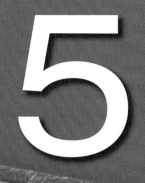

5 The Muscular System

Body movements—walking, talking, chewing food, circulating blood—depend on the action of muscles. The three types of muscles—skeletal, smooth, and cardiac—are compared in Chapter 2 (see Table 2-1). In this chapter we focus on skeletal muscle, the voluntary muscles attached to bones. Our 600 or so skeletal muscles work in coordinated ways, allowing us to carry on activities and move effectively through our world.

A SKELETAL MUSCLE IS COMPOSED OF HUNDREDS OF MUSCLE FIBERS

LEARNING OBJECTIVE

1. **Describe the structure of a skeletal muscle.**

Each **skeletal muscle** is an organ made up of hundreds, sometimes thousands, of muscle cells, referred to as **muscle fibers.** Individual muscle fibers are surrounded by a connective tissue covering—the **endomysium** (en'-doe-**mis'**-ee-um). The muscle fibers are arranged in bundles known as **fascicles** (**fas'**-ih-kuls). Each fascicle is wrapped by connective tissue, the **perimysium** (per'-ih-**mis'**-ee-um).

Each muscle has a nerve supply and a system of blood vessels that supply it with nutrients and oxygen and carry away its wastes. The muscle is surrounded by a covering of connective tissue called the **epimysium** (ep'-ih-**mis'**-ee-um) (Figure 5-1). The epimysium, perimysium, and endomysium are continuous with one another. Extensions of epimysium form tough cords of connective tissue, the **tendons,** that anchor muscles to bones. The muscle is surrounded by fibrous connective tissue called **fascia** (**fash'**-ee-ah) that merges with the tissue of the tendon.

ⓠ *Quiz Yourself*

- What are fascicles?
- What is the function of perimysium? Of endomysium?

MUSCLE FIBERS ARE SPECIALIZED FOR CONTRACTION

LEARNING OBJECTIVES

2. **Describe the structure of a muscle fiber and relate its structure to its function.**
3. **List, in sequence, the events that take place during muscle contraction.**
4. **Compare the roles of glycogen, creatine phosphate, and adenosine triphosphate (ATP) in providing energy for muscle contraction.**
5. **Define muscle tone and explain why muscle tone is important.**
6. **Distinguish between isotonic and isometric contraction.**

Each skeletal muscle fiber is a spindle-shaped cell with many nuclei and with numerous mitochondria that provide energy for muscle contraction. The plasma membrane has many inward extensions that form a set of **transverse tubules (T**

tubules**).** Each muscle fiber is almost filled with threadlike structures called **myofibrils** (my-oh-**fy'**-brills) that run lengthwise through the muscle fiber. The myofibrils are composed of even smaller structures called **muscle filaments** (myofilaments) that are made of protein threads.

There are two types of muscle filaments. Thick filaments, called **myosin** (**my'**-oh-sin) **filaments,** consist mainly of the protein **myosin.** Thin filaments, called **actin filaments,** consist of the protein **actin.** Myosin and actin are contractile proteins, which means they are capable of shortening. The myosin and actin filaments are largely responsible for muscle contraction.

Myosin and actin filaments are organized into repeating units called **sarcomeres**—the basic units of muscle contraction (Figure 5-2). Hundreds of sarcomeres connected end to end make up a myofibril. Sarcomeres are joined at their ends by an interweaving of filaments called the **Z line.** Each sarcomere consists of overlapping myosin and actin filaments. The filaments overlap lengthwise in the muscle fibers, producing the pattern of transverse bands, or **striations,** characteristic of striated muscle. (Recall from Chapter 2 that skeletal and cardiac muscle are both striated.) Muscle bands are designated by the letters *A, H,* and *I.*

Muscle Contraction Occurs When Actin and Myosin Filaments Slide Past Each Other

Movement of the body occurs when muscles pull on bones. A muscle pulls on a bone by contracting, or shortening. A muscle contracts when its fibers contract. Neither the actin nor myosin filaments change in length. The length of the muscle shortens as the filaments increase their overlap. You might think of an extension ladder. The overall ladder length changes as the ends get closer or farther apart, but the length of each ladder section stays the same.

A **motor nerve** is a nerve that signals a muscle to contract. The motor neurons (nerve cells) that make up a motor nerve transmit impulses (messages) to muscle fibers (Figure 5-3). Each motor neuron signals from one to several hundred muscle fibers. The junction of a nerve and muscle fiber is called a **neuromuscular junction.**

We can summarize the process of muscle contraction as follows:

1. A motor neuron releases the neurotransmitter acetylcholine (as'-eh-til-**koe'**-leen), which is a signaling molecule. Acetylcholine is released into the synaptic cleft (a small space) between the motor neuron and muscle fiber. Acetylcholine diffuses across the synaptic cleft and combines with receptors on the surface of the muscle fiber. This causes depolarization, a decrease in the electric charge difference across the plasma membrane of the muscle fiber. Depolarization may cause an electrical impulse, or **action potential,** to be generated in the muscle fiber. Excess acetylcholine is broken
Text continues on p. 83.

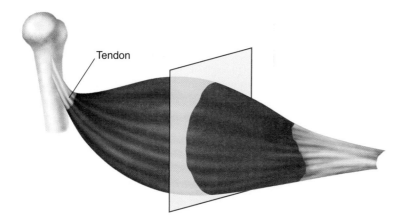

(A) The muscle is attached to bone by a tendon.

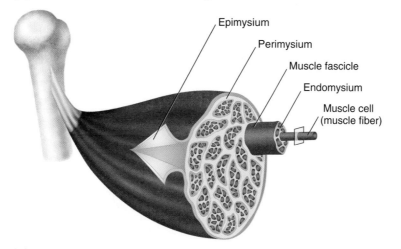

(B) The muscle is surrounded by a connective tissue covering—the epimysium. The muscle consists of fascicles—bundles of muscle fibers. Each fascicle is wrapped in connective tissue—the perimysium. Individual muscle fibers are surrounded by endomysium.

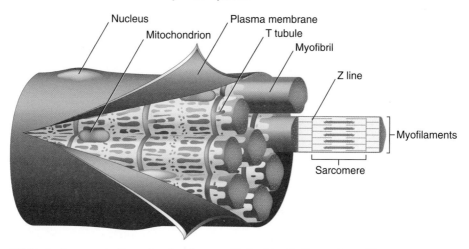

(C) Part of a muscle fiber showing the myofibrils. Myofibrils are threadlike structures composed of actin and myosin filaments. One myofibril is magnified and shown in detail to illustrate the filaments. The regular pattern of overlapping filaments gives skeletal and cardiac muscle their striated appearance. The Z lines mark the ends of the sarcomeres.

FIGURE 5-1 • Muscle structure. A skeletal muscle consists of fascicles (bundles) of muscle fibers. Each fiber is a cell containing myofibrils that consist of actin and myosin filaments. The filaments are organized into repeating units called sarcomeres.

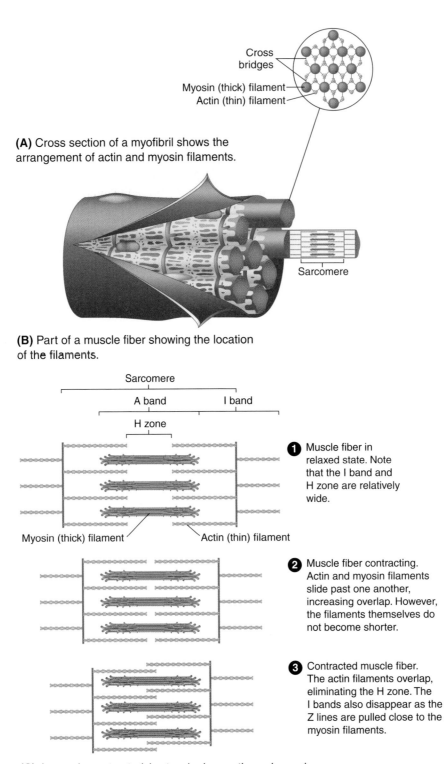

(A) Cross section of a myofibril shows the arrangement of actin and myosin filaments.

(B) Part of a muscle fiber showing the location of the filaments.

1 Muscle fiber in relaxed state. Note that the I band and H zone are relatively wide.

2 Muscle fiber contracting. Actin and myosin filaments slide past one another, increasing overlap. However, the filaments themselves do not become shorter.

3 Contracted muscle fiber. The actin filaments overlap, eliminating the H zone. The I bands also disappear as the Z lines are pulled close to the myosin filaments.

(C) A muscle contracts (shortens) when actin and myosin filaments slide past one another. The amount of overlap between actin and myosin filaments increases.

FIGURE 5-2 • Muscle contraction. Myofibrils are threadlike structures in the muscle fiber; they contain actin and myosin filaments. Muscle bands, produced by the overlapping of the filaments, are designated by the letters *A*, *H*, and *I*. The filaments themselves do not become shorter, but the *I* band and *H* zone decrease as the filaments slide past each other.

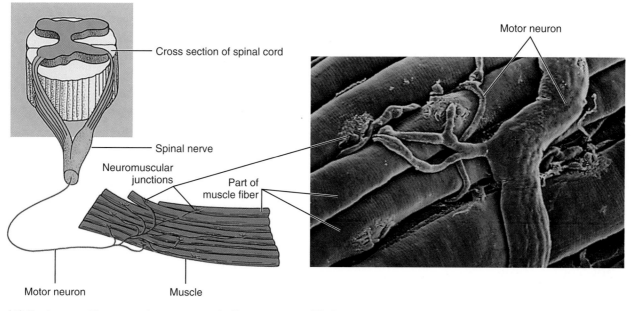

(A) Each nerve fiber controls many muscle fibers.

(B) Scanning electron micrograph of neuromuscular junctions (100x). Note how the motor neuron branches to innervate several muscle fibers.

FIGURE 5-3 • Nerve fibers from a motor nerve transmit impulses to muscle fibers. (**B** adapted from Uehara Y, Desaki J, Fujiwara T: Vascular autonomic plexuses and skeletal neuromuscular junctions: a scanning electron microscopic study, *Biomed Res* 2[Suppl]: 139-143, 1981.)

down by an enzyme called acetylcholinesterase (as'-eh-til-**ko'**-lih-nes'-ter-ase).

2. In a muscle fiber, an action potential is a wave of depolarization (impulse) that travels along the plasma membrane and spreads through the T tubules. Depolarization of the T tubules triggers release of stored calcium ions from the endoplasmic reticulum.

3. Calcium ions bind to a protein on the actin filament, causing it to change shape. This change exposes binding sites on the actin filament.

4. The energy storage molecule ATP provides the energy for muscle contraction. When the muscle is at rest (not contracting), ATP is bound to the myosin. At the same time that the binding sites are exposed, ATP is split. This reaction produces adenosine diphosphate (ADP) and inorganic phosphate. When ATP is split, energy is released and myosin is energized. The energized myosin attaches to the binding site on the actin filament, forming a cross bridge that links the myosin and actin filaments.

5. The release of inorganic phosphate from the myosin causes the cross bridges to flex. This is the power stroke.

6. The actin filament is pulled closer to the center of the sarcomere, shortening the muscle. ADP is released.

7. A new ATP molecule binds to the myosin, and the myosin detaches from the actin filament. If sufficient calcium ions are available, the process is repeated with a second, then third set of binding sites, and so on.

One way to visualize the process of muscle contraction is to imagine the myosin heads engaging "hand-over-hand" with the actin filaments. When many sarcomeres contract simultaneously, they produce the contraction of the muscle as a whole. When impulses from the motor neuron stop, the muscle fiber returns to its resting state.

Muscle Contraction Requires Energy

The immediate source of energy for muscle contraction comes from ATP. However, large amounts of ATP cannot be stored. After the first few seconds of strenuous activity, the muscle uses up its supply of ATP. Fortunately, muscle cells have a backup energy storage compound called **creatine phosphate.** This compound can be stockpiled, and its stored energy is transferred to ATP as needed.

During vigorous exercise, muscle cells soon use up their supply of creatine phosphate. As ATP and creatine phosphate stores are depleted, muscle cells must replenish their supply of these high-energy compounds. The energy for making creatine phosphate and ATP comes from fuel molecules. **Glucose,** a simple sugar, is stored in muscle cells in the form of a large energy storage molecule called **glycogen.** As needed, glycogen is degraded, yielding glucose, which is then broken down in cellular respiration. (Recall that cellular respiration requires oxygen.) When sufficient oxygen is available, enough energy is captured from the glucose to produce needed quantities of ATP and creatine phosphate.

During strenuous exercise, sufficient oxygen may not be available to meet the needs of the rapidly metabolizing muscle cells. Under these conditions, muscle cells are capable of breaking down fuel anaerobically (without oxygen) for short periods. However, anaerobic metabolism does not yield very much ATP. The depletion of ATP results in weaker contractions and **muscle fatigue.**

A waste product, called **lactic acid,** is produced during anaerobic metabolism of glucose. Lactic acid buildup contributes to muscle fatigue. During muscle exertion, an **oxygen debt** develops. The period of rapid breathing that typically follows strenuous exercise pays back the oxygen debt by breaking down lactic acid.

Muscle Tone Is a State of Partial Contraction

Even when we are not moving, our muscles are in a state of partial contraction known as **muscle tone.** Messages from nerve cells continuously stimulate muscle fibers so that at any given moment some fibers are contracted. Muscle tone is an unconscious process that helps keep muscles prepared for action. Muscle tone is also responsible for helping the muscles of the abdominal wall hold the internal organs in place and is important in maintaining posture. When the motor nerve to a muscle is cut, the muscle loses tone and becomes limp, or flaccid.

Two Types of Contraction Are Isotonic and Isometric

When you lift a heavy object or bend your elbow, muscles shorten and thicken as they contract. Muscle tone remains the same. We usually think of muscle contraction in terms of this type of contraction, called **isotonic contraction.** In contrast, if you push against a table or wall, no movement results. Muscle length does not appreciably change, but muscle tension may increase greatly. This type of muscle contraction is referred to as **isometric contraction** (Figure 5-4). Muscle tone is maintained by isometric contraction. Both isometric and isotonic contraction play roles in most body movements.

Quiz Yourself

- In what ways is a muscle fiber adapted for its function?
- What role do calcium ions play in muscle contraction?
- What is the immediate source of energy for muscle contraction?
- How is isometric contraction different from isotonic contraction?

MUSCLES WORK ANTAGONISTICALLY TO ONE ANOTHER

LEARNING OBJECTIVE

7. **Explain how muscles work antagonistically to one another.**

Muscles can only pull; they cannot push. Skeletal muscles produce movements by pulling on tendons, which in turn pull on bones. Most muscles pass across a joint and are attached to the bones that form the joint. When the muscle contracts, it draws one bone toward or away from the bone with which it articulates. The attachment of the muscle to the less movable bone is called its **origin.** The attachment of the muscle to the more movable bone is its **insertion.**

When you flex your elbow, your biceps contract, pulling the radius (and thus your forearm) upward so that you can touch your shoulder (Figure 5-5). Your biceps cannot push your radius back down, however. To move your forearm down again, the triceps muscle contracts, pulling on the ulna. Thus the biceps and triceps work **antagonistically** to one another. What one does, the other can undo.

The muscle that contracts to produce a particular action is known as the **agonist,** or **prime mover.** The muscle that produces the opposite movement is the **antagonist.** When the prime mover is contracting, the antagonist is relaxed. Generally, movements are accomplished by groups of muscles working together, so several prime movers and several antagonists may take part in any action. Note that muscles that are prime movers in one movement may be antagonists in another.

Synergists (sin′-er-gists) and **fixators** are muscles that help the prime mover by reducing unnecessary movement. Synergists stabilize joints so that undesirable movement does not occur. Fixators stabilize the origin of a prime mover so that its force is fully directed on the bone on which it inserts.

Quiz Yourself

- In muscle lingo, what is the function of an antagonist?

WE CAN STUDY MUSCLES IN FUNCTIONAL GROUPS

LEARNING OBJECTIVE

8. **Locate and give the actions of the principal muscles as described in Table 5-1.**

Several common shapes of muscles are shown in Figure 5-6, p. 89. Many of the superficial muscles are shown in *Text continues on p. 88.*

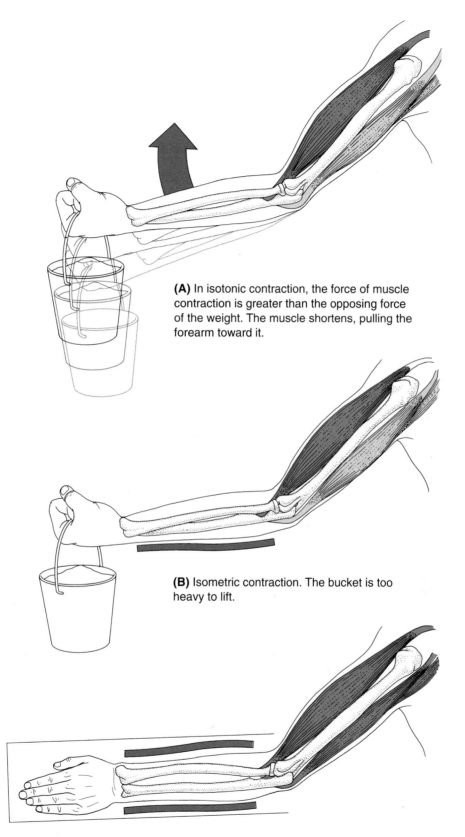

(A) In isotonic contraction, the force of muscle contraction is greater than the opposing force of the weight. The muscle shortens, pulling the forearm toward it.

(B) Isometric contraction. The bucket is too heavy to lift.

(C) Isometric contraction. The hand is pressing against a wall, but cannot move the wall.

FIGURE 5-4 • Isotonic and isometric contraction. **(B)** and **(C)** show two forms of isometric contraction. The force of muscle contraction is met by an equal opposing force. The tension within the muscle increases, but the muscle cannot shorten and no movement occurs.

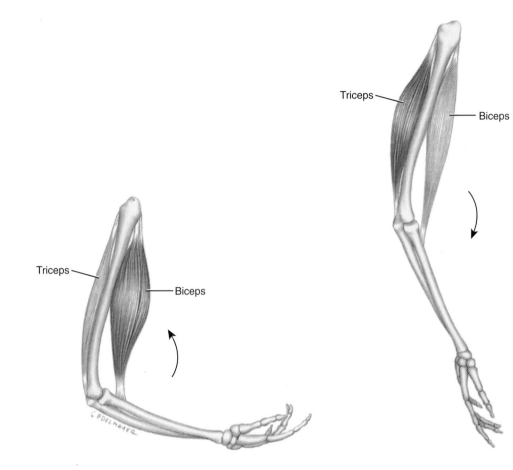

(A) In flexion, the biceps is the agonist and the triceps is the antagonist.

(B) In extension, the triceps is the agonist and the biceps is the antagonist.

FIGURE 5-5 • The antagonistic arrangement of the biceps and triceps muscles.

TABLE 5-1	SELECTED MUSCLES—FUNCTIONAL GROUPS		
Muscle	**Action**	**Origin**	**Insertion**
FACIAL MUSCLES			
Orbicularis oculi (or-bik′-u-lar′-is **ok′**-u-li)	Closes eyes; these are sphincter muscles of eyelids	Frontal bone; maxilla	Eyelids
Frontalis (fron-**tal′**-is)	Raises brows; moves entire scalp backwards	Occipital	Skin of scalp and face
Orbicularis oris	Closes lips; protrudes lips	Tissue around lips	Lips
Zygomatic (zy-go-**mat′**-ik)	Elevates upper corners of mouth	Malar (zygomatic)	Corners of mouth
CHEWING MUSCLES			
Digastric (di-**gas′**-trik)	Opens mouth; can elevate hyoid	Mastoid process of temporal	Hyoid; mandible
Buccinator (**buk′**-sih-nay′-tor)	Flattens cheek (as in whistling)	Lateral side of mandible	Maxilla
Masseter (mas-**see′**-ter)	Raises jaw; mastication	Maxilla (zygomatic arch)	Ramus of mandible
Temporalis (tem-po-**ra′**-lis)	Raises jaw; mastication	Temporal bone	Coronoid process of mandible

TABLE 5-1	SELECTED MUSCLES—FUNCTIONAL GROUPS—cont'd		
Muscle	**Action**	**Origin**	**Insertion**
MUSCLES OF THE HEAD AND TRUNK			
Sternocleidomastoid (ster-no-kly'-do-**mas'**-toid) (paired)	Contraction of both muscles flexes neck; contractions of one muscle rotates head to opposite side	Sternum and clavicle	Mastoid process of occipital
Trapezius (trah-**pee'**-zee-us) (paired)	Adducts scapula and rotates it; draws shoulder upward; extends neck laterally	Occipital bone and thoracic vertebrae	Scapula
External oblique	Contains the abdominal viscera; increases intra-abdominal pressure (as in defecation); contraction compresses abdomen	Lateral surface of lower 8 ribs	Linea alba (midline connective tissue), iliac crest
Transversus abdominis (trans-**ver'**-sus ab-**dom'**-ih-nus)	Compresses abdominal contents	Cartilages of lower 6 ribs; iliac crest	Linea alba, pubis, xiphoid process
Rectus abdominis (**rec'**-tus ab-**dom'**-ih-nus)	Flexes trunk; compresses abdominal contents	Pubis	Xiphoid process of sternum and costal cartilages of ribs 5 through 7
Pectoralis (pek-tah-**ray'**-lis) minor	Pulls scapula forward and downward	Ribs 2 through 5	Coracoid process of scapula
Serratus (ser-**ray'**-tus) anterior	Pulls scapula forward and downward	Upper 8 ribs	Scapula
MUSCLES USED IN BREATHING			
External intercostals	Elevate ribs	Inferior borders of ribs	Superior borders of ribs
Internal intercostals	Depress ribs	Inferior borders of ribs	Superior borders of ribs
Diaphragm	Increases volume of chest cavity in inspiration	Xiphoid process, internal surfaces of lower 6 ribs and first 3 lumbar vertebrae	Central tendon of diaphragm
MUSCLES THAT MOVE THE ARM			
Pectoralis (pek-to-**ray'**-lis) major	Adducts, rotates arm medially	Clavicle, sternum	Humerus
Teres major	Adducts, rotates arm medially	Scapula	Humerus
Latissimus (lah-**tis'**-i-mus) dorsi	Adducts, rotates arm medially; lowers shoulder	Spines of thoracic vertebrae; ilium, ribs	Humerus
Deltoid	Abducts upper arm	Clavicle, scapula	Humerus
MUSCLES THAT MOVE THE FOREARM			
Biceps brachii (**bray'**-kee-i)	Flexes elbow; supinates forearm	Scapula	Radius
Brachialis	Flexes elbow	Humerus	Ulna
Brachioradialis	Flexes elbow	Humerus	Radius
Triceps brachii	Extends elbow	Scapula, humerus	Ulna

Continued

TABLE 5-1	SELECTED MUSCLES—FUNCTIONAL GROUPS—cont'd		
Muscle	**Action**	**Origin**	**Insertion**
MUSCLES THAT MOVE THE THIGH			
Iliacus	Flexes and rotates thigh	Ilium	Femur
Gluteus maximus (**gloo'**-te-us **mak'**-si-mus)	Extends and rotates thigh laterally; tilts pelvis	Sacrum, coccyx, ilium	Femur
Gluteus medius	Abducts, rotates thigh medially	Ilium	Femur
Gluteus minimus	Abducts, rotates thigh laterally	Ilium	Femur
Abductor longus and magnus	Adducts, flexes, rotates thigh	Symphysis pubis; pubis, ischium	Femur
Gracilis (grah-**sill'**-is)	Adducts thigh; flexes knee	Pubis	Tibia
MUSCLES THAT MOVE THE LEG			
Sartorius (sar-**tore'**-ee-us)	Flexes knee and thigh; abducts, rotates thigh laterally	Ilium	Tibia
Quadriceps femoris (**kwod'**-rih-seps **fem'**-or-is)	Extends leg at knee	Ilium, femur	Tibia
Biceps femoris	Flexes knee; extends thigh	Ischium, femur	Tibia, fibula
MUSCLES THAT MOVE THE FOOT AND ANKLE			
Tibialis (tib-ee-**a'**-lis) anterior	Dorsiflexes foot	Tibia	Metatarsals
Peroneus (per-o-**nee'**-us)	Plantarflexes and everts foot	Fibula, tibia	Metatarsals
Gastrocnemius (gas-trok-**nee'**-me-us)	Plantarflexes foot; flexes knees	Femur	Calcaneus
Soleus (**so'**-lee-us)	Plantarflexes foot	Tibia, fibula	Calcaneus

Figures 5-7, p. 90 and 5-8, p. 91. Although every muscle is important, including them all is beyond the scope of this book. Instead, we have selected some functional groups of muscles and present them in Table 5-1 along with their actions, origins, and insertions. (Also see Figures 5-9 through 5-11, p. 92.)

Quiz Yourself

- What is the function of the external intercostal muscles?
- What is the function of the triceps brachii?
- What is the function of the quadriceps femoris?

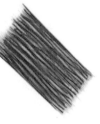

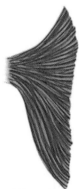

Fusiform
(spindle-shaped)   Rhomboidal   Rectangular   Triangular

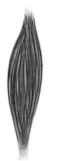
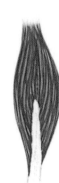
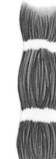
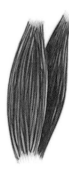

Penniform
(pennate)   Bipenniform
                 (bipennate)   Multiple bellies   Two-headed

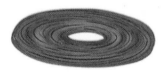
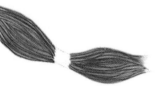

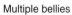

Sphincter   Two bellies

FIGURE 5-6 • Some common muscle shapes.

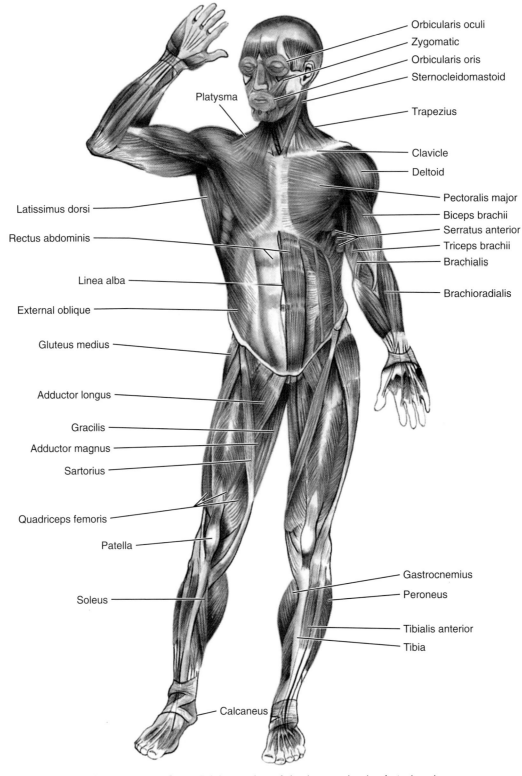

FIGURE 5-7 • Superficial muscles of the human body. Anterior view.

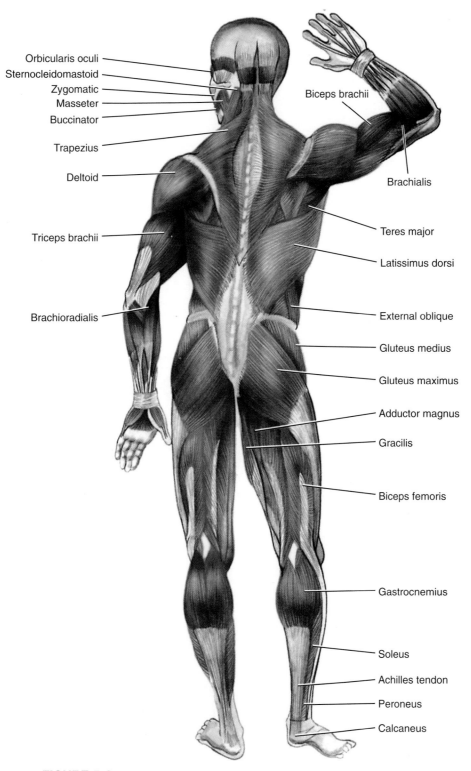

Orbicularis oculi
Sternocleidomastoid
Zygomatic
Masseter
Buccinator
Trapezius
Deltoid
Triceps brachii
Brachioradialis

Biceps brachii
Brachialis
Teres major
Latissimus dorsi
External oblique
Gluteus medius
Gluteus maximus
Adductor magnus
Gracilis
Biceps femoris
Gastrocnemius
Soleus
Achilles tendon
Peroneus
Calcaneus

FIGURE 5-8 • Superficial muscles of the human body. Posterior view.

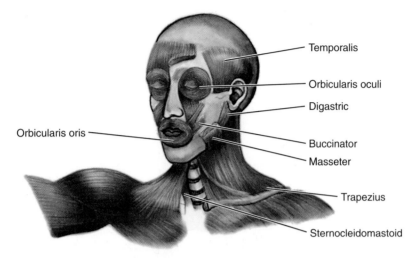

FIGURE 5-9 • Some muscles of the head and anterior neck.

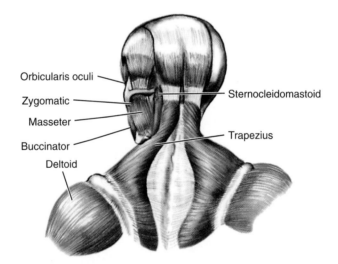

FIGURE 5-10 • Some superficial muscles of the head, neck, and back.

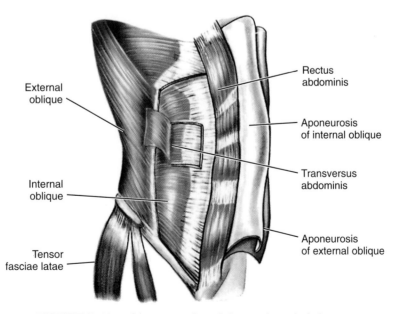

FIGURE 5-11 • Some muscles of the trunk and abdomen.

LO 1. Describe the structure of a skeletal muscle.
- A skeletal muscle consists of hundreds of muscle fibers arranged in fascicles. Each muscle fiber is wrapped in a covering of connective tissue called an endomysium. The fascicle is surrounded by a perimysium, and the entire muscle is covered by an epimysium. Tough cords of connective tissue, the tendons, extend from the epimysium and anchor muscles to bones.

LO 2. Describe the structure of a muscle fiber and relate its structure to its function.
- Muscle fibers are specialized for contraction. Each muscle fiber is filled with threadlike structures, the **myofibrils.** The myofibrils are composed of thick **myosin filaments** and thin **actin filaments.** Myosin and actin filaments are organized into repeating units called **sarcomeres.**
- The **Z line** represents the interweaving of muscle filaments where they join at their ends. The filaments overlap lengthwise, producing a pattern of **striations,** characteristic of striated muscle. Muscle contraction occurs when the actin and myosin filaments slide past one another.

LO 3. List, in sequence, the events that take place during muscle contraction.
A. **Acetylcholine,** a neurotransmitter released by the neurons of a **motor nerve,** signals the muscle fiber to contract. Acetylcholine causes **depolarization,** a decrease in the electric charge difference across the plasma membrane. Depolarization may generate an **action potential,** an electrical impulse, in the muscle fiber.
B. The action potential is a wave of depolarization that travels along the plasma membrane and spreads through the **T tubules,** inward extensions of the plasma membrane. Depolarization stimulates the release of stored calcium ions.
C. Calcium ions bind to a protein on the actin filament, causing it to change shape and expose **binding sites.**
D. **ATP** is split, producing **ADP** and inorganic phosphate. This reaction releases energy; which energizes the myosin. The energized myosin binds to active sites on the actin filament, forming **cross bridges** that link the myosin and actin filaments.

E. Inorganic phosphate is released from the myosin, which causes the cross bridges to flex. This is the power stroke.
F. The actin filament is pulled closer to the center of the sarcomere, shortening the muscle (contraction). ADP is released.
G. A new ATP binds to the myosin, and the myosin detaches from the actin filament.

LO 4. Compare the roles of glycogen, creatine phosphate, and adenosine triphosphate (ATP) in providing energy for muscle contraction.
- The immediate source of energy for muscle contraction is ATP.
- **Creatine phosphate** is an energy storage molecule found in muscle fibers. Its energy can be transferred to ATP.
- Fuel molecules such as **glucose** provide the energy for making creatine phosphate and ATP. Glucose can be stored in muscle fibers as **glycogen.**
- During vigorous exercise, muscle cells can break down glucose without oxygen (i.e., anaerobically). A waste product called **lactic acid** is produced and can cause **muscle fatigue.** During exertion, muscle fibers incur an **oxygen debt,** which is paid back during the period of rapid breathing that follows strenuous exercise.

LO 5. Define muscle tone and explain why muscle tone is important.
- **Muscle tone** is the state of partial contraction that keeps muscle prepared for action.

LO 6. Distinguish between isotonic and isometric contraction.
- In **isotonic contraction,** muscles shorten and thicken as they contract; in **isometric contraction,** muscle length does not change much but muscle tension may increase greatly.

LO 7. Explain how muscles work antagonistically to one another.
- Muscles work antagonistically to one another. The muscle that contracts to produce a particular action is the **agonist,** or **prime mover;** the muscle that produces the opposite action is the **antagonist.**

LO 8. Locate and give the actions of the principal muscles as indicated in Table 5-1.
- Use Table 5-1 to review the functional groups of muscles in the body.

LO = Learning Objective

CHAPTER QUIZ

Fill in the Blank

1. Muscle cells are referred to as muscle _____.

2. The _____ is the connective tissue covering around the muscle.

3. Cords of connective tissue that connect muscles to bones are called _____.

4. Thick filaments consist mainly of the protein _____; thin filaments consist of _____.

5. A muscle is stimulated to contract by acetylcholine released by a _____ _____.

6. An action potential in muscle stimulates the release of _____.

7. The immediate source of energy for muscle contraction is _____.

8. Creatine phosphate is a compound that stores _____.

9. The state of partial contraction that exists in a muscle even when we are not moving it is called _____ _____.

10. A muscle that opposes an agonist (prime mover) is called a(n) _____.

11. Synergists are muscles that stabilize _____.

Multiple Choice

12. The striations in striated muscle result from: a. creatine phosphate; b. ATP breakdown; c. the overlapping of actin and myosin filaments; d. the pattern of isometric contraction characteristic of these muscles.

13. Myosin binds to actin, forming cross bridges. What happens next? a. acetylcholine is released; b. calcium ions stimulate a process that leads to exposure of active sites; c. filaments slide past each other/muscle fiber shortens; d. myosin is energized.

14. Glycogen is: a. produced by actin; b. an energy storage molecule; c. depleted within 1 second of strenuous activity; d. causes oxygen debt when depleted.

15. A muscle used in chewing is the: a. triceps brachii; b. gluteus maximus; c. quadriceps femoris; d. masseter.

16. A muscle that extends the thigh is the: a. gluteus maximus; b. deltoid; c. quadriceps femoris; d. gastrocnemius.

17. A muscle that flexes the trunk is the: a. external oblique; b. rectus abdominis; c. quadriceps femoris; d. gastrocnemius.

18. A muscle that extends the elbow is the: a. triceps brachii; b. gluteus maximus; c. quadriceps femoris; d. masseter.

19. A muscle that extends the leg at the knee is the: a. biceps femoris; b. deltoid; c. quadriceps femoris; d. gastrocnemius.

20. A muscle that plantarflexes the foot is the: a. sartorius; b. deltoid; c. quadriceps femoris; d. soleus.

REVIEW QUESTIONS

1. We can think of each muscle as an organ. Explain why.

2. What are actin and myosin filaments? Why are they important?

3. What are the functions of acetylcholine? Creatine phosphate? Glycogen?

4. List and describe the steps in muscle contraction.

5. What happens when the motor nerve to a muscle is cut?

6. Give two examples of the antagonistic action of muscles.

7. List four abdominal muscles and describe their functions.

8. Which muscles function in breathing?

9. Identify two muscles that move the arm; identify three muscles that move the forearm.

10. Label the diagram. (See Figures 5-6 and 5-7 to check your answers.)

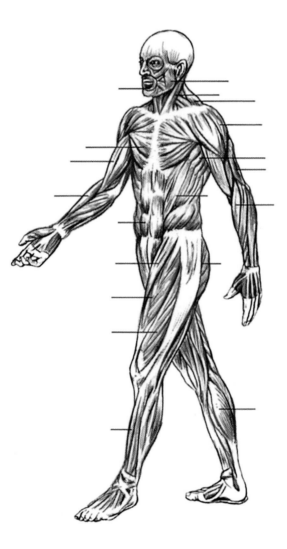

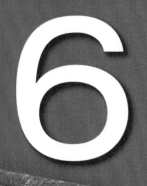

6 The Central Nervous System

Chapter Outline

The nervous system coordinates the activities of the other body systems and links us with the outside world. This regulatory system enables us to detect and respond to **stimuli**—changes that occur either within the body or in the outside environment. Together with the endocrine system, the nervous system works continuously to maintain homeostasis.

THE NERVOUS SYSTEM HAS TWO MAIN DIVISIONS

LEARNING OBJECTIVE

1. **Distinguish between the central nervous system and the peripheral nervous system and describe each.**

The two main divisions of the nervous system are the **central nervous system (CNS)** and the **peripheral nervous system (PNS)** (Figure 6-1). The CNS consists of the **brain** and **spinal cord.** Serving as the principal control center of the body, these organs integrate incoming information and determine appropriate responses.

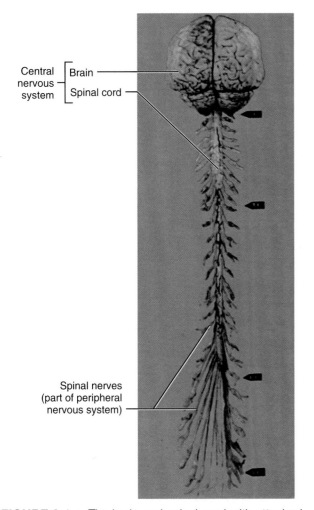

FIGURE 6-1 • The brain and spinal cord with attached spinal nerve roots, photographed from the posterior aspect. The nerves that extend caudally from the lower region of the cord have been fanned out on the left. (Dissection by Dr. M.C.E. Hutchinson, Department of Anatomy, Guy's Hospital Medical School, London. From Standring S, editor: *Gray's Anatomy,* ed 39, Edinburgh, 2005, Churchill Livingstone.)

The PNS is made up of the *sensory receptors*—for example, the visual receptors in the eyes and the auditory receptors in the ears—and the *nerves,* which are the communication lines to and from the CNS. Twelve pairs of **cranial nerves** link the brain, and 31 pairs of **spinal nerves** link the spinal cord with the sensory receptors and with other parts of the body. The nerves continually inform the CNS of changing conditions and then transmit its "decisions" to appropriate muscles and glands that make the adjustments needed to maintain homeostasis.

For convenience, the PNS may be subdivided into **somatic** and **autonomic** divisions. Sensory receptors and nerves concerned with changes in the outside environment are somatic; those that regulate the internal environment are autonomic. Both systems have (1) **afferent nerves,** also called *sensory nerves,* which transmit messages from receptors to the CNS, and (2) **efferent nerves,** also called *motor nerves,* which transmit information back from the CNS to the structures that must respond. The autonomic system has two kinds of efferent pathways—sympathetic and parasympathetic nerves. These are discussed in Chapter 7.

Quiz Yourself

- What are the components of the CNS?
- What are the components of the PNS?

NEURONS AND GLIAL CELLS ARE THE CELLS OF THE NERVOUS SYSTEM

LEARNING OBJECTIVE

2. **Relate the function of neurons to their structure, and give the functions of glial cells.**

Two types of cells unique to the nervous system are neurons and glial cells. **Neurons (new′-rons)** are highly specialized to receive and transmit electrical and chemical signals. The electrical signals are called **neural impulses,** or **action potentials**. Until recently biologists thought that new neurons are not produced after birth. Recently researchers have demonstrated that new neurons are produced in the developing brain of the child and adolescent and in several regions of the adult brain.

The neuron is distinguished by its long processes, which are threadlike extensions of the cytoplasm. The nucleus and most of the organelles are contained in the main part of the cell, the **cell body** (Figure 6-2). Two types of nerve processes are dendrites and axons. **Dendrites (den′-drites)** are highly branched fibers that extend from the cell body. Dendrites are specialized to *receive* neural impulses and transmit them to the cell body. Typically, a single **axon (ak′-son)** transmits neural messages *from* the cell body toward another neuron (or toward a muscle

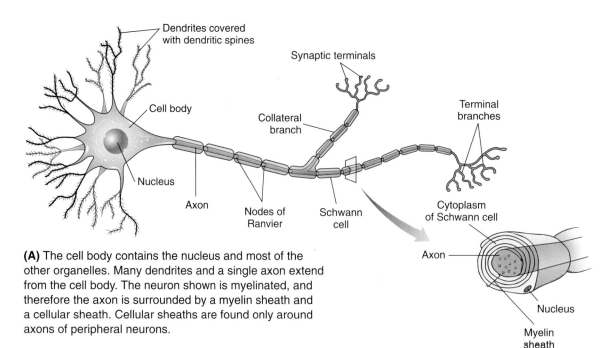

(A) The cell body contains the nucleus and most of the other organelles. Many dendrites and a single axon extend from the cell body. The neuron shown is myelinated, and therefore the axon is surrounded by a myelin sheath and a cellular sheath. Cellular sheaths are found only around axons of peripheral neurons.

(B) A Schwann cell wraps its plasma membrane around the axon many times, forming the insulating myelin sheath. The rest of the Schwann cell surrounding the myelin sheath forms the cellular sheath. Gaps in the myelin sheath occur between Schwann cells. At these gaps, called nodes of Ranvier, the axon is not insulated with myelin.

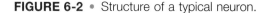

FIGURE 6-2 • Structure of a typical neuron.

or gland). An axon may give off **collateral branches.** At its distal end, the axon divides extensively, forming many **terminal branches** that end in **synaptic terminals**. The synaptic terminals release **neurotransmitters** (new-row-**trans′**-mit-ers), chemical compounds that transmit signals from one neuron to another (or from a neuron to a muscle or gland).

Axons of many neurons of the PNS are covered by two sheaths—an inner **myelin** (**my′**-eh-lin) **sheath** and an outer **cellular sheath,** or **neurilemma** (new-rih-**lem′**-ma). Both coverings are formed by support cells known as Schwann (shvon) cells. The cellular sheath is important in the repair of injured neurons. Myelin, a white fatty substance, is an excellent electrical insulator that speeds the conduction of nerve impulses. Myelin is responsible for the white color of the *white matter* of the brain and spinal cord and of myelinated peripheral nerves.

In the disease *multiple sclerosis,* patches of myelin deteriorate at irregular intervals along the axons of neurons in the CNS. The myelin is replaced by scar tissue. This damage interferes with the transmission of impulses and the victim experiences loss of coordination, tremor, and partial or complete paralysis of parts of the body.

Glial cells protect and support the neurons. They account for about 90% of the cells in the human CNS. Until recently biologists thought that glial cells were rather passive cells that

support and protect neurons. Researchers have discovered that glial cells communicate with one another and with neurons. They also carry out major regulatory functions. For example, one type of glial cell (astrocyte) helps regulate the composition of the extracellular fluid (the fluid outside of the cells) in the CNS by removing excess potassium ions.

Quiz Yourself

- What is the function of dendrites? Of synaptic terminals?
- What are some functions of glial cells?

BUNDLES OF AXONS MAKE UP NERVES

LEARNING OBJECTIVE

3. **Distinguish between nerve and tract; ganglion and nucleus.**

A **nerve** is a large bundle of axons wrapped in connective tissue. We can compare a nerve to a telephone cable. The axons are like the individual wires, and the myelin, cellular, and connective tissue sheaths are like the insulation. The cell bodies attached to the axons of a nerve are often grouped together in a mass known as a **ganglion.** Many ganglia are located just outside the spinal cord; some are located closer to the organs they innervate.

Within the CNS, bundles of axons are not usually called nerves. They are known as **tracts** or **pathways.** Masses of cell bodies located in the CNS are referred to as **nuclei** rather than ganglia.

Quiz Yourself

- What is a nerve? How does it differ from a pathway?
- What is a ganglion? A pathway?

APPROPRIATE RESPONSES DEPEND ON NEURAL SIGNALING

LEARNING OBJECTIVE

4. Briefly describe the basic processes essential for neural signaling—reception, transmission, integration, and response.

Imagine that you are driving down the street and the traffic light on the corner ahead turns red. Automatically you step on the brake and bring your vehicle to a smooth stop. Each day you respond to hundreds of such stimuli. Even very simple responses require **neural signaling**—communication among neurons. The following sequence of events is typical:

1. **Reception.** First, you must receive the information that the traffic light has turned red. In this example, reception of the information that the light is red is received by visual receptors in the eyes.
2. **Transmission.** The transmission of a neural impulse is the process of sending messages along a neuron, from one neuron to another, or from a neuron to a muscle or gland. **Afferent (sensory) neurons** in the PNS *transmit* information to **interneurons** in the CNS.
3. **Integration.** In the CNS, the information provided by the afferent neurons is sorted and interpreted as a "red light" and an appropriate response is determined. This process is known as *integration.*
4. **Transmission.** Interneurons transmit information to appropriate **efferent (motor) neurons.** Efferent neurons then transmit the message to the **effectors**—the muscles and glands.
5. **Actual response.** Muscles and glands are referred to as *effectors* because they cause an effect in response to messages from the nervous system. In our example, the message directs specific muscles to contract. You lift your foot from the gas pedal and press down on the brake.

Neural messages travel over sequences of neurons. Neurons are arranged so that the axon of one neuron signals the dendrites of other neurons. A junction between two neurons is called a synapse (**sin′**-aps). At a synapse, neurons are separated by a tiny gap known as the synaptic cleft. Neurotransmitters conduct the message across the synaptic cleft.

Quiz Yourself

- What is reception? Integration?
- What is the sequence of events by which a message is transmitted through the nervous system?

NEURONS TRANSMIT INFORMATION WITH ELECTRICAL SIGNALS

LEARNING OBJECTIVES

5. Contrast an action potential with the resting potential of a neuron. (Describe each.)
6. Compare continuous conduction and saltatory conduction.

Most cells have a difference in electrical charge across the plasma membrane—a more negative electrical charge inside the cell compared with the electrical charge of the extracellular fluid outside. The plasma membrane is said to be electrically **polarized.** This means that one side (or pole) has a different charge from the other side. When electrical charges are separated in this way, a potential energy difference exists across the membrane.

The difference in electrical charge across the plasma membrane produces an *electrical gradient.* Voltage is the force that causes charged particles to flow between two points. The voltage measured across the plasma membrane is referred to as the **membrane potential.** If the charges are permitted to come together, they have the ability to do work. Thus the cell can be thought of as a biological battery. In excitable cells such as neurons and muscle cells, the membrane potential can be rapidly changed and such changes can transmit signals to other cells.

The Neuron Has a Resting Potential

The membrane potential in a resting (not excited) neuron (or muscle cell) is its **resting potential.** The resting potential is expressed in units called *millivolts* (mV). (A millivolt equals one thousandth of a volt.) Like other cells that can produce electrical signals, the neuron has a resting potential of

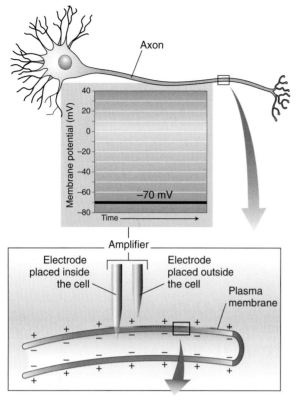

(A) Measuring the resting potential of a neuron. The difference in electrical charge across the plasma membrane can be measured by placing one electrode just inside the neuron and a second electrode in the extracellular fluid just outside the plasma membrane. In a resting (nonconducting) neuron, the axon is negatively charged compared with the surrounding extracellular fluid.

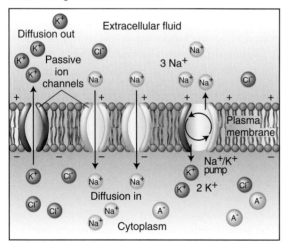

(B) Permeability of the plasma membrane of the neuron. The membrane is less permeable to sodium ions (Na^+) than to potassium ions (K^+). Potassium ions diffuse out along their concentration gradient and are largely responsible for the voltage across the membrane. Sodium–potassium pumps in the plasma membrane actively pump Na^+ out of the cell and pump K^+ in. Negatively charged chloride ions (Cl^-) and large anions (A^-) such as proteins contribute to the negative charge.

FIGURE 6-3 • Resting potential of a neuron.

about 70 mV. By convention this is expressed as −70 mV because the inner environment of the plasma membrane is negatively charged compared with the extracellular fluid (Figure 6-3).

The magnitude of the resting potential is determined by (1) differences in concentrations of specific ions (mainly positively charged sodium and potassium ions) inside the cell relative to the extracellular fluid and (2) selective permeability of the plasma membrane to these ions. Ions pass through specific **passive ion channels** in the plasma membrane. Potassium ions (K^+) leak out more readily than sodium ions (Na^+) can leak in. Chloride ions (Cl^-) accumulate along the inner surface of the plasma membrane. Proteins, which are too large to cross the plasma membrane, contribute negative charges. The gradients that determine the resting potential are maintained by sodium-potassium pumps in the plasma membrane. These pumps continuously transport Na^+ out of the neuron and transport K^+ in.

An Action Potential Is a Wave of Depolarization

Neurons are excitable cells. They have the ability to respond to stimuli and to convert stimuli into nerve impulses. An electrical, chemical, or mechanical stimulus may alter the resting potential by increasing the membrane's permeability to sodium. If the neuron membrane is only slightly stimulated, only a local excitation may occur in the membrane.

When a stimulus causes sodium ions to move into the neuron, the membrane potential becomes less negative (closer to zero) than the resting level. The membrane is described as **depolarized.** Because depolarization brings a neuron closer to transmitting a neural impulse, it is *excitatory*. In contrast, when a stimulus affects the permeability of the neuron plasma membrane in a way that causes the membrane potential to become more negative than the resting potential, the membrane is **hyperpolarized.** Hyperpolarization decreases the ability of the neuron to generate a neural impulse and is described as *inhibitory*.

When a stimulus is sufficiently strong, **voltage-activated ion channels** in the plasma membrane open. Na^+ enter the neuron through specific channels that have gates. The Na^+ depolarize the membrane (Figure 6-4). When the voltage across the membrane is decreased to a critical point, called the **threshold level,** a neural impulse, or **action potential,** is generated. Figure 6-4 illustrates an action potential that has been recorded by placing one electrode just inside an axon and one just outside. The action potential is a wave of depolarization that moves down the axon.

As the action potential moves down the axon, **repolarization** occurs behind it; changes in the permeability of ion channels bring the membrane back to its relatively negative state. Sodium ion channels close and K^+ channels open, allowing K^+ to leave the neuron. During the millisecond or so in which it is depolarized, the axon membrane is in an **absolute refractory period:** it cannot transmit another action potential

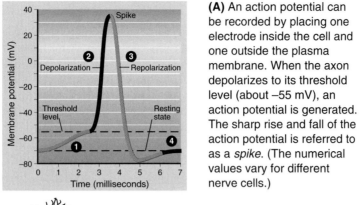

(A) An action potential can be recorded by placing one electrode inside the cell and one outside the plasma membrane. When the axon depolarizes to its threshold level (about −55 mV), an action potential is generated. The sharp rise and fall of the action potential is referred to as a *spike*. (The numerical values vary for different nerve cells.)

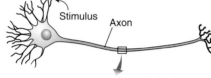

(B) When the voltage reaches threshold level, voltage-activated sodium channels open, allowing Na⁺ to pass into the cell. An action potential is transmitted as a wave of depolarization that travels down the axon. (Activation gates on the cytoplasmic end of the Na⁺ channels open when a neuron is stimulated. These gates close slowly after a brief time period. The Na⁺ channels are open only during the brief period when both activation and inactivation gates are open.)

(C) As the action potential progresses along the axon, repolarization occurs quickly behind it. Repolarization begins when the Na⁺ channels close and voltage-activated K⁺ channels open, permitting K⁺ to leave the cell.

FIGURE 6-4 • Transmission of an action potential along the axon.

no matter how great a stimulus is applied. This is because the voltage-activated Na$^+$ channels are inactivated. Until their gates are reset, they cannot be reopened. When enough Na$^+$ channel gates have been reset, the neuron enters a **relative refractory period** that lasts for a few additional milliseconds. During this period, the axon can transmit impulses, but the threshold is higher. Even with the limits imposed by their refractory periods, most neurons can transmit several hundred impulses per second.

The action potential is an **all-or-none response;** no variation exists in the strength of a single impulse. The membrane potential either exceeds threshold level and transmits an action potential or it does not. The smooth, progressive transmission of a neural impulse just described is called **continuous conduction.** This type of conduction occurs in unmyelinated neurons. Neural transmission is different and more rapid in myelinated neurons.

Myelin acts as an effective electrical insulator around the axon. However, the nodes of Ranvier are not myelinated. At these nodes, the axon plasma membrane makes direct contact with the surrounding extracellular fluid. Voltage-activated sodium and potassium ion channels are concentrated at these nodes, and ion movement across the membrane occurs only at the nodes. Because the ion activity at the active node depolarizes the next node along the axon, the action potential jumps along the axon from one node of Ranvier to the next (Figure 6-5). This type of neural transmission is known as **saltatory conduction** (from the Latin word *saltus,* which means "to leap"). Saltatory conduction is faster and requires less energy than does continuous conduction.

Quiz Yourself

- Why is an action potential described as a wave of depolarization?
- How is saltatory conduction different from continuous conduction?

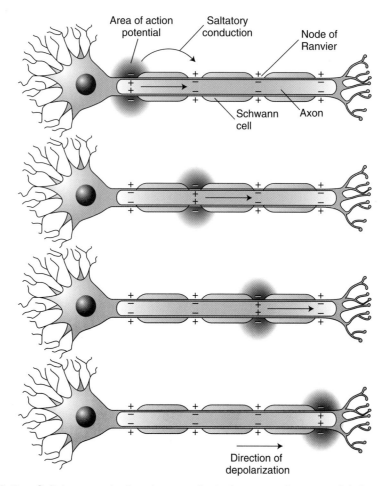

FIGURE 6-5 • Saltatory conduction. In a myelinated axon, action potentials leap along from one node of Ranvier to the next. This diagram is highly simplified. A typical neuron might have hundreds of nodes of Ranvier.

NEURONS SIGNAL OTHER CELLS ACROSS SYNAPSES

LEARNING OBJECTIVES

7. **Describe the transmission of a signal across a synapse. (Draw a diagram to support your description.)**
8. **Describe the actions of the neurotransmitters discussed in this chapter.**

Neurons are organized in specific pathways. A synapse is a junction between two neurons or between a neuron and a muscle (or gland). A neuron that *terminates* at a specific synapse is referred to as a **presynaptic neuron,** whereas a neuron that *begins* at a synapse is known as a **postsynaptic neuron** (Figure 6-6). Note that these terms are relative to a specific synapse. A neuron that is postsynaptic with respect to one synapse may be presynaptic to the next synapse in the sequence.

A presynaptic neuron is separated from a postsynaptic neuron by a **synaptic cleft,** a small space (less than one

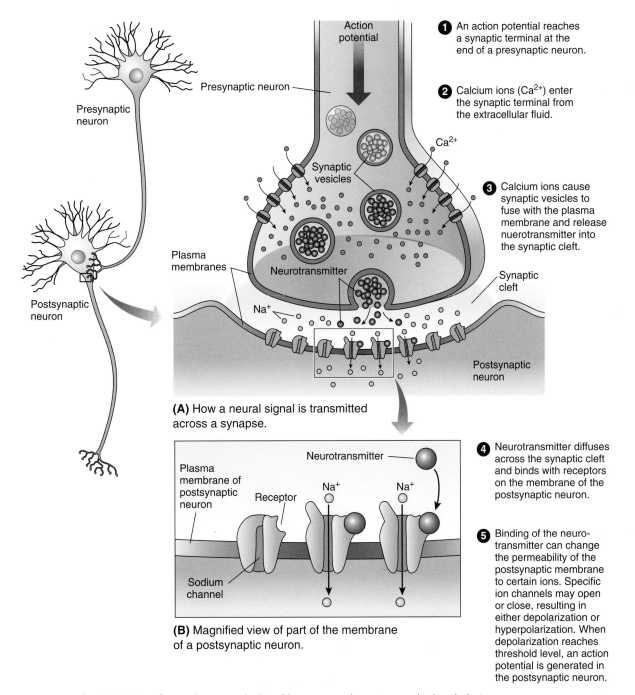

1 An action potential reaches a synaptic terminal at the end of a presynaptic neuron.

2 Calcium ions (Ca^{2+}) enter the synaptic terminal from the extracellular fluid.

3 Calcium ions cause synaptic vesicles to fuse with the plasma membrane and release nuerotransmitter into the synaptic cleft.

(A) How a neural signal is transmitted across a synapse.

4 Neurotransmitter diffuses across the synaptic cleft and binds with receptors on the membrane of the postsynaptic neuron.

5 Binding of the neurotransmitter can change the permeability of the postsynaptic membrane to certain ions. Specific ion channels may open or close, resulting in either depolarization or hyperpolarization. When depolarization reaches threshold level, an action potential is generated in the postsynaptic neuron.

(B) Magnified view of part of the membrane of a postsynaptic neuron.

FIGURE 6-6 • Synaptic transmission. Neurotransmitters transmit signals between neurons or from a neuron to an effector.

millionth of an inch). Because depolarization is a property of the plasma membrane, when an action potential reaches the end of the axon it is unable to jump across the synaptic cleft. The problem is solved by converting the electrical signal into a chemical signal.

Neurons Signal Other Cells With Neurotransmitters

Neurotransmitters are chemical messengers that transmit the neural signal across the synapse and signal other neurons or muscle or gland cells. More than 60 different chemical compounds are known to function as neurotransmitters. A few are described in Table 6-1. Some neurotransmitters (sometimes called neuromodulators) modify the effects of other neurotransmitters. For example, they may amplify or dampen the response of the postsynaptic cell.

In Chapter 5 we discussed **acetylcholine**—a neurotransmitter released from motor neurons that triggers muscle contraction. Acetylcholine is also released by some neurons in the brain and in the autonomic nervous system (see Chapter 7). Cells that release this neurotransmitter are referred to as **cholinergic neurons.**

Neurons that release **norepinephrine** are called **adrenergic neurons.** Norepinephrine and the neurotransmitter **dopamine** are **catecholamines.** Norepinephrine, dopamine, and **serotonin** belong to a class of compounds called **biogenic amines.** These compounds affect mood, and their imbalance

TABLE 6-1 SELECTED NEUROTRANSMITTERS

Substance	Source	Actions	Comments
ACETYLCHOLINE			
	Some neurons in the brain and certain neurons in the autonomic nervous system; motor neurons	Excitatory effect on skeletal muscle; inhibitory effect on cardiac muscle	Inactivated by acetylcholinesterase
CATECHOLAMINES			
Norepinephrine	Neurons in both the central and autonomic nervous systems	Excitatory or inhibitory effect; involved in dreaming	Mainly inactivated by reuptake into the axon terminal; also inactivated by enzymes; level in brain affects mood
Dopamine	CNS	Helps maintain balance between inhibition and excitation of neurons; important in motor functions	Level in brain affects mood; amount reduced in Parkinson's disease; abnormal amounts in schizophrenia and attention deficit disorder
Serotonin (5-hydroxytryptamine, 5-HT)	CNS	Excitatory effect on pathways that control muscle action; inhibitory effect on pathways involved in sensations	Highest level of secretion during alert states, lowest level during sleep; serotonin pathways also function in regulation of food intake and affect mood
AMINO ACIDS			
Glutamate	Brain	Major excitatory neurotransmitter in the brain	Functions in memory and learning
GABA	Inhibitory interneurons in CNS	Inhibitory effect on pathways in the CNS	Actions enhanced by barbiturates and benzodiazepines
NEUROPEPTIDES			
Endorphins (opioids)	Brain	Pain regulation	Morphine-like properties
Enkephalins (opioids)	Brain	Pain regulation	Morphine-like properties
Substance P	Sensory neurons	Pain regulation	
GASEOUS NEUROTRANSMITTER			
Nitric oxide	Most neurons?	Transmits signals in opposite direction from other neurotransmitters (i.e., from postsynaptic to presynaptic neuron)	Plays role in learning; modulates sensory and motor responses

has been linked to several mental disorders, including major depression, attention deficit disorder, and schizophrenia. Antidepressants and many other mood-affecting drugs work by altering the levels of biogenic amines in the brain.

Certain amino acids also serve as neurotransmitters. **Glutamate** is a major excitatory neurotransmitter in the brain. Gamma-aminobutyric acid, commonly referred to as **GABA,** inhibits interneurons in the CNS.

Opiate drugs, for example, morphine and codeine, are powerful analgesics—drugs that relieve pain without causing loss of consciousness. The body makes its own opioids, called **endorphins** and **enkephalins.** These compounds (e.g., beta-endorphin) bind to receptors in the brain (the same receptors to which opiate drugs bind) and block pain signals. Opioids modulate the effects of other neurotransmitters, including **substance P,** which activates the pathways that transmit pain signals.

Nitric oxide (NO), a signaling molecule that has been the focus of much recent research, is a gas. NO is a *retrograde messenger* at some synapses. It transmits information from the postsynaptic neuron to the presynaptic neuron—the opposite direction of other neurotransmitters.

Neurotransmitters Bind With Receptors on Postsynaptic Neurons

Neurotransmitters are stored in the synaptic terminals within small membrane-bounded sacs called **synaptic vesicles.** Each time an action potential reaches a synaptic terminal, calcium ions from the extracellular fluid flow into the synaptic terminal. The calcium ions cause synaptic vesicles to fuse with the presynaptic membrane and release neurotransmitter molecules into the synaptic cleft.

Neurotransmitter molecules diffuse across the synaptic cleft and combine with specific **receptors** on the plasma membrane of postsynaptic cells (see Figure 6-6). These receptors are found on dendrites and cell bodies of postsynaptic neurons and on the plasma membranes of muscle fibers and gland cells. Identification of neurotransmitter receptors is an area of intense biomedical research.

Many neurotransmitter receptors are chemically activated ion channels. When activated, they change the permeability of the membrane to sodium and other ions. When a sufficient number of receptors are activated, the postsynaptic neuron may reach its threshold level. Depolarization occurs, and the neuron transmits an action potential.

If repolarization of a postsynaptic cell is to occur quickly, excess neurotransmitter in the synaptic cleft must be removed. Some neurotransmitters are inactivated by enzymes. For example, excess acetylcholine is degraded by the enzyme *acetylcholinesterase.* Other neurotransmitters, for example, the catecholamines, are actively transported back into the synaptic terminals—a process known as **reuptake.** These neurotransmitters are repackaged in vesicles and recycled. Many drugs inhibit the reuptake of neurotransmitters. For example, some antidepressants (selective serotonin reuptake inhibitors, or

SSRIs) work by inhibiting the reuptake of serotonin, thus increasing its concentration in the synaptic cleft. Some antidepressants also inhibit the reuptake of dopamine. Cocaine inhibits the reuptake of dopamine.

Neurotransmitter Receptors Can Send Excitatory or Inhibitory Signals

Depending on the type of postsynaptic receptor with which it combines, the same neurotransmitter can have different effects. For example, acetylcholine has an excitatory effect on skeletal muscle. It opens sodium ion channels, which increases the permeability of the muscle fiber membrane to Na^+. The influx of Na^+ depolarizes the membrane, leading to contraction. In contrast, acetylcholine has an inhibitory effect on cardiac muscle, resulting in a decreased heart rate. A postsynaptic neuron may have receptors for several types of neurotransmitters. Some of its receptors may be excitatory, and others may be inhibitory.

A change in membrane potential that brings the neuron closer to firing is called an **excitatory postsynaptic potential (EPSP).** A neurotransmitter-receptor combination that hyperpolarizes the postsynaptic membrane takes the neuron farther away from the firing level. This is referred to as an **inhibitory postsynaptic potential (IPSP).**

Each EPSP or IPSP is a graded potential that varies in magnitude depending on the strength of the stimulus applied. One EPSP is usually too weak to trigger an action potential by itself. Its effect is below threshold level. Even though subthreshold EPSPs do not produce an action potential, they do affect the membrane potential. EPSPs may be added together, a process known as **summation.**

⊚ *Quiz Yourself*

- What happens after a neurotransmitter is released?
- What is the action of serotonin? Of GABA?

NEURAL IMPULSES MUST BE INTEGRATED

LEARNING OBJECTIVE

9. **Define neural integration and describe how a postsynaptic neuron integrates incoming stimuli and "decides" whether to fire.**

Neural integration is the process of summing incoming signals. Each neuron may synapse with hundreds of other neurons. EPSPs and IPSPs are produced continually in postsynaptic neurons, and IPSPs cancel the effects of some of the EPSPs.

It is important to remember that each EPSP and IPSP is *not* an all-or-none response. It does not travel like an action potential. Rather, each is a *graded* response that may be added to or subtracted from other EPSPs and IPSPs. As the neuron membrane continuously updates its molecular tabulations, the neuron may be inhibited or brought to threshold level. This mechanism provides for integration of hundreds of signals (EPSPs and IPSPs) before an all-or-none action potential is actually transmitted along the axon of a postsynaptic neuron. Local responses permit the neuron and the entire nervous system a far greater range of response than would be the case if every EPSP generated an action potential.

Where does neural integration take place? Every neuron sorts through (on a molecular level) the hundreds and thousands of bits of information continually bombarding it. Because more than 90% of the neurons in the body are located in the CNS, most neural integration takes place there, within the brain and spinal cord. These neurons are responsible for making most of the "decisions."

Quiz Yourself

- What is neural integration?
- How does an EPSP differ from an action potential?

THE HUMAN BRAIN IS THE MOST COMPLEX MECHANISM KNOWN

LEARNING OBJECTIVES

10. Describe the structure and functions of the main parts of the brain: medulla, pons, midbrain, diencephalon (thalamus and hypothalamus), cerebellum, cerebrum. (Be able to label the main structures of the brain on a diagram.)
11. Describe the principal areas and functions associated with the lobes of the cerebrum and the limbic system.

The human brain, a soft, wrinkled mass of tissue, is a highly complex, adaptive system. Each of its 25 billion neurons is connected to thousands of other neurons. It is no wonder that scientists have barely begun to unravel the tangled neural circuits that govern human physiology and behavior.

What we do know is that at any moment millions of neural messages are flashing through the brain. They bring information to the brain about the state of the body and transmit "decisions" back to the organs maintaining an appropriate heart rate, blood pressure, respiration rate, temperature, muscle tone, and blood chemistry. At the same time, the brain receives and responds to hundreds of messages from the outer environment—for example, a ringing telephone, the aroma of a steak dinner, the sounds of traffic, and the printed words on this page.

Brain cells require a continuous supply of oxygen and glucose. The brain is so dependent on its blood supply that when it is deprived of it, consciousness may be lost very quickly

and irreversible damage may occur within a few minutes. In fact, the most common cause of brain damage is a stroke, or *cerebrovascular accident (CVA)*. In a CVA, a portion of the brain is deprived of its blood supply (often because a blood vessel has been blocked by a blood clot).

The main divisions of the brain are the medulla, pons, midbrain, diencephalon (which includes the thalamus and hypothalamus), cerebellum, and cerebrum (Figures 6-7 and 6-8 and Table 6-2). The medulla, pons, and midbrain make up the **brainstem**—the elongated portion of the brain that looks like a stalk for the cerebrum. The brain is a hollow organ. Its fluid-filled spaces are called **ventricles** (Figure 6-9).

The Medulla Contains Vital Centers

More formally known as the **medulla oblongata** (meh-**dul'**-ah ob'-long-**gah'**-tah), the medulla is the most posterior portion of the brainstem. It is continuous with the spinal cord (see Figure 6-8). Its cavity, the **fourth ventricle,** is continuous with the central canal of the spinal cord. The medulla consists of white matter and gray matter. The white matter consists mainly of nerve tracts passing between the spinal cord and the various portions of the brain. Because of the medulla's position, all nerve tracts carrying messages from the spinal cord to the brain must pass through it. Similarly, all the motor tracts transmitting messages back from the decision-making parts of the brain pass through the medulla. The gray matter of the medulla consists mainly of various nuclei (groups of cell bodies). Most of the motor fibers cross within the medulla. This explains why the right side of the brain controls the movement of the left side of the body and vice versa.

The **reticular formation** is a network of neurons that extends from the spinal cord through the medulla and upward through the brainstem and thalamus. The reticular formation receives sensory information that enters the spinal cord and brainstem and influences the level of arousal; it is important in keeping the cerebrum conscious and alert.

The medulla contains discrete nuclei that serve as vital centers. These include the following:

1. **Cardiac centers** that control heart rate
2. **Vasomotor centers** that help regulate blood pressure by controlling the diameter of the blood vessels
3. **Respiratory centers** that initiate and regulate breathing

Centers for other reflex actions such as vomiting, sneezing, coughing, and swallowing also are found within the medulla. Four cranial nerves, designated *cranial nerves IX through XII,* originate within the medulla, and their nuclei are located there.

The Pons Is a Bridge to Other Parts of the Brain

The **pons** forms a bulge on the anterior (ventral) surface of the brainstem. The pons is just superior to the medulla, with

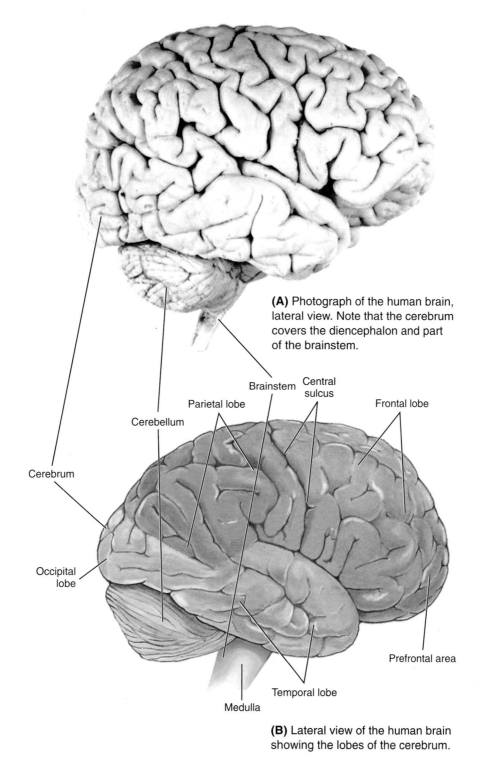

(A) Photograph of the human brain, lateral view. Note that the cerebrum covers the diencephalon and part of the brainstem.

(B) Lateral view of the human brain showing the lobes of the cerebrum.

FIGURE 6-7 • Structure of the human brain. (**A** from Williams P, Warwick R, editors: *Gray's Anatomy*, ed 36, Edinburgh, 1980, Churchill Livingstone.)

TABLE 6-2	DIVISIONS OF THE BRAIN	
	Description	**Functions**
Medulla	Most inferior portion of the brainstem; continuous with spinal cord; its white matter consists of nerve tracts passing between the spinal cord and various parts of the brain; its gray matter consists of nuclei; contains nuclei of cranial nerves IX through XII,* its cavity is the fourth ventricle	Contains vital centers that regulate heartbeat, respiration, and blood pressure; contains reflex centers that control swallowing, coughing, sneezing, and vomiting; relays messages to the other parts of the brain
Pons	Consists mainly of nerve tracts passing between the medulla and other parts of the brain; forms a bulge on the anterior surface of the brainstem; contains respiratory centers and nuclei of cranial nerves V through VIII	Connects various parts of the brain; helps regulate respiration and sleep
Midbrain	Just superior to the pons; cavity is the cerebral aqueduct; within midbrain are nuclei of cranial nerves III and IV	Regulates visual and auditory reflexes
Diencephalon		
Thalamus	At top of brainstem; contains many important nuclei	Main sensory relay center between spinal cord and cerebrum; incoming messages are sorted and partially interpreted here before being relayed to the appropriate centers in the cerebrum
Hypothalamus	Forms ventral floor of third ventricle; contains many nuclei; optic chiasma marks the crossing of the optic nerves; connected to the pituitary gland	Contains centers for control of body temperature, appetite, and water balance; regulates pituitary gland and links nervous and endocrine systems; helps control autonomic system; involved in some emotional and sexual responses
Cerebellum	Second largest part of the brain; superior to the fourth ventricle; consists of two hemispheres	Responsible for smooth, coordinated movement; maintains posture and muscle tone; helps maintain equilibrium
Cerebrum	Largest, most prominent part of the brain; longitudinal fissure divides the cerebrum into right and left hemispheres, each containing a lateral ventricle; each hemisphere is divided into lobes: frontal, parietal, occipital, and temporal	Center of consciousness, intellect, memory, and language; receives and interprets sensory information from sense organs; controls motor functions
Cerebral cortex	Convoluted, outer layer of gray matter covering the cerebrum; functionally divided into:	
	1. Sensory areas	Receive incoming sensory information from eyes, ears, touch and pressure receptors, and other sense organs; sensory association areas interpret incoming sensory information
	2. Motor areas	Control voluntary movement and certain types of involuntary movement
	3. Association areas	Connect sensory and motor areas; responsible for thought, learning, memory, language, judgment, and personality
White matter	Consists of myelinated axons that connect various regions of the brain; these axons are arranged into tracts (bundles); the basal ganglia are located within the white matter	Connects the following: 1. Neurons within same hemisphere 2. Right and left hemispheres (corpus callosum) 3. Cerebrum with other parts of brain and spinal cord (e.g., the fornix connects the cerebrum with the thalamus)

*Cranial nerves are discussed in Table 7-1.

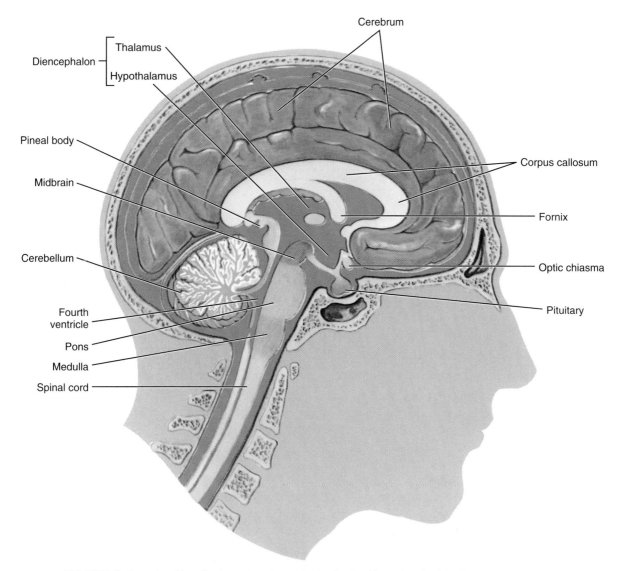

FIGURE 6-8 • A midsagittal section through the brain. Note that in this view structures normally covered by the cerebrum are exposed.

which it is continuous; its posterior surface is hidden by the cerebellum. The word *pons* means *bridge,* and indeed the pons serves as a link connecting various parts of the brain. In fact, the pons consists mainly of nerve fibers passing between the medulla and other parts of the brain. The pons also contains centers that help regulate respiration and sleep. Centers for the reflexes mediated by cranial nerves V through VII are located within the pons.

The Midbrain Contains Centers for Visual and Auditory Reflexes

The **midbrain,** the shortest portion of the brainstem, extends from the pons to the diencephalon. Its cavity, the **cerebral aqueduct** (seh-**ree′**-bral **ah′**-kweh-duct), connects the third and fourth ventricles. Anteriorly (ventrally), the midbrain

consists of large bundles of neurons connecting the cerebrum with lower portions of the brain and with the spinal cord.

The roof of the midbrain consists of four rounded bodies that serve as reflex centers for visual and auditory (ear) reflexes. For example, constriction of the pupil in response to light is controlled by this area of the midbrain. The nuclei of cranial nerves III and IV are found in the midbrain.

The Diencephalon Includes the Thalamus and the Hypothalamus

The **diencephalon** (dye-en-**sef′**-ah-lon) is the part of the brain between the cerebrum and the midbrain. Its cavity is the third ventricle (see Figure 6-9). Two important regions of the diencephalon are the thalamus and hypothalamus.

The **thalamus** (**thal′**-ah-mus), a major relay center, consists of two oval masses—one located on each side of the third

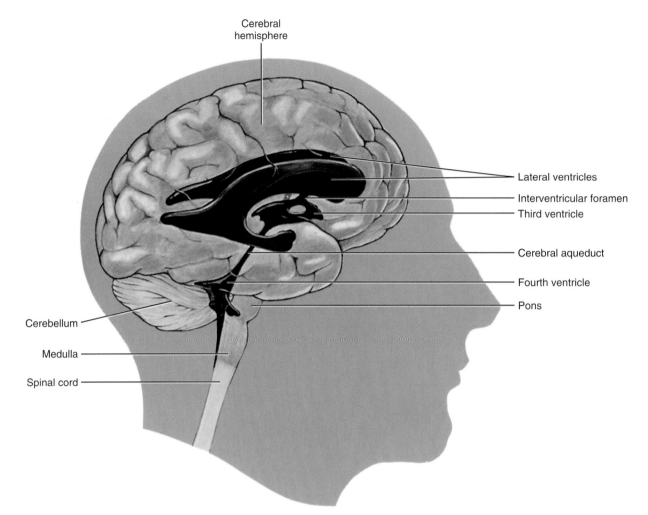

Cerebral hemisphere

Lateral ventricles

Interventricular foramen

Third ventricle

Cerebral aqueduct

Fourth ventricle

Pons

Cerebellum

Medulla

Spinal cord

FIGURE 6-9 • The ventricles of the brain, lateral view.

ventricle. Nuclei in the thalamus serve as relay stations for all sensory information (except smell) to the cerebrum. Afferent neurons coming from the sense organs synapse within these nuclei. We become vaguely aware of sensory input when it reaches the thalamus. If sensory areas of the cerebrum are destroyed, an individual can still be conscious of pain, temperature, touch, and pressure. The thalamus plays a gating role by determining whether sensory information is sent on into the cerebrum, where we become more acutely aware of it.

The thalamus is also concerned with movement. It integrates motor information from the cerebellum (and basal ganglia) and transmits messages to motor areas in the cerebrum.

The **hypothalamus** (hy'-poe-**thal'**-ah-mus) lies below the thalamus. The many nuclei within the hypothalamus help regulate homeostasis and reproductive behavior. Afferent and efferent neurons connect these centers with all other parts of the CNS. A stalk of tissue connects the pituitary gland (an important endocrine gland) to the hypothalamus. The optic chiasma (crossing) is located in the floor of the hypothalamus. This prominent X-shaped structure is formed by the crossing of part of each optic nerve.

Although the hypothalamus makes up less than 1% of the total volume of the brain, it helps regulate an impressive number of mechanisms essential to maintaining homeostasis. Here are some of its functions:

1. The hypothalamus is sometimes called the *control center of the autonomic system* because it is the most important relay station between the cerebral cortex and the lower autonomic centers. For example, stimulation of certain areas in the hypothalamus results in a decrease in heart rate. In this role the hypothalamus serves as an important link between "mind" (cerebrum) and "body" (physiological mechanisms).

2. The hypothalamus is the link between the nervous and endocrine systems. It produces several releasing hormones that regulate the secretion of hormones from the anterior lobe of the pituitary gland. In addition, the hypothalamus manufactures two hormones—antidiuretic hormone (ADH, controls rate of water reabsorption by the kidney) and oxytocin. (Oxytocin stimulates contraction of the uterus during childbirth and release of milk from the breast.) ADH and oxytocin are stored in the posterior lobe

of the pituitary gland and are released from the pituitary gland when needed.

3. The hypothalamus helps maintain fluid balance. ADH produced by its cells regulates the volume of water excreted by the kidneys. In addition, a thirst center in the hypothalamus lets us know when we need fluids.
4. The hypothalamus regulates body temperature.
5. The appetite and satiety (fullness) centers within the hypothalamus regulate food intake.
6. The hypothalamus influences sexual behavior and the affective (emotional) aspects of sensory input. Centers there help us decide whether something is pleasant or painful, influencing us to maintain behaviors that are rewarding. Thus the hypothalamus helps determine emotional and motivational states.
7. The hypothalamus, along with the brainstem, regulates sleep-wake cycles, or **circadian rhythms.** The **suprachiasmatic** (soo-pruh-kie-as-**mat′**-ik) **nucleus** in the hypothalamus is the most important of the body's biological clocks.

The Cerebellum Is Responsible for Coordination of Movement

The second largest part of the brain, the **cerebellum** (ser-eh-**bel′**-um), consists of two lateral masses called *hemispheres* and a connecting portion. The outer layer of the cerebellum, called the *cerebellar cortex,* consists of gray matter; beneath it, the cerebellum is composed mainly of white matter.

The cerebellum is responsible for coordination of movements. We can list the following among its main functions:

1. The cerebellum helps make movements smooth instead of jerky and steady rather than trembling. When the cerebellum is damaged, movements essential in running, walking, writing, talking, and many other activities become uncoordinated.
2. The cerebellum helps maintain muscle tone and posture.
3. Impulses from the vestibular apparatus (organ of balance) in the inner ear are continuously delivered to the cerebellum, which uses that information to help maintain equilibrium.
4. The cerebellum is important in learning motor skills.
5. Recent studies indicate that the cerebellum receives information from sensory association areas in the cerebrum and is important in cognitive function, including language.

The Cerebrum Is the Largest Part of the Brain

The **cerebrum** (seh-**ree′**-brum) is the largest and most prominent part of the human brain. It controls motor activities, interprets sensation, and serves as the center of intellect, memory, language, and consciousness. The cerebrum is also important in expression of emotion. For convenience we can divide the functions performed by the cerebrum into three main categories:

1. **Sensory functions.** The cerebrum receives information from the sensory receptors and then interprets these messages so that we "know" what we are seeing, hearing, tasting, smelling, or feeling. These functions are carried out by areas of the cerebrum known as **sensory areas.**
2. **Motor functions.** The **motor areas** of the cerebrum are responsible for all voluntary movement and for some involuntary movement.
3. **Association functions.** The **association areas** link the sensory and motor areas. Association areas are responsible for all of the intellectual activities of the brain. These include thought, reasoning, judgment, learning, memory storage and recall, and language abilities.

In the embryo the cerebrum grows rapidly, enlarging out of proportion to the rest of the brain. It grows backward over the brainstem and also folds on itself, forming convolutions, or gyri (**jye′**-ree) (singular—gyrus). The convolutions are separated by shallow grooves, called sulci (**sul′**-si) and by deep grooves called **fissures.** The **longitudinal fissure** partially divides the cerebrum into right and left halves—the right and left cerebral hemispheres (Figure 6-10). The cerebrum is separated from the cerebellum by the **transverse fissure.**

The thin outer layer of the cerebrum consists of gray matter and is called the **cerebral cortex. Gray matter** consists of the cell bodies of neurons and of unmyelinated fibers. Beneath the gray matter, the cerebrum consists of **white matter,** which is composed of myelinated nerve fibers. Deep within the white matter lie the **basal ganglia**—paired nuclei that play an important role in movement. The two cavities within the cerebrum are the **lateral ventricles.**

The myelinated neurons that make up the white matter of the cerebrum transmit impulses between neurons in the cerebrum and connect the cerebrum with other parts of the nervous system. A large band of white matter, the **corpus callosum,** connects the right and left hemispheres. The **fornix** connects the cortex with the thalamus.

Fissures and sulci divide each cerebral hemisphere into four major lobes named after the bones that protect them: frontal, parietal, occipital, and temporal (see Figures 6-10 and 6-11). Each frontal lobe is separated from a parietal lobe by a **central sulcus.** Investigators have drawn maps of the brain indicating which area is most responsible for each function.

Some of the principal functions of the lobes follow:

1. **Frontal lobe.** The anterior portion of each frontal lobe is an association area known as the **prefrontal area.** This area is responsible for executive functions such as considering consequences of behavior and planning actions accordingly. Just anterior to the central sulcus lies the **precentral gyrus** of the frontal lobe. Because voluntary movements of skeletal muscles are controlled from this area, it is known as the **primary motor area.** One part of the frontal lobe, **Broca's**

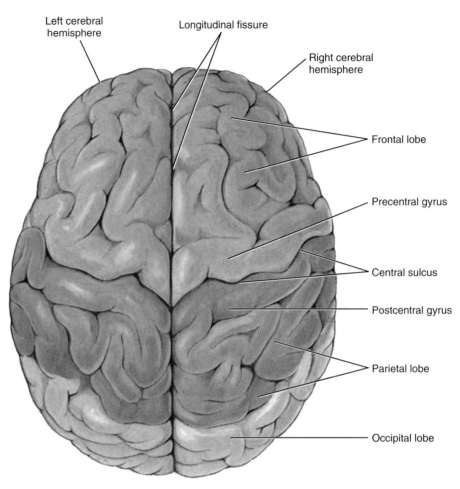

Left cerebral hemisphere

Longitudinal fissure

Right cerebral hemisphere

Frontal lobe

Precentral gyrus

Central sulcus

Postcentral gyrus

Parietal lobe

Occipital lobe

FIGURE 6-10 • Superior view of the cerebrum.

speech area, is concerned with directing the formation of words.

2. **Parietal lobe.** The parietal lobe has a **general sensory area** located in the **postcentral gyrus** (just posterior to the central sulcus). The general sensory area receives information from the sensory receptors in the skin and joints. Sensory association areas in the parietal lobe receive and integrate information about visual, auditory, and taste sensations from other areas of the cortex and thalamus. Through this integration process, persons become aware of themselves in relation to their environment. They are able to interpret characteristics of objects that they feel with their hands and to comprehend spoken and written language.

3. **Occipital lobe.** The occipital lobe receives information about what we see from the thalamus and integrates the information to formulate an appropriate response. The area that receives the visual information is known as the **primary visual area;** the portion that integrates the information is the **visual association area.**

4. **Temporal lobe.** The **primary auditory area** and the **auditory association area** are located in the temporal lobe. These areas are centers for reception and integration of auditory messages. Part of the temporal lobe is concerned with emotion, personality, and behavior.

The Limbic System Affects Emotional Aspects of Behavior

The **limbic system,** an action system of the brain, is a group of interconnected nuclei involved in memory and in the regulation of emotion. This system of neurons evaluates rewards and is important in motivation. It also plays a role in sexual behavior, biological rhythms, and autonomic responses. The limbic system includes parts of the cerebrum (parts of the frontal lobe and temporal lobe), parts of the thalamus and hypothalamus, several nuclei in the midbrain, and the neural pathways that connect these structures (Figure 6-12).

Two very important limbic regions are the **hippocampus** (hip-oh-**camp′**-us) and the **amygdala** (ah-**mig′**-duh-lah), both located below the cortex in the temporal lobe. The hippocampus is involved in the formation and retrieval of memories. It helps us file our experiences in categories so that similar memories can be stored together. The amygdala filters incoming sensory information and evaluates its importance in terms of emotional needs and survival.

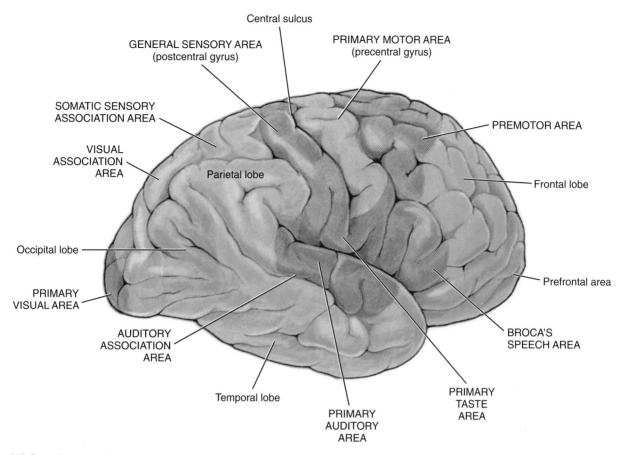

Central sulcus

GENERAL SENSORY AREA
(postcentral gyrus)

PRIMARY MOTOR AREA
(precentral gyrus)

SOMATIC SENSORY
ASSOCIATION AREA

PREMOTOR AREA

VISUAL
ASSOCIATION
AREA

Parietal lobe

Frontal lobe

Occipital lobe

Prefrontal area

PRIMARY
VISUAL AREA

AUDITORY
ASSOCIATION
AREA

BROCA'S
SPEECH AREA

Temporal lobe

PRIMARY
AUDITORY
AREA

PRIMARY
TASTE
AREA

(A) Specific parts of the cerebral cortex perform specific functions.

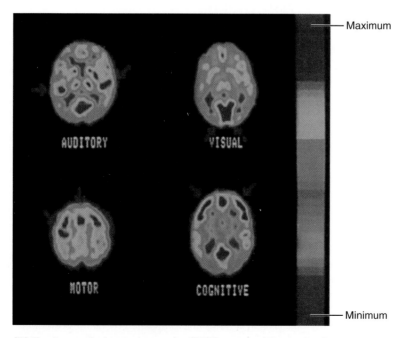

Maximum

Minimum

(B) Positon emission tomography (PET) scans of the brain. Specific areas of the brain "light up" on PET scans as an individual performs various tasks. When a specific region of the brain is more active, more blood flows to the area. PET scans detect the magnitude of blood flow. Thus, PET scans are pictures of the brain at work at specific tasks.

FIGURE 6-11 • Functional areas of the cerebrum. (**B** from Phelps ME, Mazziotta JC: Positron emission tomography: human brain function and biochemistry. *Science* 228:799-805, 1985. Reprinted with permission from AAAS.)

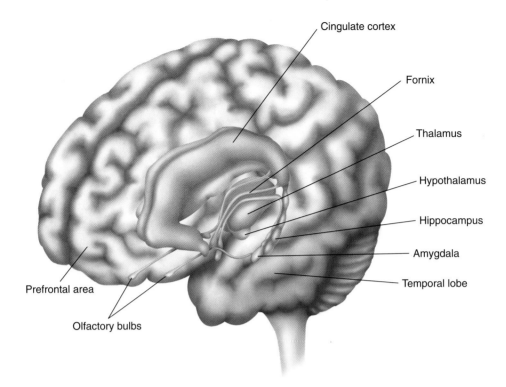

Cingulate cortex

Fornix

Thalamus

Hypothalamus

Hippocampus

Amygdala

Temporal lobe

Prefrontal area

Olfactory bulbs

FIGURE 6-12 • The limbic system.

Parts of the limbic system are essential in the process of an infant's bonding with a caregiver during the first year of life. The quality of early *attachment* between child and caregiver affects brain development and future behavior. The development of a secure attachment bond is the foundation for future emotional and social connections between the child and other human beings.

Learning Involves Many Areas of the Brain

Learning is the process by which we acquire information as a result of experience. **Memory** is the process by which information is encoded, stored, and retrieved. Memories are integrated in many areas of the brain, including the association areas of the cerebral cortex and parts of the limbic system. Memories are stored throughout the cerebrum.

For learning to occur, changes must take place in the nervous system, particularly at synapses. **Synaptic plasticity** refers to the ability of the nervous system to modify synapses during learning and remembering. Researchers have shown that long-term memory storage involves activation of certain genes and long-term functional changes at synapses.

Quiz Yourself

• What are five functions of the hypothalamus?
• What are the functions of the frontal lobe?
• Why is the limbic system important?

THE SPINAL CORD TRANSMITS INFORMATION TO AND FROM THE BRAIN

LEARNING OBJECTIVES

12. List two functions of the spinal cord and describe its structure.
13. Trace in sequence the structures through which signals are transmitted in a withdrawal reflex. (Draw and label a diagram of a withdrawal reflex.)

The spinal cord has two main functions: (1) it transmits information to and from the brain and (2) it controls many reflex activities of the body. The spinal cord is a slightly flattened, hollow cylinder that extends downward from the brain. It extends caudally to the level of the second lumbar vertebra. The spinal cord occupies the vertebral canal of the vertebral column.

Several fissures (deep grooves) divide the spinal cord into regions. The deepest groove, the **anterior median fissure,** lies in the mid anterior line. Opposite this, on the posterior (dorsal) surface, is the shallower **posterior (dorsal) fissure.** When we examine a cross section through the spinal cord, we can see a small central canal surrounded by an area of gray matter. The gray matter is shaped somewhat like the letter "H" (Figure 6-13). Outside the gray matter, the spinal cord is composed of white matter.

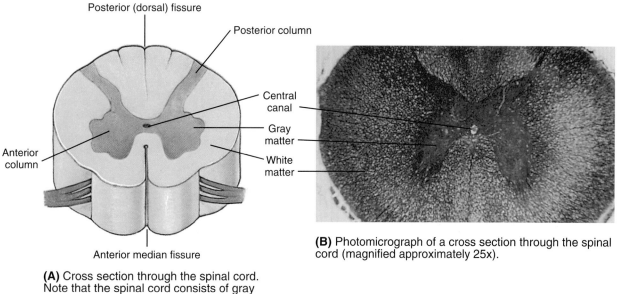

(A) Cross section through the spinal cord. Note that the spinal cord consists of gray and white matter.

(B) Photomicrograph of a cross section through the spinal cord (magnified approximately 25x).

FIGURE 6-13 • Structure of the spinal cord.

The gray matter of the spinal cord is subdivided into columns. The anterior (ventral) portions of the letter H are the anterior columns; the posterior (dorsal) regions are the posterior columns. The white matter consists of myelinated axons arranged in bundles, called *tracts* or *pathways*. **Ascending tracts** transmit sensory information up the spinal cord to the brain. **Descending tracts** transmit impulses (the "decisions") from the brain back down the spinal cord to efferent nerves.

A **reflex action** is a predictable, automatic response to a specific stimulus. Most of the internal activities of the body are regulated by reflex actions. A good example is the regulation of body temperature. A change in body temperature stimulates the temperature-regulating center of the hypothalamus to mobilize homeostatic mechanisms that bring body temperature back to normal.

Many responses to external stimuli, such as withdrawing from painful stimuli, are also reflex actions. Let us examine a withdrawal reflex, which is a protective response. Like all neural responses, a reflex pathway has five steps: (1) reception of the stimulus, (2) transmission of information to the CNS, (3) integration (interpretation and determination of an appropriate response), (4) transmission of information from the CNS to a muscle, and (5) the actual response.

Withdrawal reflexes require the participation of three sets of neurons (Figure 6-14). Imagine that you accidentally rest your hand on a hot stove. Almost instantly, and before you become consciously aware of the pain, you jerk your hand away. Pain receptors (dendrites of sensory neurons) have sent messages through afferent (sensory) neurons to the spinal cord. There, each neuron synapses with an interneuron—a neuron within the CNS that links sensory and motor neurons. Integration takes place. Then, impulses sent via efferent (motor) neurons to muscles in the arm and hand instruct these muscles to contract, jerking the hand away from the harmful stimulus.

At the same time that the interneuron sends a message to the motor neuron, it may also dispatch a message up the spinal cord to the conscious areas of the brain. Almost at the same time that you withdraw your hand, you become aware of your plight and can make the conscious decision to hold your burned hand under cold water. None of this is part of the reflex action, however. Some reflex actions (e.g., the pupil reflex of the eye) do involve parts of the brain. However, these are parts of the brain that have nothing to do with conscious thought.

We can consciously inhibit or facilitate some reflexes. An example is the reflex that empties the urinary bladder when it fills with urine. In babies, urination occurs by reflex action whenever the bladder becomes full. In early childhood we learn to facilitate the reflex by consciously stimulating it before the bladder pressure reaches the critical level. We also learn to inhibit the reflex consciously so that we do not urinate when the bladder becomes full at an inconvenient time or place.

Quiz Yourself

- What are the two main functions of the spinal cord?
- What are ascending tracts?
- What are the five steps in a withdrawal reflex?

THE CENTRAL NERVOUS SYSTEM IS WELL PROTECTED

LEARNING OBJECTIVES

14. **Describe the structures that protect the brain and spinal cord.**

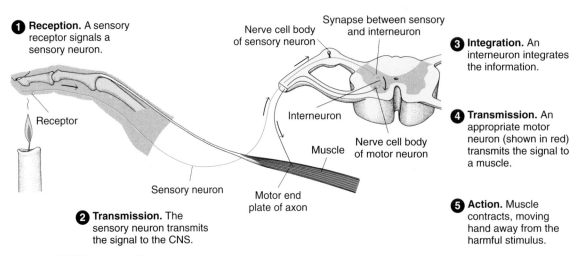

1 Reception. A sensory receptor signals a sensory neuron.

Receptor

2 Transmission. The sensory neuron transmits the signal to the CNS.

Sensory neuron

Nerve cell body of sensory neuron

Synapse between sensory and interneuron

Interneuron

Muscle

Motor end plate of axon

Nerve cell body of motor neuron

3 Integration. An interneuron integrates the information.

4 Transmission. An appropriate motor neuron (shown in red) transmits the signal to a muscle.

5 Action. Muscle contracts, moving hand away from the harmful stimulus.

FIGURE 6-14 • The withdrawal reflex shown here involves a chain of three neurons. An afferent (sensory) neuron transmits the message from the receptor to the CNS, where it synapses with an interneuron. Then an appropriate efferent (motor) neuron *(red)* transmits an impulse to the muscles that move the hand away from the flame (the response).

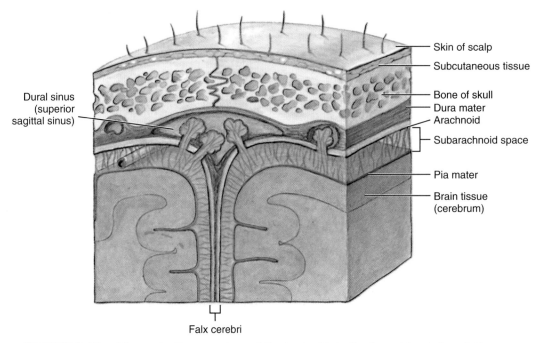

Dural sinus (superior sagittal sinus)

Skin of scalp
Subcutaneous tissue
Bone of skull
Dura mater
Arachnoid
Subarachnoid space
Pia mater
Brain tissue (cerebrum)

Falx cerebri

FIGURE 6-15 • The protective coverings of the brain. Note the large blood sinus between two layers of the dura mater. Blood leaving the brain flows into sinuses and then circulates to the larger jugular veins in the neck. The falx cerebri is the partition between the cerebral hemispheres.

The soft, fragile brain and spinal cord are the most carefully protected organs in the body. Both are encased in bone, covered by three layers of connective tissue, and bathed in a cushioning fluid.

The Meninges Are Connective Tissue Coverings

The three connective tissue layers covering the brain and spinal cord are the **meninges** (meh-**nin′**-jeez). The outermost of the meninges is the **dura mater** (**doo′**-rah **may′**-ter), a tough, double-layered membrane (Figure 6-15). Inside the skull, the two layers of the dura mater are separated in some regions by large blood vessels called **sinuses.** These sinuses receive blood leaving the brain and deliver it to the jugular veins in the neck.

The dura mater forms four partitions (septa) that subdivide the cranium into compartments. The largest of these partitions (the falx cerebri) dips down between the cerebral hemispheres.

The second of the meninges is the **arachnoid** (ah-**rak′**-noyd)—a thin, delicate membrane. Threadlike fibers of the arachnoid extend like the threads of a web through the **subarachnoid space** to the innermost meningeal layer—the **pia mater** (**pee′**-ah **may′**-ter). The pia mater is a very thin membrane that adheres closely to the brain and spinal cord, following each curve or indentation of tissue. It has many blood vessels.

Meningitis, an inflammation of the meninges, is usually caused by infection by bacteria or viruses. Bacterial meningitis has a high mortality rate if not treated. Viral meningitis is usually a self-limited disease from which the patient recovers fully. However, some viruses that cause meningitis can spread, causing inflammation of the brain itself. This more serious illness is *encephalitis.*

The Cerebrospinal Fluid Cushions the Central Nervous System

The shock-absorbing **cerebrospinal fluid (CSF)** fills the ventricles, the cavities within the brain, and the **subarachnoid space,** the space between the arachnoid layer and the pia mater (Figure 6-16). Most of the CSF is produced by clusters of capillaries, the **choroid** (**koe′**-royd) **plexuses,** which project from the pia mater into the ventricles.

The CSF circulates through the ventricles and then passes into the subarachnoid space. Finally, it is reabsorbed into the blood through structures called **arachnoid villi.** These structures project from the arachnoid layer into large blood sinuses within the dura mater.

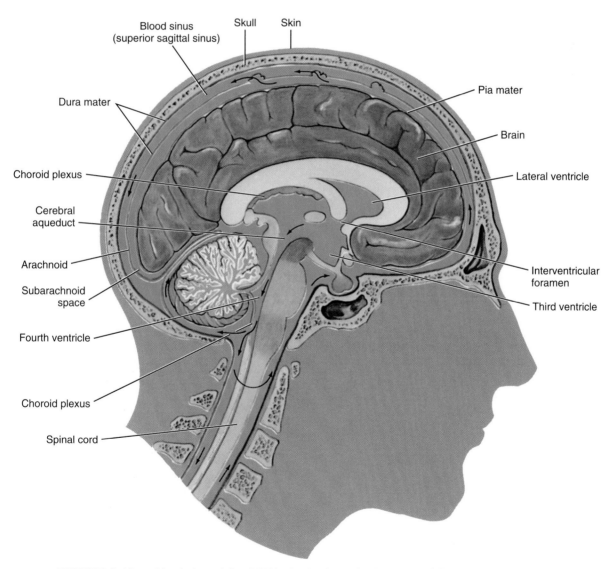

FIGURE 6-16 • Circulation of the CSF in the brain and spinal cord. CSF is produced by the choroid plexuses located in the ventricles. It circulates through the ventricles and subarachnoid space. CSF is continuously produced and continuously reabsorbed into the blood of the dural sinuses.

The brain actually floats in the CSF, which protects it against mechanical injury. CSF also dissolves and transports substances filtered from the blood. It serves as a medium for the exchange of nutrients and waste products between the blood and the brain.

A normal volume of CSF is essential to normal nervous system function. Blockage of CSF flow or abnormally rapid production can result in *hydrocephalus,* which means literally "water in the head." As CSF accumulates, the resulting pressure can cause enlargement of the skull in children and, eventually, brain damage; in severe cases, mental retardation may result. In infants and children, hydrocephalus most commonly results from a birth defect. Surgical placement of a shunt permits excess fluid to drain into a vein.

The dura mater and arachnoid extend below the level of the spinal cord. Thus a needle can be safely inserted into the subarachnoid space between the level of the third and fourth lumbar vertebrae. This procedure, called a *lumbar puncture,* can be used to measure CSF pressure or to withdraw small amounts of CSF without damaging the cord itself. Analysis of this fluid can be helpful in diagnosing certain CNS disorders. For example, blood in the CSF may provide a clue in the diagnosis of cerebral (brain) hemorrhage. When indicated, lumbar puncture is often followed by computed tomography scanning.

Injections of an anesthetic into the subarachnoid space block neural transmission from sensory neurons. In *spinal anesthesia* the patient remains awake but feels no pain in the lower part of the body.

Quiz Yourself

- What are the three meninges?
- What are the functions of cerebrospinal fluid?

SUMMARY

LO 1. Distinguish between the central nervous system and the peripheral nervous system and describe each.
- The two principal divisions of the nervous system are the **central nervous system (CNS)** and the **peripheral nervous system (PNS).** The CNS consists of the **brain** and **spinal cord.**
- The PNS consists of **somatic** and **autonomic divisions.** Two types of efferent nerves in the autonomic system are sympathetic and parasympathetic nerves.

LO 2. Relate the function of neurons to their structure, and give the functions of glial cells.
- **Neurons** transmit signals. A neuron is made up of a **cell body** that contains the nucleus, **dendrites** that transmit signals to the cell body, and an **axon** that transmits signals away from the cell body. Axons may be covered by both a **myelin sheath** and a **cellular sheath. Synaptic terminals** at the ends of axons release **neurotransmitters,** chemical compounds that transmit signals from one neuron to another, or from a neuron to a muscle or gland.
- **Glial cells** protect and support the neurons, signal neurons, and carry out regulatory functions.

LO 3. Distinguish between nerve and tract, ganglion and nucleus.
- A **nerve** is a bundle of axons located outside the CNS. A **tract** or **pathway** is a bundle of axons located within the CNS.
- A **ganglion** is a mass of cell bodies located outside the CNS. A **nucleus** is a mass of cell bodies located inside the CNS.

LO 4. Briefly describe the basic processes essential for neural signaling—reception, transmission, integration, and response.
- Every response requires **neural signaling** and involves a sequence of five steps:
  A. **Reception**—a stimulus is received by sensory receptors.
  B. **Transmission**—information is conducted to the CNS by **afferent (sensory) neurons.**
  C. **Integration**—information is sorted and interpreted so that an appropriate response can be determined.
  D. **Transmission**—a message is delivered from the CNS by **efferent neurons** to the appropriate muscle or gland.
  E. **Actual response**—the muscle contracts (or gland secretes), producing the actual response to the stimulus.

LO = Learning Objective

LO 5. Contrast an action potential with the resting potential of a neuron. (Describe each.)
- Neurons transmit information with electrical signals. The **resting potential** of a neuron is the voltage measured across the plasma membrane of a neuron that is not transmitting a message.
- The magnitude of the resting potential is determined by (1) differences in concentrations of specific ions (mainly Na⁺ and K⁺) inside the cell relative to the extracellular fluid, and (2) the permeability of the plasma membrane to these ions. **Sodium-potassium pumps** in the plasma membrane help maintain the resting potential.
- An excitatory stimulus increases the membrane's permeability to sodium ions. When Na⁺ move into the neuron, the membrane potential **depolarizes**—becomes less negative than the resting level. Depolarization brings the membrane closer to its **threshold level**—the critical point at which it fires.
- When a stimulus is inhibitory, it changes the permeability of the membrane in a way that causes the membrane potential to become more negative than the resting potential. The membrane is **hyperpolarized,** which brings it farther away from its threshold level.
- When the voltage across a neuron plasma membrane reaches threshold level, **voltage-activated ion channels** open, allowing Na⁺ to flow into the neuron. An **action potential** is a wave of depolarization that moves along the axon.
- As the action potential moves down the axon, **repolarization** occurs behind it; changes in ion channels bring the membrane back to its relatively negative state.
- During the millisecond or so in which it is depolarized, the axon membrane is in an **absolute refractory period:** it cannot transmit another action potential, no matter how great a stimulus is applied. When enough Na⁺ channel gates have been reset, the neuron enters a **relative refractory period** that lasts for a few additional milliseconds. During this period, the axon can transmit impulses but the threshold is higher.

LO 6. Compare continuous conduction with saltatory conduction.
- **Continuous conduction** is the smooth, progressive transmission of neural impulses that occurs in unmyelinated neurons. In **saltatory conduction,** the action potential jumps along the axon from one node of Ranvier to the next. Saltatory conduction is faster and requires less energy than continuous conduction.

LO 7. Describe the transmission of a signal across a synapse. (Draw a diagram to support your description.)
- Neurons signal other cells across **synapses,** the junction between two neurons (or between a neuron and muscle fiber or gland cell). When an action potential reaches the end of the axon of a **presynaptic neuron,** neurotransmitter is released from **synaptic vesicles.**
- Neurotransmitter diffuses across the synapse and binds to **receptors** in the plasma membrane of the **postsynaptic neuron.** These receptors are chemically activated ion channels that can change the permeability of the membrane. When enough receptors are activated, the postsynaptic neuron transmits an action potential.
- A change in membrane potential that brings the neuron closer to firing is called an **excitatory postsynaptic potential (EPSP).** A neurotransmitter-receptor combination that hyperpolarizes the postsynaptic membrane is referred to as an **inhibitory postsynaptic potential (IPSP).** In **summation,** EPSPs and IPSPs are added and subtracted.

LO 8. Describe the actions of the neurotransmitters discussed in this chapter.
- Neurotransmitters include acetylcholine, norepinephrine, serotonin, dopamine, endorphins, enkephalins, substance P, and nitric oxide. Their actions are described in Table 6-1.

LO 9. Define neural integration and describe how a postsynaptic neuron integrates incoming stimuli and "decides" whether to fire.
- **Neural integration** is the process of summing incoming signals. Each EPSP and IPSP is a graded response that can be added or subtracted from other EPSPs and IPSPs. The molecular tabulations determine whether a neuron is brought to threshold level or is inhibited.

LO 10. Describe the structure and functions of the main parts of the brain: medulla, pons, midbrain, diencephalon (thalamus and hypothalamus), cerebellum, cerebrum. (Be able to label the main structures of the brain on a diagram.)
- The medulla, pons, and midbrain make up the **brainstem.** The **medulla oblongata,** the lowest part of the brainstem, contains nerve tracts passing from the spinal cord to the brain and tracts descending from the brain to the spinal cord. The medulla contains vital centers that control respiration, heart rate, and blood pressure.

- The **pons** serves as a bridge connecting various parts of the brain and helps to regulate respiration. The **midbrain** controls certain visual and auditory reflexes.
- The **diencephalon** includes the thalamus and hypothalamus. The **thalamus** is a major relay station for all sensory information (except smell) going to the cerebrum. The thalamus also integrates motor information.
- The **hypothalamus** serves as a link between the nervous and endocrine systems and a link between the cerebrum and the lower autonomic centers. It helps regulate temperature, helps maintain fluid balance, influences emotional and sexual behavior, and regulates appetite. The hypothalamus also helps regulate **circadian rhythms** (sleep-wake cycles). The **suprachiasmatic nucleus** is the principal biological clock.
- The **cerebellum** makes movements smooth and coordinated, maintains posture and equilibrium, and is important in learning motor skills.
- The **cerebrum** has sensory, motor, and association functions. The cerebrum is folded on itself, forming **convolutions,** or **gyri.** The convolutions are separated by shallow grooves called **sulci** and by deep grooves called **fissures.**
- The cerebrum is divided into right and left **cerebral hemispheres** by the **longitudinal fissure.** The cerebrum is separated from the cerebellum by the **transverse fissure.**
- The thin outer layer of **gray matter** is the **cerebral cortex.** Beneath it lies **white matter.** The **basal ganglia,** paired nuclei that play an important role in movement, are located within the white matter. The two cavities within the cerebrum are the **lateral ventricles.**

LO 11. Describe the principal areas and functions associated with the lobes of the cerebrum and the limbic system.
- Each hemisphere is divided into four major lobes. The **frontal lobes** include the **prefrontal area,** which is responsible for executive functions; the **primary motor area;** and **Broca's speech area,** which controls the ability to speak. **Synaptic plasticity** permits changes to occur at synapses so that learning and remembering can occur.

- The **parietal lobe** is responsible for integrating information about touch and about visual, auditory, and taste sensations. The **occipital lobes** contain the visual centers and the **temporal lobes** contain the centers for hearing.
- The **limbic system** is involved in learning and in the emotional aspects of behavior.

LO 12. List two functions of the spinal cord and describe its structure.
- The spinal cord, which is continuous with the medulla, extends to the level of the second lumbar vertebra. The spinal cord has a central canal surrounded by gray matter and an outer portion of white matter. **Ascending tracts** transmit sensory information up the spinal cord to the brain. **Descending tracts** transmit information from the brain down the spinal cord to efferent nerves.
- The spinal cord functions as a reflex control center and transmits information back and forth between the brain and the peripheral nerves.

LO 13. Trace in sequence the structures through which signals are transmitted in a withdrawal reflex. (Draw and label a diagram of a withdrawal reflex.)
- In a **reflex action,** a stimulus results in a predictable, automatic response. A **withdrawal reflex** requires an afferent (sensory) neuron that transmits signals to the CNS, an interneuron in the CNS, and an efferent (motor) neuron that transmits signals from the CNS to a muscle or gland.

LO 14. Describe the structures that protect the brain and spinal cord.
- The brain and spinal cord are protected by bone, **cerebrospinal fluid (CSF),** and three connective tissue coverings called meninges—the **dura mater, arachnoid,** and **pia mater.** The CSF is produced by clusters of capillaries, the **choroid plexuses.** The CSF circulates through the ventricles, passes into the subarachnoid space, and is reabsorbed into the blood by the **arachnoid villi.**

CHAPTER QUIZ

Fill in the Blank

1. The CNS consists of the _____ and the _____.

2. Sensory receptors and nerves belong to the _____ nervous system.

3. The supporting cells of nervous tissue are called _____ cells.

4. Cells that are specialized to transmit nerve impulses are called _____.

5. The nucleus of a neuron is located within the _____ _____.

6. The fiber of a neuron specialized to transmit impulses away from the cell body is the _____.

7. A mass of cell bodies outside the CNS is termed a _____; within the CNS it is called a _____.

8. The first step in any type of neural action is _____ of a stimulus.

9. The junction between two neurons is called a(n) _____.

10. The cavities within the brain are called _____.

11. The medulla, pons, and midbrain make up the _____.

12. The central canal of the spinal cord is surrounded by an area of _____ matter.

13. _____ tracts transmit sensory information up the spinal cord to the brain.

14. Three types of neurons that participate in a withdrawal reflex are afferent neurons, _____, and _____ neurons.

15. The outermost of the meninges is the tough _____ _____.

16. The ventricles of the brain contain _____ _____.

Multiple Choice

17. Sodium-potassium pumps: a. help maintain the hyperpolarized state of the resting neuron; b. pump potassium ions out of the neuron; c. help maintain the resting potential of a neuron; d. are activated by strong voltage.

18. An action potential: a. is an all-or-none-response; b. depends on the presence of myelin in the neuron; c. is accelerated by norepinephrine; d. is the mechanism of neural signaling across synapses.

19. The part of the brain that helps maintain posture and equilibrium is the: a. medulla; b. cerebellum; c. cerebrum; d. thalamus.

20. The part of the brain that controls voluntary movement is the: a. medulla; b. cerebellum; c. cerebrum; d. hypothalamus.

21. The part of the brain that links the nervous and endocrine systems is the: a. medulla; b. thalamus; c. cerebrum; d. hypothalamus.

22. Visual information is integrated in the: a. occipital lobes; b. frontal lobes; c. temporal lobes; d. parietal lobes.

REVIEW QUESTIONS

1. What are the main divisions of the nervous system?

2. What is the main function of the nervous system?

3. How is a neuron adapted to perform its function?

4. What is a nerve? What is a tract?

5. Imagine that you awake from your sleep and you smell smoke. What processes take place in your nervous system that allow you to respond? (Hint: in your answer, include reception, transmission, integration, and response.)

6. What is an action potential? Describe the sequence of events leading to transmission of an action potential, describe the action potential, and explain refractory periods.

7. How are neural messages generally transmitted from one neuron to another? Give the functions of acetylcholine, catecholamines, and nitric oxide.

8. What is neural integration? Describe the process.

9. List the main parts of the brain and give the functions of each.

10. Identify the part of the brain most closely associated with each of the following functions: (a) regulation of body temperature; (b) regulation of heart rate; (c) reflex center for pupil constriction; (d) interpretation of language; (e) emotional aspects of behavior.

11. In which part of the cerebrum would you find the basal ganglia? Broca's speech area? Motor cortex? Primary visual area?

12. What is synaptic plasticity?

13. What are the functions of the spinal cord?

14. Imagine that you have just stepped on something sharp. What happens in your nervous system? Draw a diagram of a withdrawal reflex pathway, label its parts, and relate the diagram to your description.

15. What structures protect the brain and spinal cord?

16. Label the diagram. (See Figure 6-8 to check your answers.)

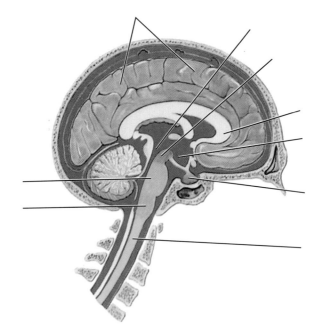

7 The Peripheral Nervous System

Chapter Outline

I. The somatic division responds to changes in the outside world

    A. The cranial nerves link the brain with sensory receptors and muscles

    B. The spinal nerves link the spinal cord with various structures

        1. Each spinal nerve divides into branches

        2. The ventral branches form plexuses

II. The autonomic division maintains internal balance

    A. The sympathetic system mobilizes energy

    B. The parasympathetic system conserves and restores energy

    C. Sympathetic and parasympathetic nerves have opposite effects on many organs

The peripheral nervous system (PNS) is made up of the sensory receptors, the nerves that link the sensory receptors with the central nervous system (CNS), and the nerves that link the CNS with effectors—the muscles and glands. That portion of the PNS that keeps the body in adjustment with the outside world is the somatic division. The nerves and receptors that maintain internal balance make up the autonomic division.

THE SOMATIC DIVISION RESPONDS TO CHANGES IN THE OUTSIDE WORLD

LEARNING OBJECTIVES

1. Describe the components of the somatic division of the nervous system.
2. List the cranial nerves and give the functions of each.
3. Describe the structure of a typical spinal nerve.
4. Name and describe the major plexuses.

The somatic division includes the sensory receptors that react to changes in the outside world (see Chapter 8), the afferent neurons that keep the CNS informed of those changes, and the efferent neurons that tell the muscles to respond. The afferent and efferent neurons of the somatic division, like those of the autonomic division, are part of the cranial and spinal nerves.

The Cranial Nerves Link the Brain With Sensory Receptors and Muscles

Twelve pairs of **cranial nerves** emerge from the brain (Figure 7-1). Cranial nerves transmit information to the brain from sensory receptors. Then they transmit orders in the form of neural signals from the CNS to muscles and glands. Cranial nerves are designated by Roman numerals and by name. The numbers indicate the sequence in which the nerves emerge from the brain. Table 7-1 lists the cranial nerves, their distributions, and their functions. Some cranial nerves consist only of sensory (afferent) fibers, but most are mixed nerves, consisting of both sensory and motor (efferent) neurons.

The Spinal Nerves Link the Spinal Cord With Various Structures

Thirty-one pairs of **spinal nerves** emerge from the spinal cord. They are all mixed nerves that (1) transmit sensory information to the spinal cord through their afferent neurons and (2)

TABLE 7-1	THE CRANIAL NERVES		
Number	Name	Origin of Sensory Fibers	Effector Innervated by Motor Fibers
I	Olfactory	Olfactory epithelium of nose (smell)	None
II	Optic	Retina of eye (vision)	None
III	Oculomotor	Proprioceptors* of eyeball muscles	Muscles that move eyeball; muscles that change shape of lens; muscles that constrict pupil
IV	Trochlear	Proprioceptors* of eyeball muscles	Muscles that move eyeball
V	Trigeminal	Teeth and skin of face	Some muscles used in chewing
VI	Abducens	Proprioceptors* of eyeball muscles	Muscles that move eyeball
VII	Facial	Taste buds of anterior part of tongue	Muscles used for facial expression; submaxillary and sublingual salivary glands
VIII	Vestibulocochlear (auditory)		None
	Vestibular branch	Semicircular canals of inner ear (senses of movement, balance, and rotation)	
	Cochlear branch	Cochlea of inner ear (hearing)	
IX	Glossopharyngeal	Taste buds of posterior third of tongue and lining of pharynx	Parotid salivary gland; muscles of pharynx used in swallowing
X	Vagus	Nerve endings in many of the internal organs (e.g., lungs, stomach, aorta, larynx)	Parasympathetic fibers to heart, stomach, small intestine, larynx, esophagus, and other organs
XI	Spinal accessory	Muscles of shoulder	Muscles of neck and shoulder
XII	Hypoglossal	Muscles of tongue	Muscles of tongue

*Proprioceptors are receptors located in muscles, tendons, or joints that provide information about body position and movement (discussed in Chapter 8).

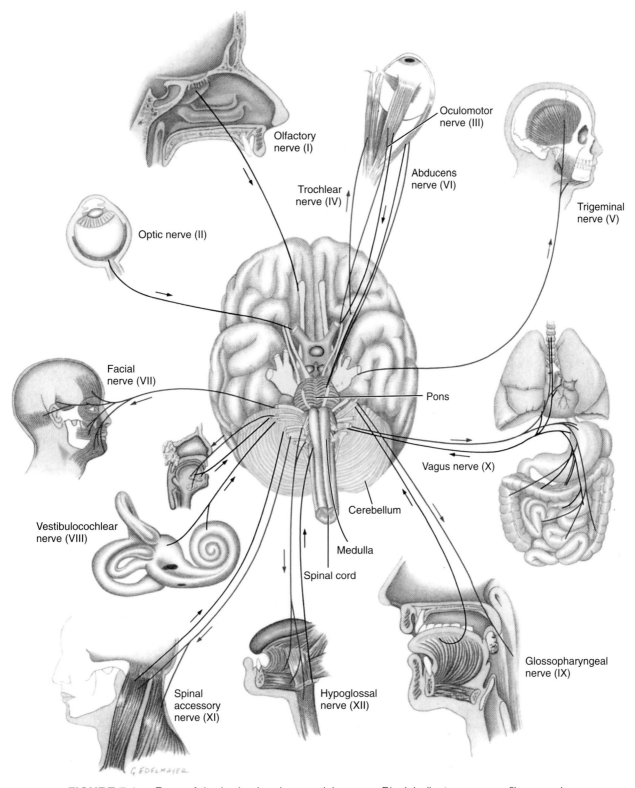

FIGURE 7-1 • Base of the brain showing cranial nerves. *Black* indicates sensory fibers; *red* indicates motor fibers.

transmit information from the spinal cord to the various parts of the body through their efferent neurons.

Spinal nerves are named for the general region of the vertebral column from which they originate and are numbered in sequence. There are 8 pairs of **cervical spinal nerves,** numbered C1 to C8; 12 pairs of **thoracic spinal nerves,** numbered T1 to T12; 5 pairs of **lumbar spinal nerves,** numbered L1 to L5; 5 pairs of **sacral spinal nerves,** numbered S1 to S5; and 1 pair of **coccygeal spinal nerves** (Figure 7-2).

Each spinal nerve has two points of attachment with the spinal cord. The **dorsal root** consists only of afferent (sensory) fibers that transmit information from the sensory receptors to the spinal cord (Figure 7-3). Just before the dorsal root joins the spinal cord, it is marked by a swelling, the **spinal ganglion,** which consists of the cell bodies of the sensory neurons. The **ventral root** consists only of efferent (motor) fibers leaving the cord. Cell bodies of the motor neurons are located within the gray matter of the cord. Dorsal and ventral roots join to form the spinal nerve (see Figure 7-3).

Each Spinal Nerve Divides Into Branches

Just after a spinal nerve emerges from the vertebral column, it divides into branches (see Figure 7-3). The **dorsal (posterior) branch** of each nerve supplies the muscles and skin of the posterior part of the body in that region. The dorsal branch divides and gives rise to various nerves. The **ventral (anterior) branch** innervates the anterior and lateral body trunk in that area and the limbs.

The Ventral Branches Form Plexuses

The ventral branches of most of the spinal nerves do not pass directly to the body structures they innervate. Instead, the ventral branches of several spinal nerves interconnect, forming networks called **plexuses.** Each plexus is a tangled network of fibers from all of the spinal nerves involved. The nerves that emerge from a plexus consist of neurons that originated in several different spinal nerves. Nerves that emerge from a plexus may be named for the region of the body that they innervate.

The main plexuses are the cervical plexus, the brachial plexus, the lumbar plexus, and the sacral plexus (see Figure 7-2).

1. The **cervical plexus** is located deep within the neck. It receives sensory information from the back of the head, neck, shoulder, and upper chest. It sends impulses to the skin and muscles of part of the head, the neck, and upper shoulders. The **phrenic nerve,** which sends impulses to the diaphragm, exits from this plexus.
2. The **brachial plexus** is located deep within the shoulder. It supplies the lower part of the shoulder, the arm, and the hand. Two of the nerves that emerge from this plexus are the *ulnar* (funny bone) and the *radial.*
3. The **lumbar plexus** is located in the lumbar region of the back. It supplies the lower abdominal wall, thigh, and exter-

nal genital structures. The *femoral nerve* is the largest nerve arising from this plexus.
4. The **sacral plexus** supplies the buttock, thigh, leg, and foot. The main branch of the sacral plexus is the **sciatic nerve,** which is the largest nerve in the body.

Quiz Yourself

- What is the function of cranial nerve II? Of cranial nerve X?
- What makes up the dorsal root of a spinal nerve?
- What is the function of the brachial plexus?

THE AUTONOMIC DIVISION MAINTAINS INTERNAL BALANCE

LEARNING OBJECTIVES

5. Compare and contrast the autonomic division with the somatic division.
6. Describe a reflex pathway in the autonomic division.
7. Compare and contrast the sympathetic system with the parasympathetic system.
8. Compare the effect of sympathetic stimulation with that of parasympathetic stimulation on specific organs such as the heart and the digestive tract.

While the somatic system works to keep the body in adjustment with the outside world, the autonomic division works to maintain homeostasis within the body. For instance, it functions to maintain body temperature within a narrow range and to regulate heart rate and blood pressure. The autonomic division acts on smooth muscle, cardiac muscle, and glands.

Like the somatic division, the autonomic division is organized into reflex pathways (Figure 7-4). Receptors within the organs relay information via afferent nerves to the CNS. The information is integrated at various levels. Then the decision is transmitted along efferent nerves to the appropriate muscles or glands. The efferent portion of the autonomic division is subdivided into sympathetic and parasympathetic systems. Table 7-2 compares several characteristics of these systems.

Recall that in the somatic division a single efferent neuron is found between the CNS and the muscle. In the autonomic division *two* efferent neurons are found between the CNS and the muscle or gland it innervates. The first neuron synapses with the second within a ganglion.

The Sympathetic System Mobilizes Energy

The sympathetic system prepares the body for action. It is most active during stressful situations. For example, the sympathetic system dominates when you are rushing to class or taking a test.

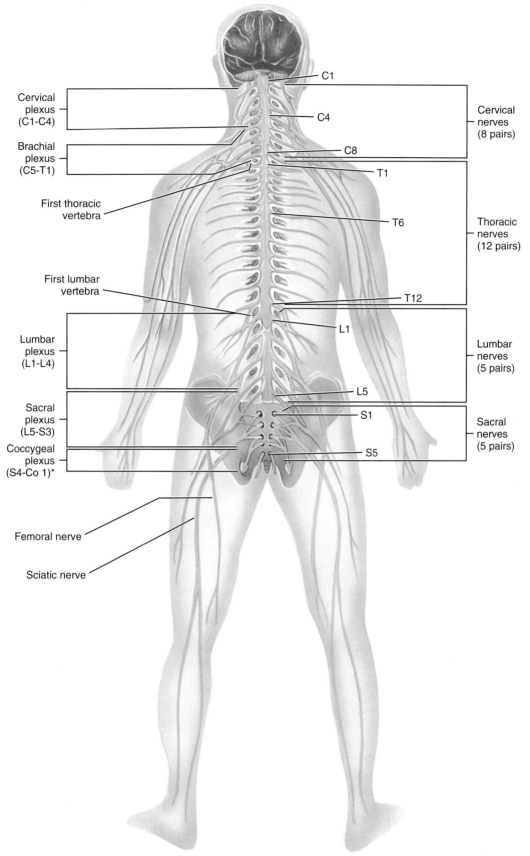

Cervical
plexus
(C1-C4)

Brachial
plexus
(C5-T1)

First thoracic
vertebra

First lumbar
vertebra

Lumbar
plexus
(L1-L4)

Sacral
plexus
(L5-S3)

Coccygeal
plexus
(S4-Co 1)*

Femoral nerve

Sciatic nerve

C1

C4

C8

T1

T6

T12

L1

L5

S1

S5

Cervical
nerves
(8 pairs)

Thoracic
nerves
(12 pairs)

Lumbar
nerves
(5 pairs)

Sacral
nerves
(5 pairs)

*Co 1 is not shown in this figure.

FIGURE 7-2 • Posterior view of the spinal cord showing the spinal nerves and some
of their major branches and plexuses. Spinal nerves are named for the general region
of the vertebral column from which they originate, and they are numbered in sequence.
C, Cervical; *T*, thoracic; *L*, lumbar; *S*, sacral; *Co*, coccygeal.

Neurons of the sympathetic system emerge from the thoracic and lumbar regions of the spinal cord. Efferent sympathetic neurons pass through a branch of a spinal nerve—the autonomic branch. Then they pass into the ganglia of the **paravertebral sympathetic ganglion chain.** This chain is a series of ganglia located along the length of the vertebral column (Figure 7-5). Most of the first efferent neurons end within the ganglia and synapse there with the second efferent neurons in the sequence.

Axons of some of the second efferent neurons leave the ganglion as various sympathetic nerves. They innervate blood vessels and organs in the head, neck, and thoracic region. Other sympathetic nerves innervate sweat glands.

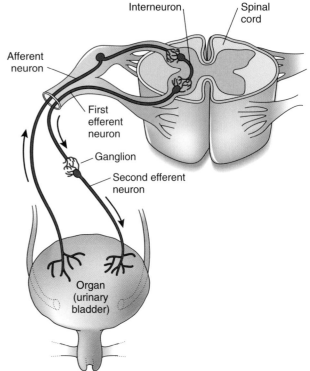

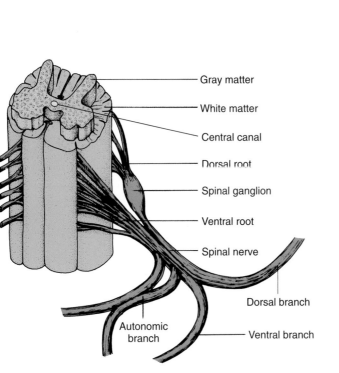

FIGURE 7-3 • Dorsal and ventral roots join to form a spinal nerve. The spinal nerve divides into several branches.

FIGURE 7-4 • An autonomic reflex. An afferent neuron transmits impulses from a receptor in an organ to the CNS. Interneurons in the CNS integrate the information. Then a sequence of two efferent neurons (preganglionic and postganglionic) transmits impulses to the smooth muscle of the organ. Note that the two efferent neurons synapse within a ganglion.

TABLE 7-2	COMPARISON OF SYMPATHETIC AND PARASYMPATHETIC SYSTEMS	
Effector	**Sympathetic System**	**Parasympathetic System**
General effect	Prepares body to cope with stressful situations	Restores body to resting state after stressful situation; actively maintains normal body functions
Extent of effect	Widespread throughout body	Localized
Neurotransmitters released	Preganglionic: acetylcholine Postganglionic: norepinephrine (usually)	Acetylcholine
Duration of effect	Lasting	Brief
Outflow from CNS	Thoracic and lumbar nerves from spinal cord	Cranial nerves and sacral nerves from spinal cord
Location of ganglia	Chain and collateral ganglia	Terminal ganglia
Number of postganglionic fibers with which each preganglionic fiber synapses	Many	Few

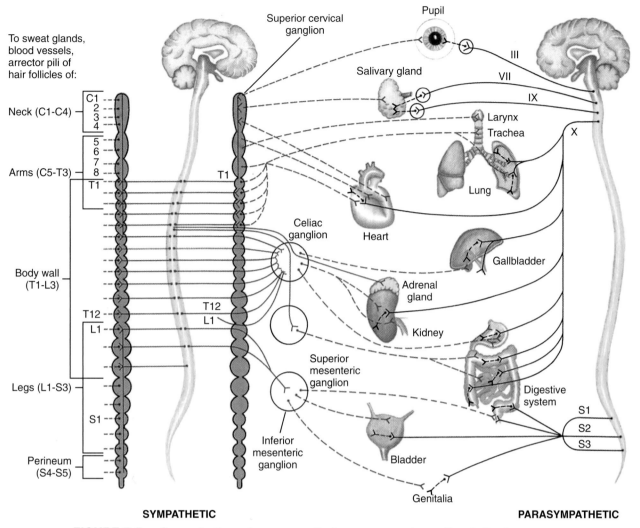

FIGURE 7-5 • Sympathetic and parasympathetic nervous systems. For clarity, the sympathetic system has been divided. Nerves going to the body wall are shown on one side of the spinal cord, and nerves going to the internal organs are shown on the other side. Complex as it appears, this diagram has been greatly simplified. *Red lines* represent sympathetic nerves, *black lines* represent parasympathetic nerves, and *dotted lines* represent postganglionic (second efferent) neurons. *C,* Cervical; *T,* thoracic; *L,* lumbar; *S,* sacral.

Some of the first efferent neurons do not end in the ganglia of the paravertebral chain but instead pass on to ganglia located in the abdomen. These ganglia are known as **collateral ganglia.** Efferent neurons emerging from the collateral ganglia innervate smooth muscles and glands of the abdominal and pelvic organs and their blood vessels. These include organs of the digestive, urinary, and reproductive systems.

The first efferent neurons are referred to as **preganglionic neurons,** and the second efferent neurons are **postganglionic neurons.** Preganglionic neurons of the sympathetic system release the neurotransmitter **acetylcholine;** for this reason they are referred to as **cholinergic.** The postganglionic neurons release **norepinephrine** and are referred to as **adrenergic.**

The Parasympathetic System Conserves and Restores Energy

The parasympathetic system helps return the body to resting conditions. This system is most active during periods of calm and physical rest—for example, when you are relaxing in front of the television set. Its activities result in conserving and restoring energy. Neurons of the parasympathetic system emerge from the brain as part of cranial nerves and from the sacral region of the spinal cord. About 75% of all parasympathetic fibers are in the **vagus nerves.**

The first efferent neurons synapse with the second efferent neurons in **terminal ganglia** located near or within the walls of the organs they innervate. Neurons from the cranial region innervate the eye, structures of the head, and thoracic and abdominal organs. Branches of the vagus innervate the heart, lungs, liver, pancreas, esophagus, stomach, small intestine, and upper portion of the large intestine (see Figure 7-5).

The parasympathetic nerves that emerge from the sacral region form the *pelvic nerves*. They innervate the lower portion of the large intestine, urinary system, and reproductive system. The parasympathetic nerves do not innervate the blood vessels or sweat glands.

Both preganglionic and postganglionic fibers of the parasympathetic system are cholinergic. They release the neurotransmitter *acetylcholine*.

Sympathetic and Parasympathetic Nerves Have Opposite Effects on Many Organs

Many organs are innervated by both sympathetic and parasympathetic nerves. In general, these systems have opposite effects. Sympathetic nerves typically stimulate organs and mobilize energy, whereas parasympathetic nerves signal organs to conserve and restore energy. For example, sympathetic nerves increase both the rate and force of contraction of the heart. Parasympathetic nerves have opposite effects; they decrease the heart rate and its strength of contraction (pumping effectiveness) (Figures 7-5 and 7-6). The digestive system is mainly under parasympathetic control. Parasympathetic stimulation increases its activity. Sympathetic stimulation is not necessary for the normal function of the digestive system, but strong sympathetic stimulation does inhibit the movement of food through the digestive tract. Table 7-3 summarizes some autonomic effects on various organs.

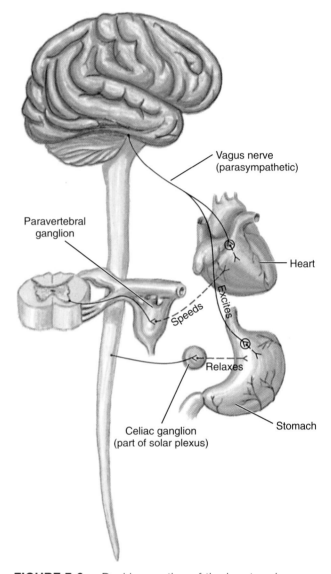

FIGURE 7-6 • Dual innervation of the heart and stomach by sympathetic and parasympathetic nerves. Sympathetic nerves are shown in *red*. Postganglionic (second efferent) neurons are indicated by *red dotted lines*.

TABLE 7-3	COMPARISON OF SYMPATHETIC AND PARASYMPATHETIC ACTIONS ON SELECTED EFFECTORS*	
Organ	**Sympathetic System**	**Parasympathetic System**
Heart	Increases rate and strength of contraction	Decreases rate; no direct effect on strength of contraction
Bronchial tubes	Dilates	Constricts
Iris of eye	Dilates pupil	Constricts pupil
Sex organs (male)	Constricts blood vessels; ejaculation	Dilates blood vessels; erection
Blood vessels	Generally constricts	No innervation for many
Sweat glands	Stimulates	No innervation
Intestine	Inhibits motility	Stimulates motility and secretion
Liver	Stimulates glycogenolysis (conversion of glycogen to glucose)	No effect
Adipose tissue	Stimulates free fatty acid release from fat cells	No effect
Adrenal medulla	Stimulates secretion of epinephrine and norepinephrine	No effect
Salivary glands	Stimulates a thick, viscous secretion	Stimulates a profuse, watery secretion

*Refer to Figure 7-5 as you study this table. Note that many other examples could be added to this list.

SUMMARY

LO 1. Describe the components of the somatic division of the nervous system.

- The **peripheral nervous system (PNS)** consists of the sensory receptors, the nerves that link the sensory receptors with the central nervous system (CNS), and the nerves that link the CNS with effectors, which are the muscles and glands. The **somatic division** is the part of the PNS that keeps the body in adjustment with the external environment. It consists of sensory receptors and nerves.

LO 2. List the cranial nerves and give the functions of each.

- Twelve pairs of **cranial nerves** link the brain with sensory receptors and effectors. Table 7-1 lists the cranial nerves and describes their functions.

LO 3. Describe the structure of a typical spinal nerve.

- Thirty-one pairs of **spinal nerves** link the spinal cord with sensory receptors and effectors. There are 8 pairs of **cervical spinal nerves,** 12 pairs of **thoracic spinal nerves,** 5 pairs of **lumbar spinal nerves,** 5 pairs of **sacral spinal nerves,** and 1 pair of **coccygeal spinal nerves.**

- Each spinal nerve has a **dorsal root** consisting of sensory fibers and a **ventral root** consisting of motor fibers. The dorsal and ventral roots join to form a spinal nerve. The cell bodies of sensory neurons are found in the **spinal ganglion,** visible as an enlargement of the dorsal root just before it joins the spinal cord.

- Each spinal nerve branches. The **dorsal branch** supplies the skin and muscles of the dorsal part of the body; the **ventral branch** supplies the ventral and lateral body trunk.

LO 4. Name and describe the major plexuses.

- The ventral branches of several spinal nerves join to form a **plexus.** The principal plexuses are the **cervical plexus,** which serves the head, neck, and shoulders; the **brachial plexus,** which supplies the shoulder, arm, and hand; the **lumbar plexus,** which supplies the lower abdominal wall, thigh, and genitals; and the **sacral plexus,** which supplies the buttock, thigh, leg, and foot.

LO = Learning Objective

LO 5. **Compare and contrast the autonomic division with the somatic division.**

- The somatic division of the PNS keeps the body in adjustment with the external environment. The **autonomic division** works to maintain a steady state within the internal environment.

LO 6. **Describe a reflex pathway in the autonomic division.**

- Afferent fibers of the autonomic division run through cranial and spinal nerves, along with somatic fibers. The efferent portion of the autonomic division is divided into sympathetic and parasympathetic systems; their neurons also are part of certain spinal and cranial nerves.

LO 7. **Compare and contrast the sympathetic system with the parasympathetic system.**

- The **sympathetic system** emerges from the spinal cord at the thoracic and lumbar regions. The sympathetic system regulates activities that mobilize energy and is especially important when the body is under stress.
- A typical sympathetic pathway might consist of the following: a **preganglionic neuron** (the first efferent neuron) emerges from the spinal cord and ends in a ganglion of the **paravertebral sympathetic ganglion chain.** The preganglionic neuron is **cholinergic;** it releases **acetylcholine.** It synapses with a **postgangli-** onic neuron (the second efferent neuron), which branches forming a nerve that innervates smooth muscle or sweat glands. The postganglionic neuron is **adrenergic;** it releases **norepinephrine.** Some first efferent neurons end in **collateral ganglia** in the abdomen.

- The **parasympathetic system** consists of nerves that emerge from the brain and from the sacral region of the spinal cord. The parasympathetic system works to restore energy and is dominant during periods of relaxation.
- The first efferent neuron (the preganglionic neuron) in the chain synapses with the second (the postganglionic neuron) in **terminal ganglia** located near or within the walls of the organs they innervate. Preganglionic and postganglionic neurons release acetylcholine.

LO 8. **Compare the effect of sympathetic stimulation with that of parasympathetic stimulation on specific organs such as the heart and the digestive tract.**

- Some organs are innervated by both sympathetic and parasympathetic nerves. In general, these systems have opposite effects. Sympathetic nerves typically stimulate organs and mobilize energy, whereas parasympathetic nerves signal organs to conserve and restore energy. For example, sympathetic nerves accelerate heart rate, whereas parasympathetic (vagus) nerves decrease heart rate.

CHAPTER QUIZ

Fill in the Blank

1. The part of the PNS that keeps the body in adjustment with the external environment is the _____ division.

2. The second cranial nerve is the _____ nerve; the tenth cranial nerve is the _____ nerve.

3. The vestibulocochlear nerve is responsible for equilibrium and _____.

4. There are _____ pairs of cervical spinal nerves and _____ pairs of thoracic spinal nerves.

5. The dorsal root of a spinal nerve consists of _____ fibers.

6. The ventral branches of several spinal nerves may interconnect to form a _____.

7. The portion of the PNS that functions to maintain a steady state within the internal environment is the _____ division.

8. The rate and force of contraction of the heart are increased by its _____ nerves.

9. The digestive system is stimulated by _____ nerves.

10. An autonomic nerve that emerges from the brain or sacral region of the spinal cord would be a _____ nerve.

Multiple Choice

11. A spinal ganglion would be found: a. on the cervical plexus; b. on the ventral branch of a spinal nerve; c. on the dorsal root of a spinal nerve; d. at the end of a preganglionic neuron of the sympathetic system.

12. Spinal nerves: a. are mainly motor nerves; b. transmit sensory information to the spinal cord; c. transmit motor information to the spinal cord; d. consist of both preganglionic and postganglionic neurons.

13. Norepinephrine is released by: a. postganglionic neurons of the sympathetic system; b. postganglionic neurons of the parasympathetic system; c. preganglionic neurons of the sympathetic system; d. preganglionic neurons of the parasympathetic system.

14. Neurons that release acetylcholine are referred to as: a. adrenergic; b. cholinergic; c. preganglionic; d. terminal.

REVIEW QUESTIONS

1. Contrast the somatic and autonomic divisions of the nervous system.

2. List the cranial nerves and their principal functions.

3. What two structures join to form a spinal nerve?

4. Name the four main plexuses and identify the structures they innervate.

5. Compare sympathetic and parasympathetic systems.

6. Give two specific examples of how sympathetic and parasympathetic systems work together to maintain homeostasis.

7. Label the diagram. (See Figure 7-3 to check your answers.)

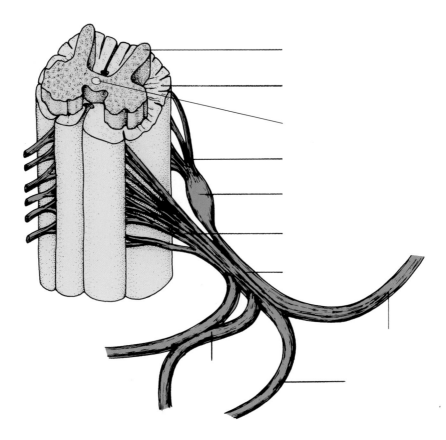

8

The Sense Organs

Chapter Outline

I. Sensory receptors transduce the energy of a stimulus into electrical signals

    A. Sensory receptors produce receptor potentials
    B. We can differentiate between seeing a dog and tasting a cookie
    C. Sensory receptors adapt to stimuli
    D. The mind constructs sensory perceptions

II. Sensory receptors respond to different types of energy

III. The eye contains photoreceptors

    A. The eye is well protected
    B. The eye is enclosed by three specialized tissue layers
    C. The eyes form a sharp image
    D. The retina contains light-sensitive rods and cones
    E. The optic nerves transmit signals to the brain

IV. The ear functions in hearing and equilibrium

    A. The outer ear conducts sound waves to the middle ear
    B. The middle ear amplifies sound waves
    C. The inner ear contains mechanoreceptors
        1. The cochlea contains the receptors for hearing
        2. Sounds differ in pitch, loudness, and quality
    D. The vestibule and semicircular canals help maintain equilibrium

V. Chemoreceptors sense smell and taste

    A. Chemoreceptors in the nasal cavity sense odorants
    B. Taste buds detect dissolved food molecules

VI. The general senses are widespread through the body

    A. Tactile receptors are located in the skin
    B. Temperature receptors are nerve endings
    C. Pain sensation is a protective mechanism
    D. Proprioceptors inform us of our position

We are continuously bombarded with sensory information about the internal environment and the world outside. Any detectable change in the environment—internal or external—is called a **stimulus** (plural—stimuli). We detect stimuli through our sensory receptors. These receptors connect us with the outside environment and also transmit signals about internal changes that threaten homeostasis.

SENSORY RECEPTORS TRANSDUCE THE ENERGY OF A STIMULUS INTO ELECTRICAL SIGNALS

LEARNING OBJECTIVE

1. **Describe how a sensory receptor functions. (Include sensory reception, energy transduction, receptor potential, sensory adaptation, and perception.)**

How we respond to changes in our environment depends both on receptors that sense changes in the *outside* world (cold versus hot, bitterness versus sweetness, pain versus pleasure) and on the internal receptors that sense changes *inside* the body. Information is transmitted to the central nervous system (CNS), which signals effectors to make appropriate adjustments.

A sensory receptor may be a specialized ending of a sensory (afferent) neuron or one or more specialized cells in close contact with a sensory neuron. A receptor absorbs energy from the stimulus. The energy may be in any one of several forms, including light, sound, heat, and pressure. Sensory receptors **transduce** (convert) the energy of a stimulus into electrical signals. Recall that electrical signals are the information currency of the nervous system.

Sensory receptors, along with other types of cells, make up complex **sense organs:** eyes, ears, nose, and taste buds. A human taste bud, for example, consists of modified epithelial cells that detect chemicals dissolved in saliva. In addition to the senses of sight, hearing, equilibrium, smell, taste, and touch, the body has many internal sensors that maintain homeostatic balance. For example, certain blood vessels have receptors that maintain a normal balance of oxygen and carbon dioxide.

Sensory Receptors Produce Receptor Potentials

Sensory processing involves several steps: (1) a sensory receptor absorbs a small amount of energy from some stimulus in the environment, (2) the sensory receptor converts the energy of the stimulus into electrical energy—the process known as **energy transduction,** (3) a change in membrane potential occurs and produces a **receptor potential**—a depolarization or hyperpolarization of the membrane, (4) the receptor potential may generate action potentials in a sensory neuron, and (5) the sensory neuron transmits signals to the CNS, where integration takes place. A receptor potential is a *graded response,* which means that the extent of change depends on the energy of the stimulus. (Recall that excitatory postsynaptic potentials, or EPSPs, are also graded responses.)

We Can Differentiate Between Seeing a Dog and Tasting a Cookie

The action potentials generated by seeing a dog or by tasting a cookie are the same. Our ability to distinguish between these stimuli depends both on the sensory receptor and on the brain. Each sensory receptor is connected by neurons to a particular area of the brain. Each type of receptor normally responds to only one type of stimulus, for example, sound, light, chemicals (taste and smell), or touch. When a message arrives in the brain from a particular receptor, the brain "knows" the type of stimulus that has occurred.

The brain decodes incoming sensory messages. Signals from a sensory receptor may differ in the total number of sensory neurons transmitting impulses and the specific neurons transmitting action potentials. The number of action potentials transmitted by a given neuron is also important. The intensity of a stimulus is coded by the frequency of action potentials transmitted by a given fiber. For example, an intense pain would involve a greater frequency of action potentials (and a greater number of action potentials) than would a mild pain.

Sensory Receptors Adapt to Stimuli

You may have noticed how quickly you adapt to an unpleasant odor. After a few minutes, you may hardly notice it. Many sensory receptors do not continue to respond at the initial rate, even if the stimulus continues at the same intensity. With time, the response to a continued, constant stimulus decreases. This decrease in frequency of action potentials in a sensory neuron even though the stimulus is maintained is called **sensory adaptation.**

The Mind Constructs Sensory Perceptions

Sensory perception is the process of selecting, interpreting, and organizing sensory information. The brain interprets sensations by converting them to perceptions of the stimuli received by our sensory receptors. We construct sensory perceptions by comparing our sensory experience with our memories of past experiences. Individuals may perceive incoming stimuli in different ways. For example, if you grew up with large dogs as pets, your perception of a friend's German shepherd may be very different from that of someone who was bitten by a dog as a young child.

Quiz Yourself

- What is a receptor potential?
- What steps must take place in sensory processing?
- What is sensory adaptation?

SENSORY RECEPTORS RESPOND TO DIFFERENT TYPES OF ENERGY

LEARNING OBJECTIVE

2. **Classify sensory receptors according to the type of energy they transduce.**

We receive information about the environment in various energy forms. Sensory receptors transduce these types of energy into electrical energy that can result in action potentials. Each kind of sensory receptor is especially sensitive to one particular form of energy. For example, photoreceptors in the eye absorb light energy, whereas temperature receptors respond to heat. We can classify sensory receptors according to the type of energy they transduce.

Photoreceptors, located in the retina of the eye, respond to visible wavelengths of light. They transduce light energy. **Mechanoreceptors** are activated when they change shape as a result of being pushed or pulled. These receptors transduce mechanical energy—touch, pressure, gravity, stretching, and movement. Mechanoreceptors convert mechanical forces directly into electrical signals. **Chemoreceptors** transduce the energy of certain chemical compounds. **Thermoreceptors** respond to thermal infrared energy (heat). **Nociceptors** are pain receptors; they respond to stimuli that could damage the body, such as strong touch, pressure, heat, temperature extremes, and damaging chemicals.

⊚ *Quiz Yourself*

- What type of energy do mechanoreceptors transduce?
- What type of energy do photoreceptors transduce?

THE EYE CONTAINS PHOTORECEPTORS

LEARNING OBJECTIVE

3. **Describe the anatomy of the eye and give the function of each structure. (Include a description of the visual pathway.)**

Vision is our dominant and most refined sense. Our eyes allow us to appreciate a world of many colors and shapes. The position of the eyes in front of the head allows both eyes to focus on the same object. The information they receive overlaps and the same visual information strikes the light-sensitive areas (retinas) of the eye at the same time. We call this **binocular vision.** This type of vision helps us judge distances and depth.

The Eye Is Well Protected

The eye is an extremely delicate organ that is protected by its position in the body and by accessory structures. The eye and its muscles are set in the orbit formed by the skeletal bones of the face, and the eyes are cushioned by layers of fat. The eyelashes and eyelids help protect the eye anteriorly from foreign objects. When danger is perceived, the lids close by reflex action. Frequent blinking lubricates the eye and clears debris.

Even though we are not aware of the process, tears flow at all times from the **lacrimal** (lak′-rih-mal) **glands.** They pass out through the lacrimal ducts and lubricate the surface of the eye. Tears keep the eye moist and free of dust and minute objects.

The Eye Is Enclosed by Three Specialized Tissue Layers

The eyeball is formed by three layers of tissue: (1) the fibrous *sclera* and *cornea,* (2) the *choroid layer,* and (3) the *retina.* A lens, ciliary body, iris, and inner fluid-filled cavities make up the rest of the structure (Figure 8-1).

The **sclera** (skleh′-rah), the "white of the eye," is opaque and white. It is a tough, fibrous tissue, generously supplied with nerve endings. The sclera covers the entire eyeball except the anterior colored portion (iris) and pupil. The sclera joins the **cornea** (kor′-nee-ah)—the transparent layer that covers the iris and the pupil at the front of the eye. The cornea is frequently called the "window of the eye." The sclera is covered by the **conjunctiva** (kon-junk-**tie′**-vah)—a moist mucous membrane that extends as a continuous lining of the inner layer of the eyelids.

The second layer of the eyeball is the **choroid** (koe′-royd). This layer is made of black pigment cells that absorb light rays so that they are not reflected back out of the eye. Blood vessels of the choroid nourish the retina.

The **anterior cavity** between the cornea and the lens is filled with a watery substance—the **aqueous humor.** The larger **posterior cavity** between the lens and the retina is filled with a more viscous fluid—the **vitreous humor.** Both fluids are important in maintaining the shape of the eyeball by providing an internal fluid pressure. An abnormal accumulation of aqueous humor results in *glaucoma,* a disorder marked by increased pressure in the eye that can cause damage to the retina and optic nerve.

The Eyes Form a Sharp Image

The **iris,** the colored part of the eye, appears as blue, green, or brown. Its color is determined by the amount of pigment present. The iris regulates the amount of light entering the eye. It is composed of two mutually antagonistic sets of smooth muscle fibers. One set is arranged circularly and contracts to

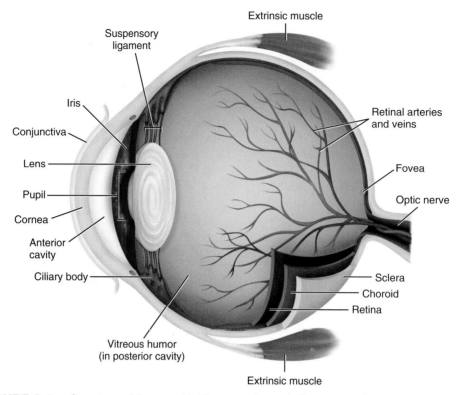

FIGURE 8-1 • Structure of the eye. Light passes through the eye to photoreceptor cells in the retina. In this lateral view, the eye is shown partly dissected to show its internal structures.

decrease the size of the pupil. The other is arranged radially and contracts to *increase* the size of the pupil.

The black spot, or opening in the center of the circular muscles of the iris, is the **pupil** of the eye. When the eye is stimulated by bright light, the circular muscle of the iris contracts, decreasing the size of the pupil. In dim light, the iris increases the size of the pupil. Certain medications and levels of consciousness may also affect the size of the pupil. For example, narcotics constrict pupils.

The **lens** of the eye is an adjustable, transparent, elastic ball that lies just behind the iris (see Figure 8-1). The lens refracts (bends) the light rays coming in and brings them to a focus on the retina. The lens is aided by the curved surface of the cornea and by the refractive properties (ability to bend light rays) of the liquids inside the eyeball.

The retina can be compared with the light-sensitive film used in a camera. The choroid layer absorbs light rays like the interior dark surface of a camera. We focus a camera by changing the distance between the lens and the film. Several processes are involved in focusing light rays on the retina. We can position the two eyeballs so they focus on a single object. Positioning the eyeballs is the function of the coordinated and precise actions of the six **extrinsic muscles** that control the movement of each eye. The extrinsic muscles of the eye originate from outside the eye. They extend from the bony structure of the orbit or the covering of the eyeball. Other processes that help focus light rays on the retina include refraction (bending) of light rays by the cornea and lens,

adjustment of the size of the pupil, and accommodation of the lens.

The eye has the power of **accommodation**—the ability to change focus for near or far vision by changing the shape of the lens (Figure 8-2). Accommodation is the function of the **ciliary** muscle. At its anterior margin, the choroid is thick and projects medially into the eyeball to form the **ciliary body,** which consists of **ciliary processes** and the **ciliary muscle.** The ciliary processes are glandlike folds that project toward the lens and secrete the aqueous humor. The lens is attached to the ciliary muscles by tiny fibers that make up the **suspensory ligament.**

To focus on objects that are near, the ciliary muscle contracts, causing the elastic lens to assume a rounder shape. To focus on more distant objects, the ciliary muscle relaxes and the lens assumes a flattened (ovoid) shape. Because of the ability of the eye to accommodate to different distances, the image is clearly focused on the retina unless there is some error in accommodation. As we grow older, the lens loses some of its elasticity and cannot adjust as well to bring objects into focus. This age-related change is called **presbyopia** (prez-bi-**oh′**-pee-ah).

The Retina Contains Light-Sensitive Rods and Cones

The **retina** (**ret′**-ih-nah), the innermost layer of the eye, contains the photoreceptors—the **rods** and **cones**. The cones are

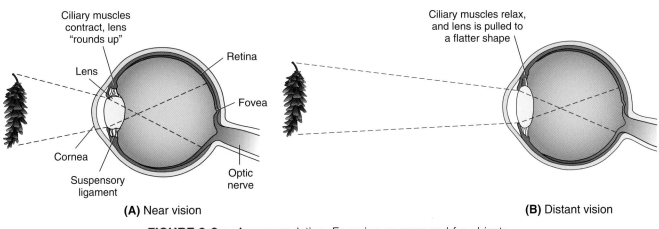

Ciliary muscles contract, lens "rounds up"

Lens

Cornea

Suspensory ligament

Retina

Fovea

Optic nerve

(A) Near vision

Ciliary muscles relax, and lens is pulled to a flatter shape

(B) Distant vision

FIGURE 8-2 • Accommodation. Focusing on near and far objects.

responsible for color vision and vision during the daytime. The rods are responsible mainly for vision in dim light or darkness. They allow us to detect shape and movement. The cones are most concentrated in the **fovea** (**foe′**-vee-ah)—a small depression in the center of the posterior region of the retina. The fovea is the region of sharpest vision.

For vision to occur, light must pass through the eye and form an image on the retina. Light must pass through several layers of connecting neurons in the retina to reach the rods and cones (Figure 8-3). Photoreceptors (rods and cones) synapse on **bipolar cells,** which make synaptic contact with **ganglion cells.** The axons of the ganglion cells extend across the surface of the retina and unite to form the **optic nerve.** The area where the optic nerve passes out of the eyeball, the **optic disc,** is known as the "blind spot"; because it lacks rods and cones, images falling on it cannot be perceived.

How is light converted into the neural signals that transmit information about environmental stimuli into pictures in the brain? The pigment **rhodopsin** in the rod cells and some very closely related pigments in the cone cells are responsible for the ability to see. When exposed to light, rhodopsin breaks down into (1) a large protein called **opsin** and (2) **retinal,** a derivative of vitamin A. The breakdown of rhodopsin leads to the transduction of light and the transmission of neural signals.

The Optic Nerves Transmit Signals to the Brain

Axons of ganglion cells in the retina form the optic nerves (cranial nerve II), which transmit information to the brain by way of complex, encoded signals. The optic nerves cross in the floor of the hypothalamus, forming an X-shaped structure—the **optic chiasm** (Figure 8-4). Some of the axons of the optic nerves cross over and then extend to the opposite side of the brain.

Axons of the optic nerves end in the **lateral geniculate nuclei** of the thalamus. From there, neurons send signals to the **primary visual cortex** in the occipital lobe of the cere-

brum. The lateral geniculate nucleus controls which information is sent to the visual cortex. Information can be transmitted from the primary visual cortex to other cortical areas for further processing. Information about touch, pain, and temperature is transmitted from the eye to the brain by the **trigeminal nerve** (cranial nerve V).

A simplified summary of the visual pathway follows:

> Light passes through the cornea → through aqueous humor → through lens → through vitreous humor → image forms on photoreceptor cells in retina → signal bipolar cells → signal ganglion cells → optic nerve transmits signals to thalamus → signals cerebral cortex → integration by visual areas of the cerebral cortex

Neurobiologists have not yet discovered all of the mechanisms by which the brain makes sense out of the visual information it receives. We do know that a large part of the association areas of the cerebrum is involved in integrating visual input. The neurons of the visual cortex are organized as a map of the external visual field.

Quiz Yourself

- What are the functions of the pupil? The lens?
- What are the functions of rods and cones?
- Through what sequence of structures do light and neural signals travel as they pass from the cornea to the visual areas of the cerebral cortex?

THE EAR FUNCTIONS IN HEARING AND EQUILIBRIUM

LEARNING OBJECTIVES

4. Describe the structures and functions of the three major parts of the ear.
5. Trace the transmission of sound through the ear.

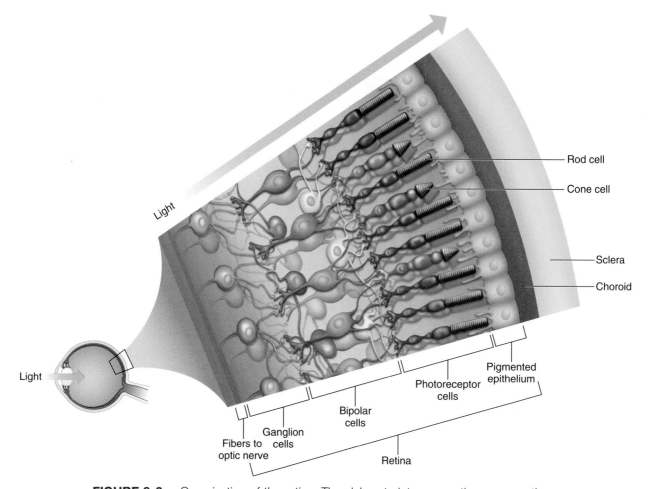

Light

Light

Rod cell

Cone cell

Sclera

Choroid

Pigmented epithelium

Photoreceptor cells

Bipolar cells

Ganglion cells

Fibers to optic nerve

Retina

FIGURE 8-3 • Organization of the retina. The elaborate interconnections among the various layers of neurons in the retina allow them to interact and to influence one another. The rods and cones, the photoreceptor cells, are located in the back of the retina. The elongated rods permit us to see shape and movement, whereas the shorter cones allow us to view our world in color. The rods and cones synapse with bipolar cells (shown in orange), which synapse with ganglion cells. Interneurons (unlabeled yellow and blue neurons) are also involved. Axons of ganglion cells make up the optic nerve.

6. **Describe the functions of the vestibule and semicircular canals.**

The ear has three major regions (Figure 8-5):

1. The outer ear includes the part we see and a canal connecting with the middle ear.
2. The middle ear contains three small bones (auditory ossicles) that conduct sound waves.
3. The inner ear contains sensory receptors for sound waves and for maintaining the equilibrium of the body.

The Outer Ear Conducts Sound Waves to the Middle Ear

The **pinna** (**pin′**-ah), the part of the **outer ear** that projects from the side of the head, surrounds the ear canal. The ear canal, more formally called the **external auditory meatus,** leads to the middle ear. The lining of this canal contains **ceruminous** (se-**roo′**-mih-nus) **glands** that secrete earwax, or **cerumen** (seh-**roo′**-men). Cerumen helps protect the lining of the canal from infection.

The **tympanic** (tim-**pan′**-ik) membrane, or eardrum, separates the middle ear and the external ear. Incoming sound waves cause this flexible membrane to vibrate, transmitting the sound waves to the middle ear.

The Middle Ear Amplifies Sound Waves

The **middle ear** is a small, moist cavity in the temporal bone containing air and three small bones, or **auditory ossicles** (**os′**-ih-kuls). At the rear of the cavity, the middle ear opens into the mastoid process of the temporal bone. This area is filled with air spaces that communicate with the middle ear

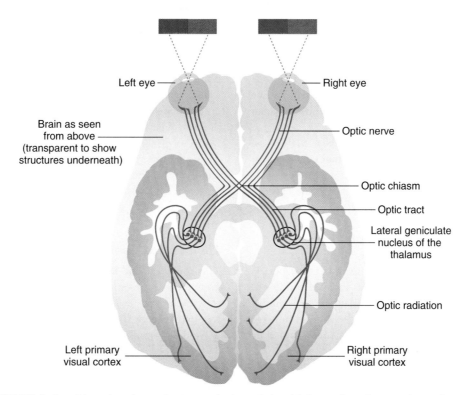

FIGURE 8-4 • Neural pathway for transmission of visual information. Axons of ganglion cells form the optic nerves. The optic nerves cross, forming the optic chiasm. Many optic nerve fibers end in the lateral geniculate nuclei of the thalamus. From there, signals are sent to the visual cortex.

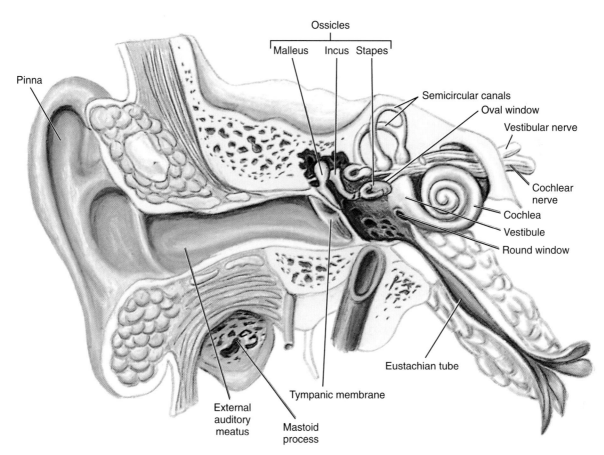

FIGURE 8-5 • Structure of the ear. The ear is adapted to direct sound waves from outside the body to receptors in the inner ear.

and help equalize pressure. Under normal circumstances the air pressure is equalized on the two sides of the tympanic membrane by the **eustachian** (u-**stay'**-kee-an) **tube.** This tube connects the middle ear and the nasopharynx (part of the throat). Bacteria in the throat can pass through the eustachian tube, leading to painful middle ear infection.

The three auditory ossicles are the **malleus** (**mal'**-ee-us) (hammer), **incus** (**ing'**-kus) (anvil), and **stapes** (**stay'**-peez) (stirrup). These tiny bones form a chain from the tympanic membrane to the **oval window**—a small membrane between the middle and inner ears. Sound waves cause vibrations of the tympanic membrane. The auditory ossicles act as three interconnected levers that help amplify the vibrations.

A very small movement in the malleus causes a larger movement in the incus and a very large movement in the stapes. As the stapes rocks back and forth, it causes the oval window to bow in and out. These vibrations pass through the oval window to the fluid in the inner ear. If sound waves were conducted directly from air to the oval window, much energy would be lost. The middle ear functions to couple sound waves in the air with the pressure waves conducted through the fluid in the inner ear.

The Inner Ear Contains Mechanoreceptors

The **inner ear** contains mechanoreceptors that convert sound waves to nerve impulses. This part of the ear also contains receptors that enable us to maintain our equilibrium. The inner ear lies inside the temporal bone. It is a **bony labyrinth** (**lab'**-ih-rinth) composed of three compartments: (1) the vestibule, which lies next to the oval window; (2) the cochlea; and (3) the semicircular canals (Figure 8-6).

The bony labyrinth contains a fluid called **perilymph** (**per'**-ih-limf). The perilymph surrounds the **membranous labyrinth**—a group of ducts and sacs that lie within the bony labyrinth. The membranous labyrinth contains a fluid called **endolymph.** The two fluids, perilymph and endolymph, are separated and have different chemical compositions. Both fluids carry vibrations through the system of canals within the inner ear.

The Cochlea Contains the Receptors for Hearing

The **cochlea** (**kok'**-lee-ah) is a snail-shaped portion of the inner ear that contains the **organs of Corti**—the sound receptors. Each organ of Corti contains sensory cells that respond to sound waves by stimulating the **cochlear nerve.** The cochlear nerve then transmits the message to the brain.

If we uncoiled the cochlea, we could easily see that it consists of three canals separated from each other by thin membranes; the canals come almost to a point at the apex. Two of these canals, or ducts, the **vestibular canal** and the **tympanic canal,** are connected at the apex of the cochlea and are filled with perilymph (Figure 8-7). The middle canal, the **cochlear duct,** is filled with endolymph and contains the organ of Corti.

Each organ of Corti contains about 18,000 **hair cells** arranged in rows that extend the length of the coiled cochlea.

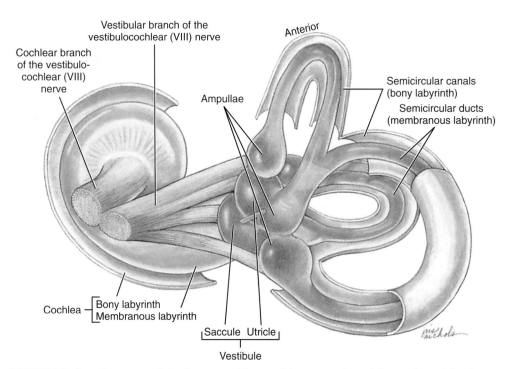

FIGURE 8-6 • Structure of the inner ear. The cochlea, saccule, utricle, and semicircular canals are located in the inner ear. The membranous labyrinth is exposed. Because this is a posterior view, the utricle and saccule can be seen. Outer white color shows bony labyrinth. Inner orange and yellow colors show the membranous labyrinth.

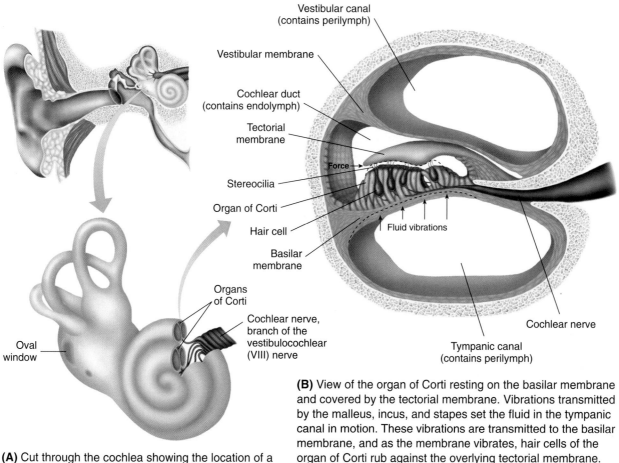

(B) View of the organ of Corti resting on the basilar membrane and covered by the tectorial membrane. Vibrations transmitted by the malleus, incus, and stapes set the fluid in the tympanic canal in motion. These vibrations are transmitted to the basilar membrane, and as the membrane vibrates, hair cells of the organ of Corti rub against the overlying tectorial membrane. This stimulation depolarizes hair cells, resulting in action potentials in the sensory neurons of the cochlear nerve.

(A) Cut through the cochlea showing the location of a couple organs of Corti. Note how neurons from each organ of Corti join to form the cochlear nerve.

FIGURE 8-7 • The cochlea is the organ of hearing.

Each hair cell is equipped with tiny projections called **stereocilia** (not true cilia) that extend into the cochlear duct. The hair cells rest on the **basilar membrane,** which separates the cochlear duct from the tympanic canal. Overhanging and in contact with the hair cells of the organ of Corti is another membrane—the **tectorial membrane.**

Sound waves in the air are transformed into pressure waves. Each pressure wave presses on the membranes separating the three canals. The pressure wave is transmitted to the tympanic canal and causes a bulging of the **round window,** a membrane at the end of the tympanic canal. The movements of the basilar membrane produced by these pulsations cause the stereocilia on the hair cells of the organ of Corti to rub against the overlying tectorial membrane. When stereocilia are bent by this contact, ion channels in the plasma membrane of the hair cells open. Depolarization may occur, and a receptor potential may be generated.

Hair cells release the neurotransmitter **glutamate,** which binds to receptors on sensory neurons that synapse on each hair cell. Glutamate binding may lead to depolarization of sensory neurons. Axons of the sensory neurons join to form the cochlear nerve, a component of cranial nerve VIII.

We can summarize the steps in the physiology of hearing as follows:

Sound waves enter external auditory meatus → tympanic membrane vibrates → malleus, incus, and stapes amplify vibrations → oval window vibrates → vibrations are conducted through perilymph → vibrations transmitted to the endolymph → basilar membrane vibrates → hair cells in the organ of Corti are stimulated → cochlear nerve transmits impulses to brain

Sounds Differ in Pitch, Loudness, and Quality

Pitch depends on frequency of sound waves, or number of vibrations per second, and is expressed as *hertz (Hz).* The human ear is equipped to register sound frequencies between about 20 and 20,000 Hz. We are most sensitive to sounds between 1000 and 4000 Hz. Dogs and some other animals can hear sounds of much higher frequencies. Low-frequency vibrations result in the sensation of low pitch, whereas high-frequency vibrations result in the sensation of high pitch. Sounds of a given frequency set up resonance waves in the cochlear fluid that cause a particular section of the basilar membrane to vibrate. The brain infers the pitch of a sound from the particular hair cells that are stimulated.

Loud sounds cause resonance waves of greater amplitude (height). The hair cells are more intensely stimulated, and the cochlear nerve then transmits a greater number of impulses per second.

Variations in the **quality** of sound, such as those evident when an oboe, a cornet, and a violin play the same note, depend on the number and kinds of overtones, or harmonics, produced. These provide stimulation to different hair cells in addition to the main stimulation common to all three instruments. Thus differences in tone quality are recognized in the *pattern* of the hair cells stimulated.

Deafness may be caused by malformation of, or injury to, the sound-transmitting mechanism of the outer, middle, or inner ear or the sound-perceiving mechanism of the inner ear. Exposure to heavily amplified music or other high-intensity sound damages the hair cells of the organ of Corti.

The Vestibule and Semicircular Canals Help Maintain Equilibrium

The **vestibule** and **semicircular canals** contain receptor cells that transmit information about the position of the body. Inside the vestibule, the membranous labyrinth is divided into two saclike chambers—the **saccule** (**sak′**-yool) and the **utricle** (**yoo′**-trih-kul). These chambers house gravity detectors in the form of small calcium carbonate ear stones called **otoliths** (Figure 8-8). Each receptor cell has a group of hair cells surrounded at the tips by a gelatinous mass called a **cupula.** The hair cells in the saccule and utricle lie in different planes.

Normally, the pull of gravity causes the otoliths to press against the stereocilia of the hair cells. This stimulates them to initiate impulses that are sent to the brain by way of sensory nerve fibers at their bases. When the head is tilted or in linear acceleration (an increase in speed when the body is moving in a straight line), otoliths press on the stereocilia of different cells. The stereocilia are deflected (bent). Deflection of the stereocilia toward the longest cilium depolarizes the hair cell. Deflection in the opposite direction hyperpolarizes the hair cell. Thus, depending on the direction of movement, the hair cells release more or less neurotransmitter. The brain interprets the neural messages so that we are aware of our position relative to the ground regardless of the position of our head.

Information about turning movements, referred to as *angular acceleration,* is provided by the three semicircular canals. Each canal, a hollow ring connected with the utricle, lies at right angles to the other two and is filled with endolymph. A small, bulblike enlargement, the ampulla, is located at one of the openings of each canal into the utricle. Within each ampulla lies a clump of hair cells called a **crista** (plural—*cristae*). These hair cells are similar to the groups of hair cells in the utricle and saccule, but no otoliths are present (Figure 8-9). The stereocilia of the hair cells of the cristae are stimulated by movements of the endolymph in the canals.

When the head is turned, there is a lag in the movement of the fluid within the canals. The stereocilia move in relation to the fluid and are stimulated by its flow. This stimulation produces not only the consciousness of rotation but also certain reflex movements in response to it. These reflexes cause the eyes and head to move in a direction opposite that of the original rotation. Because the three canals are in three different planes, head movement in any direction stimulates fluid movement in at least one of the canals.

We are used to movements in the horizontal plane but not to vertical movements (parallel to the long axis of the upright body). The motion of an elevator or of a ship pitching in a rough sea stimulates the semicircular canals in an unusual way and may cause seasickness or motion sickness, with nausea or vomiting. When a seasick person lies down, the movement stimulates the semicircular canals in a more familiar way and nausea is less likely to occur.

The response of the sensory cells in the semicircular canals is produced by the flow of endolymph within the canals as the position of the head changes. These responses in turn are transmitted to the **vestibular nerve,** which joins the *cochlear nerve* to form the **vestibulocochlear nerve** (cranial nerve VIII).

Quiz Yourself

- What is the function of the middle ear?
- How do hair cells function?
- What is the function of otoliths? Of semicircular canals?

CHEMORECEPTORS SENSE SMELL AND TASTE

LEARNING OBJECTIVE

7. **Compare the receptors of smell and taste.**

Chemoreceptors allow us to detect chemical substances in the air and in food and water. When specific chemical substances bind with chemoreceptors, a series of chemical events takes place, leading to changes in membrane permeability. If the membrane is sufficiently depolarized, action potentials are generated in sensory neurons. Unlike most neurons, both taste and smell receptors are continuously regenerated.

Chemoreceptors in the Nasal Cavity Sense Odorants

Olfaction (ohl-**fak′**-shen), the sense of smell, is the function of chemoreceptor cells in the **olfactory epithelium** lining the upper part of the nasal cavity (Figure 8-10, p. 147). These receptor cells are stimulated by **odorants,** chemical substances that can be smelled. Odorants dissolve in the mucus on the surface of the olfactory epithelium.

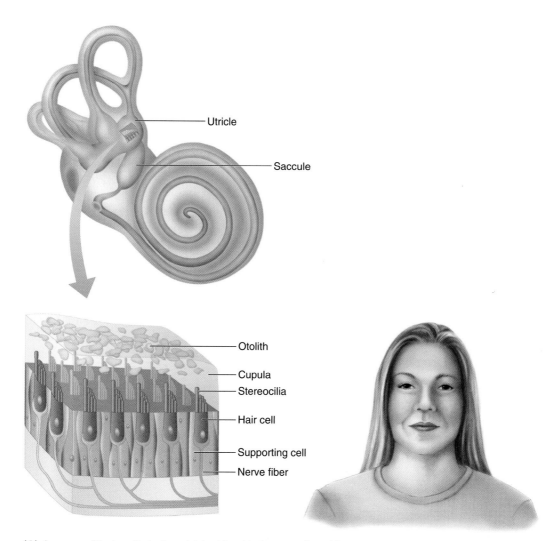

(A) A group of hair cells in the utricle. Head is in normal position.

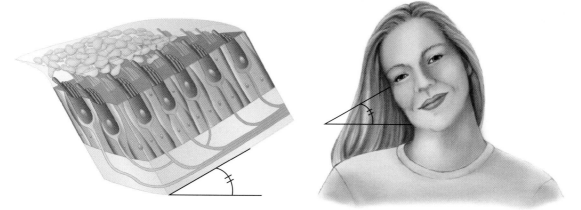

(B) When you bend your head, otoliths press on the stereocilia of different hair cells. When the stereocilia are deflected, the hair cells may be depolarized or hyperpolarized (depending on direction).

FIGURE 8-8 • Function of the saccule and utricle in maintaining posture. The saccule and utricle sense linear acceleration, allowing us to know our position relative to the ground. Compare the positions of the otoliths and hair cells in **A** with those in **B**. Changes in head position cause the force of gravity to distort the cupula, which in turn distorts the stereocilia of the hair cells. The hair cells respond by sending impulses along the vestibular nerve (part of the vestibulocochlear nerve) to the brain.

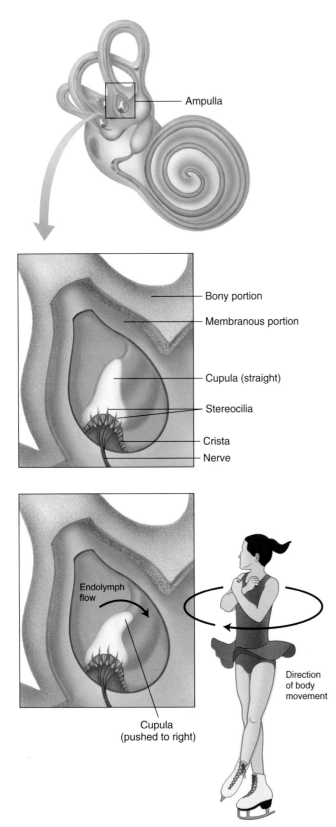

FIGURE 8-9 • Semicircular canals and equilibrium. When the head changes its rate of rotation, endolymph within the ampulla of the semicircular canal distorts the cupula. The hair cells of the cupula are bent, increasing the frequency of action potentials in sensory neurons. The vestibular nerve transmits information to the brain.

The odors detected by the olfactory epithelium are transmitted by the **olfactory nerve** (cranial nerve I) to the olfactory cortex (part of the limbic system) in the temporal lobe. (Odors are often associated with feelings and memories.) We can detect at least seven main groups of odors, and we can perceive about 10,000 different scents.

Taste Buds Detect Dissolved Food Molecules

Gustation, the sense of taste, is the job of **taste buds** on the tongue and various parts of the mouth. Taste buds are found mainly in **papillae,** tiny elevations, on the tongue (Figure 8-11). Each of the thousands of taste buds is an oval epithelial capsule containing about 100 taste receptor cells interspersed with supporting cells. The taste receptors detect chemical substances dissolved in saliva.

Traditionally, four main tastes have been recognized: sweet, sour, salty, and bitter. A fifth taste, *glutamate*, is now recognized. Glutamate is the taste responsible for the savoriness of soy sauce, anchovies, and certain aged cheeses and seafood.

Three cranial nerves—the facial (cranial nerve VII), the glossopharyngeal (cranial nerve IX), and the vagus (cranial nerve X)—transmit impulses from the taste buds to the medulla. Information is transmitted to the thalamus and then on to the gustatory area in the parietal lobe.

Both smell and taste are important in stimulating appetite and digestive juices. Much of what we think is taste is actually smell. A bad head cold decreases appetite, partly because the efficiency of the olfactory receptors is reduced by inflammation.

Quiz Yourself

- What is the function of chemoreceptors in the olfactory epithelium?
- How are olfaction and taste similar?

THE GENERAL SENSES ARE WIDESPREAD THROUGH THE BODY

LEARNING OBJECTIVES

8. Describe the tactile receptors and temperature receptors.
9. Describe the process of pain perception and explain the basis of phantom and referred pain.
10. Locate proprioceptors in the body and describe their functions.

The **general senses** include the receptors that respond to touch, pressure, vibration, pain, changes in temperature, and

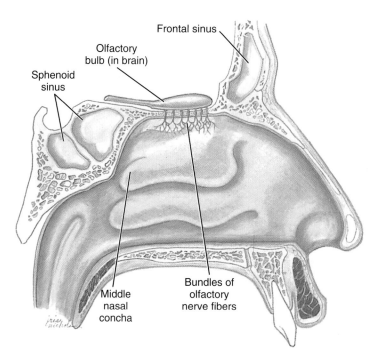

FIGURE 8-10 • Location and structure of the olfactory epithelium. The receptor cells are located within the epithelium.

muscle stretch. Most of these receptors are mechanoreceptors. Those that sense pain are nociceptors.

Tactile Receptors Are Located in the Skin

The simplest mechanoreceptors are free nerve endings (dendrites of sensory neurons) in the skin. These nerve endings detect touch and pressure when stimulated by objects that contact the body surface. Thousands of more specialized **tactile** (touch) **receptors** are also located in the skin (Figure 8-12). Some sense light touch and pressure, whereas others inform us of heavy and continuous touch and pressure. Still others respond to deep pressure.

Temperature Receptors Are Nerve Endings

Thermoreceptors are free nerve endings that allow us to detect temperature changes. Widely distributed throughout the body, thermoreceptors are especially concentrated in the lips and mouth. These receptors are highly sensitive to differences between skin temperature and the temperature of objects that come into contact with the body.

Thermoreceptors in the hypothalamus detect internal changes in temperature and receive and integrate information from thermoreceptors on the body surface. The hypothalamus then initiates homeostatic mechanisms that ensure a constant body temperature.

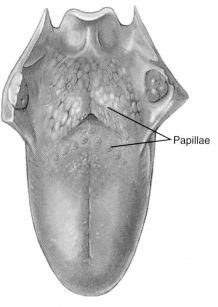

Apex of tongue

(A) Taste buds are mainly located on papillae (small elevations) on the tongue.

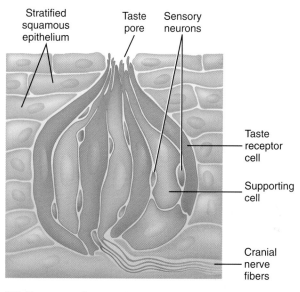

(B) Structure of a taste bud.

FIGURE 8-11 • The sense of taste.

Pain Sensation Is a Protective Mechanism

The sensation of pain is a protective mechanism that makes us aware of tissue injury. Pain receptors, called **nociceptors** (no-see-**sep**′-tors) (from the Latin, *nocere,* "to injure"), are free nerve endings (dendrites) of certain sensory neurons found in almost every tissue. Several types of nociceptors have been identified. Thermal nociceptors respond to temperature

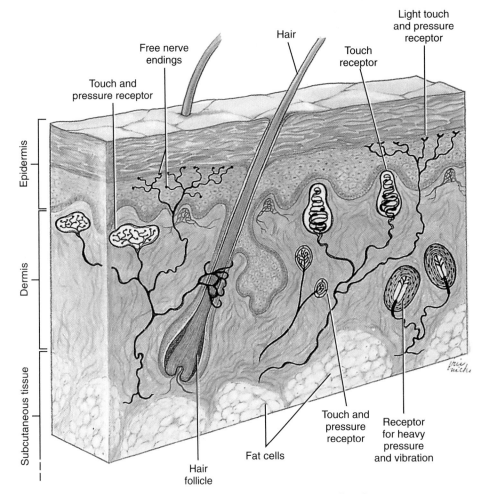

FIGURE 8-12 • Receptors in the skin sense touch, pressure, vibration, temperature change, and pain.

extremes (temperatures above 45° C or below 5° C). Mechanical nociceptors respond to strong tactile stimuli such as penetration by sharp objects or pinching. Other nociceptors respond to a variety of stimuli, including certain chemicals.

Stimulation of nociceptors does not always result in the perception of pain. We feel pain when information from nociceptors reaches the brain and is interpreted. When stimulated, nociceptors transmit signals through sensory neurons to interneurons in the spinal cord. Recall that some interneurons synapse directly with motor neurons so that a withdrawal reflex can occur before signals are transmitted to the brain. The sensory neurons release the neurotransmitter *glutamate* and several other neurotransmitters, including **substance P.**

The interneuron transmits the message to the opposite side of the spinal cord and then upward through one of five ascending pathways. The principal ascending nociceptive pathway is the *spinothalamic tract,* which transmits signals to the thalamus, where pain perception begins. From the thalamus, impulses are sent into the parietal lobes and several other cortical regions, including areas of the limbic system. The emotional aspects of pain are processed in the limbic system. When

the signals reach the cerebrum, the individual becomes fully aware of the pain and can evaluate the situation. How threatening is the stimulus? How intense is the pain? What is the most adaptive response?

The body has a variety of mechanisms for analgesia (pain control). Neurophysiologists have long known that *opiates,* such as morphine and codeine, relieve pain, and these compounds and their derivatives are widely used clinically to control pain. For example, patient-controlled morphine pumps are routinely used in many hospitals. Opiates work by blocking the release of substance P.

More than 10 opiates have now been discovered in the brain, spinal cord, and pituitary gland, including **endorphins** (for "endogenous morphine-like") such as **beta-endorphin,** and **enkephalins.** These endogenous opiates are thought to inhibit certain neurons in the spinal cord. The endogenous opiates are more effective than morphine, and several are being investigated as potential analgesic drugs.

The brain locates pain on the basis of past experience. Generally, pain at the body surface is accurately projected back to the injured area. For example, when you step on a nail, your brain perceives the pain and then projects it back to the injured foot, so that you feel pain at the site of puncture. Artificial stimulation of the leg nerves may produce a sensation of pain in the foot even though the foot is untouched. In fact, for years after an amputation, a patient may feel **phantom pain** in the missing limb. This occurs because, when the severed nerve is stimulated and sends a message to the brain, the brain "remembers" the nerve as it originally was—connected to the limb before it was missing.

Nociceptors in most internal organs are not easily activated. Pain is often not projected back to the organ that is stimulated. Instead it is *referred* to an area just under the skin that may be some distance from the organ involved. The area to which the pain is referred generally is connected to nerve fibers from the same level of the spinal cord as the organ involved. A person with angina who feels heart pain in the left arm is experiencing **referred pain.** Neurons from both the heart and the arm converge on the same neurons in the CNS. The brain interprets the incoming message as coming from the body surface because that is the more familiar origin of pain. When pain is felt both at the site of the distress and as referred pain, it may seem to spread, or *radiate,* from the organ to the superficial area.

You may have observed that rubbing the skin around an injury or pressing on the area can alleviate pain. Activating certain large sensory neurons that deliver messages about touch or pressure can stimulate interneurons in the spinal cord that release enkephalins. Thus these interneurons inhibit neurons in the pain pathway. Clinical methods have been developed for relieving pain by electrical stimulation of large sensory nerve fibers. Stimulation of the skin over a painful area with electrodes has successfully relieved pain in some patients. This procedure is called *transcutaneous electrical nerve stimulation (TENS).* Electrodes can also be implanted in the brain, allowing the patient to control chronic pain by stimulating the release of endorphins.

In *acupuncture,* a Chinese therapy for treating pain, needles are inserted to stimulate afferent neurons that inhibit pain signals. Endogenous opioids are also involved in analgesia induced by acupuncture. Studies suggest that acupuncture needles stimulate nerves deep within the muscles, which in turn stimulate certain neurons in the brain to release endorphins.

Proprioceptors Inform Us of Our Position

Proprioceptors (pro′-pre-o-**sep**′-ters) help us maintain the position of the body and its parts. Three main types of proprioceptors are **muscle spindles,** which detect muscle movement; **Golgi tendon organs,** which determine stretch in the tendons that attach muscle to bone; and **joint receptors,** which detect movement in ligaments. Impulses from the proprioceptors are important in ensuring the harmonious contractions of the several distinct muscles involved in a single movement. Without such receptors, complicated, skillful acts would be impossible.

Information from proprioceptors is transmitted rapidly to the brain so that the central nervous system is aware of the location of the parts of the body at all times. The brain coordinates this information with input from the vestibule and semicircular canals in the inner ear to maintain equilibrium and coordination of muscular activities. This provides us with a conscious awareness of body position and movement (known as *kinesthetic sense*). Proprioceptors are probably more numerous and more continually active than any of the other sensory receptors, although we are less aware of them than of most of the others.

Quiz Yourself

- To what type of energy do tactile receptors respond?
- What is phantom pain?
- What is the function of proprioceptors? Of joint receptors?

⟳   **SUMMARY**

LO 1. **Describe how a sensory receptor functions. (Include sensory reception, energy transduction, receptor potential, sensory adaptation, and perception.)**
   - **Sensory receptors** are specialized to respond to specific types of energy that stimulate them. Sensory receptors may be neuron endings or specialized receptor cells in close contact with neurons. **Sense organs** consist of sensory receptors and other types of cells.
   - Receptor cells absorb energy, **transduce** (convert) that energy into electrical energy, and produce **receptor potentials,** which are depolarizations or hyperpolarizations of the membrane.
   - **Sensory adaptation** is the decrease in frequency of action potentials in a sensory neuron even when the stimulus is maintained. It results in decreased response to that stimulus.

LO 2. **Classify sensory receptors according to the type of energy they transduce.**
   - On the basis of the type of energy they transduce, sensory receptors can be classified as **photoreceptors, mechanoreceptors, chemoreceptors, thermoreceptors,** and **nociceptors.**

LO 3. **Describe the anatomy of the eye and give the function of each structure. (Include a description of the visual pathway.)**
   - The eye is protected by its position in the orbit and by the eyelids, eyelashes, and tears, which are secreted by the **lacrimal glands.**
   - The **cornea,** the transparent layer that covers the front of the eye, is continuous with the **sclera**—a tough membrane that envelops the rest of the eyeball.
   - The internal surface of the eye is covered by a black coat, the **choroid,** which prevents light rays from scattering.
   - The **anterior cavity** is filled with **aqueous humor.** The **posterior cavity** is filled with a thicker fluid—the **vitreous humor.**
   - The **iris** regulates the amount of light entering the eye. In bright light it contracts, narrowing its opening—the **pupil;** in weak light it dilates the pupil, permitting more light to enter.
   - Light passes through the transparent, elastic lens and forms an image on the **retina.**

   - The six **extrinsic muscles** permit the eyes to move together to focus on an object.
   - The **ciliary body** consists of the **ciliary process** and the **ciliary muscle.** The lens is attached to the ciliary muscles by the **suspensory ligament.** When the ciliary muscle contracts, the lens becomes rounder. When this muscle relaxes, the lens flattens.
   - **Accommodation** is the ability to change the curvature of the lens to clearly focus on a close or far object.
   - The photoreceptors—the **rods** and **cones**—are located in the retina. Rods are sensitive to dim light and allow us to detect shape and movement but not color. Cones are sensitive to color. The cones are most concentrated in the **fovea**—the region of sharpest vision.
   - Rods and cones synapse on **bipolar cells,** which synapse on **ganglion cells.** The axons of ganglion cells join to form the **optic nerve.** The area where the optic nerve passes out of the eyeball is the optic disc. **Rhodopsin** in the rods and some closely related pigments in the cones break down when exposed to light, leading to transduction of light and the transmission of neural signals.
   - The optic nerves cross in the floor of the hypothalamus, forming the **optic chiasm.** Axons of the optic nerves end in the **lateral geniculate nucleus** of the thalamus. Neurons that synapse there transmit messages to the **primary visual cortex** in the occipital lobe of the cerebrum.

LO 4. **Describe the structures and functions of the three major parts of the ear.**
   - The ear functions in hearing and equilibrium. The **outer ear** is separated from the **middle ear** by the **tympanic membrane.** The middle ear contains three small **ossicles** (bones)—the **malleus, incus,** and **stapes**—that amplify sound waves. They extend from the tympanic membrane to the **oval window.** The **eustachian tube,** which connects the middle ear with the nasopharynx, equalizes pressure on both sides of the tympanic membrane.
   - The **inner ear** is a **bony labyrinth** composed of the cochlea, vestibule, and semicircular canals. The **perilymph** in the bony labyrinth surrounds the inner membranous labyrinth, which consists of a group of ducts and sacs. The **membranous labyrinth** contains **endolymph.**

LO = Learning Objective

- The **cochlea** contains the **organs of Corti,** which convert pressure waves to nerve impulses for transmission to the brain. **Hair cells** in the each organ of Corti have **stereocilia** that extend into the cochlear duct. The **tectorial membrane** overhangs the hair cells. The hair cells rest on the **basilar membrane.**

LO 5. **Trace the transmission of sound through the ear.**
- Sound waves pass through the external auditory meatus and cause the tympanic membrane to vibrate. In the middle ear, the malleus, incus, and stapes amplify the vibrations.
- The oval window vibrates and these vibrations are transmitted through the perilymph in the inner ear to the endolymph and cause the basilar membrane to vibrate.
- Hair cells in the organ of Corti are stimulated and the cochlear nerve transmits signals to the brain.

LO 6. **Describe the functions of the vestibule and semicircular canals.**
- The **vestibule** and **semicircular canals** are organs of equilibrium. The vestibule contains the **saccule** and the **utricle.** These structures house **otoliths,** small calcium carbonate stones that detect gravity. Each receptor cell has a group of hair cells surrounded at their tips by a gelatinous mass called a **cupula.** When the head is tilted, deflection of stereocilia by otoliths depolarizes hair cells. Information sent to the brain makes us aware of our position relative to the ground.
- The semicircular canals provide information about turning movements. **Cristae,** clumps of hair cells within each ampulla, are stimulated by movements of the endolymph.

LO 7. **Compare the receptors of smell and taste.**
- Chemoreceptors detect chemical substances in the air, and in food and water. **Olfaction,** the sense of smell, and **gustation,** the sense of taste, depend on chemoreceptors in the nose and tongue.
- **Olfactory receptors** are chemoreceptors in the **olfactory epithelium,** the lining of the upper

part of the nasal cavity. Olfactory receptors sense **odorants,** chemical substances that can be smelled. The olfactory receptors transmit impulses to the brain through the **olfactory nerve** (cranial nerve I).
- **Gustation,** or **taste,** is sensed by the **taste buds,** which are located in small elevations, called **papillae,** on the tongue. Taste receptors in the taste buds transmit signals to cranial nerves, which transmit signals to the brain.

LO 8. **Describe the tactile receptors and temperature receptors.**
- The **general senses** include receptors that respond to touch, pressure, vibrations, change in temperature, pain, and muscle stretch.
- **Tactile receptors** located in various parts of the skin respond to touch, pressure, and vibration.
- **Thermoreceptors** are free nerve endings that detect temperature changes.

LO 9. **Describe the process of pain perception and explain the basis of phantom and referred pain.**
- **Nociceptors** are free nerve endings sensitive to stimuli that may be perceived as painful. Sensory neurons transmitting messages regarding painful stimuli secrete glutamate and **substance P.** Endorphins and enkephalins are endogenous opiates that inhibit neurons that transmit pain signals in the spinal cord.
- **Phantom pain** occurs when a severed nerve is stimulated.
- **Referred pain** occurs when the brain interprets an incoming message as coming from the body surface rather than from an internal organ.

LO 10. **Locate proprioceptors in the body and describe their functions.**
- **Proprioceptors** allow us to perceive the position of the body and its parts. Three main types of proprioceptors are **muscle spindles,** which detect muscle movement; **Golgi tendon organs,** which determine stretch in tendons; and **joint receptors,** which detect movement in ligaments.

CHAPTER QUIZ

Fill in the Blank

1. Sensory receptors transduce the energy from some stimulus into _____ energy.

2. Energy transduction results in a change in membrane potential that produces a _____ potential.

3. Sensory _____ is the decrease in frequency of action potentials in a sensory neuron even though the stimulus is maintained.

4. The pigment _____ in the rod cells is responsible for our ability to see.

5. The ability to change focus for near or far vision by changing the shape of the lens is called _____.

6. The auditory ossicles are the _____, _____, and _____.

7. The organs of Corti are located in the _____ in the inner ear.

8. Otoliths are found in the _____ and _____.

9. Information about turning movements is sensed by the three _____ _____.

10. Information from receptors in the olfactory epithelium is transmitted to the brain by the _____ nerve.

11. Nociceptors sense _____.

12. Some headaches could be the result of _____ pain.

13. Proprioceptors that detect muscle movement are _____ _____.

Multiple Choice

14. The window of the eye is the: a. pupil; b. cornea; c. ciliary body; d. iris.

15. Photoreceptors that function in dim light are: a. rods; b. cones; c. rods and cones; d. ciliary processes.

16. The area of sharpest vision is the: a. fovea; b. optic disc; c. iris; d. optic chiasm.

17. Photoreceptor cells in the retina synapse directly with the: a. ganglion cells; b. bipolar cells; c. thalamus; d. optic chiasm.

18. The tectorial membrane is located in the: a. saccule; b. utricle; c. vestibule; d. organ of Corti.

19. Substance P is most associated with: a. vision; b. pain; c. touch; d. olfaction.

20. The following is *not* a general sense: a. touch; b. pressure; c. temperature; d. taste.

21. Joint receptors: a. detect movement in ligaments; b. detect movement in tendons; c. are nociceptors; d. send messages to the brain through the vestibular nerve.

REVIEW QUESTIONS

1. How do sensory receptors help us maintain homeostasis?

2. How do sensory receptors work? Describe the sequence of events that take place in sensory processing.

3. What is sensory perception?

4. Describe the layers of the eyeball. What are the functions of the pupil? Iris? Lens? Rods and cones?

5. List in sequence the structures through which light passes in the visual pathway.

6. List in sequence the steps that take place as sound waves are converted to impulses in the brain that allow us to hear.

7. What are the functions of the malleus, incus, and stapes; cochlea; organ of Corti; and cochlear nerve?

8. Compare the functions of the saccule and utricle with the functions of the semicircular canals.

9. Stimulation of nociceptors does not always result in the perception of pain. Why? What factors influence pain perception?

10. What are the functions of proprioceptors? Where are they located?

11. Label each of the diagrams. (See Figures 8-1 and 8-5 to check your answers.)

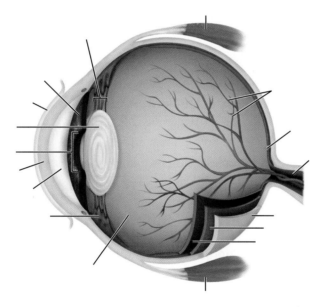

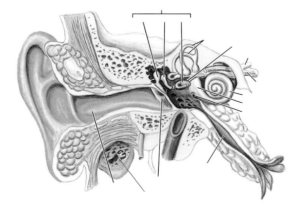

9

Endocrine Control

Chapter Outline

The **endocrine system** helps regulate growth, reproduction, use of nutrients by cells, salt and fluid balance, and metabolic rate and also helps us respond to stress. The endocrine system works with the nervous system to maintain **homeostasis**—the balanced internal environment, or steady state, of the body. Responses to nervous system stimulation tend to be rapid and brief. In contrast, responses to many *hormones* released by the endocrine system may require several hours or even longer and effects may be long lasting. **Endocrinology,** the study of the endocrine system, is an exciting field of biological research.

154

MANY TISSUES SECRETE HORMONES OR HORMONE-LIKE SUBSTANCES

LEARNING OBJECTIVES

1. **Describe the sources, transport, and general functions of hormones and hormone-like substances (for example, neurohormones and prostaglandins).**
2. **Identify the principal endocrine glands, locate them in the body, and list the hormones secreted by each gland.**

The endocrine system consists of specialized tissues and **endocrine glands,** which secrete **hormones,** chemical messengers that help regulate many body activities. Endocrine glands lack ducts. They differ from **exocrine glands** (e.g., sweat glands, gastric glands), which release their secretions into ducts. Endocrine glands release their hormones into the surrounding interstitial (tissue) fluid or into the blood. Hormones are typically transported by the blood and affect the activity of their **target cells**—the specific cells on which they act. Target cells, the cells influenced by a particular hormone, may be located in another endocrine gland or in an entirely different type of organ, such as a bone.

Endocrinologists have identified about 10 discrete endocrine glands. The principal endocrine glands are illustrated in Figure 9-1 and described in Table 9-1. Researchers have also identified specialized cells in the kidneys, heart, digestive tract, and many other organs that also release hormones or hormone-like substances.

Certain neurons, known as **neuroendocrine cells,** are an important link between the nervous and endocrine systems. Neuroendocrine cells produce **neurohormones** that are transported down axons and released into the interstitial fluid. They typically diffuse into capillaries and are transported by the blood. As you will learn, the hypothalamus produces several neurohormones.

Some local regulators, chemical messengers that act on nearby cells, are also considered hormones. **Prostaglandins** (pros′-tah-**glan′**-dins) are a group of about 16 closely related lipids that are manufactured by many different tissues in the body, including the prostate gland (where they were first identified). Prostaglandins interact with other hormones to regulate various metabolic activities. Some prostaglandins reduce blood pressure; others raise it. Various prostaglandins dilate the respiratory passageways, inhibit secretion in the stomach, cause inflammation, affect nerve function, and stimulate contraction of the uterus.

Because prostaglandins are involved in the regulation of so many metabolic processes, they have great potential for a variety of clinical uses. At present, prostaglandins are used to induce labor in pregnant women, to induce abortion, and for the prevention of ulcers in the stomach and duodenum. Some

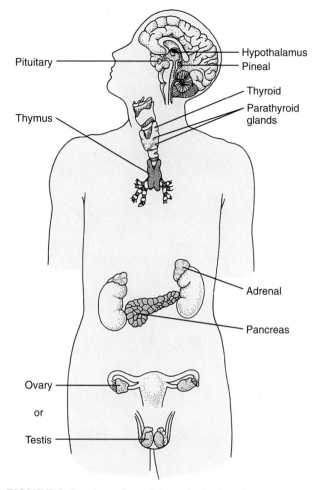

FIGURE 9-1 • Location of the principal endocrine glands. Both male and female gonads are shown.

investigators think that these substances may someday be used to treat such illnesses as asthma, arthritis, kidney disease, and some forms of cancer.

Quiz Yourself

*   What are hormones?
*   What are neurohormones?
*   What hormones are secreted by the thyroid gland? The parathyroid gland?

NEGATIVE FEEDBACK SYSTEMS REGULATE ENDOCRINE GLANDS

LEARNING OBJECTIVE

3. **Describe how endocrine glands are regulated by negative feedback systems.**

Homeostasis depends on normal concentrations of hormones. Hormone secretion is typically regulated by **negative feedback**

TABLE 9-1   SOME ENDOCRINE GLANDS AND THEIR HORMONES*

Endocrine Gland and Hormone	Target Tissue	Principal Actions
HYPOTHALAMUS		
Releasing and inhibiting hormones	Anterior lobe of pituitary	Regulate secretion of hormones by the anterior lobe of pituitary
HYPOTHALAMUS (production) **POSTERIOR LOBE OF PITUITARY** (storage and release)		
Oxytocin	Uterus	Stimulates contraction
	Mammary glands	Stimulates ejection of milk into ducts
Antidiuretic hormone (ADH)	Kidneys (collecting ducts)	Stimulates reabsorption of water; conserves water
ANTERIOR LOBE OF PITUITARY		
Growth hormone (GH)	General	Stimulates production of insulin-like growth factors (IGF); stimulates growth by promoting protein synthesis
Prolactin	Mammary glands	Stimulates milk production
Thyroid-stimulating hormone (TSH)	Thyroid gland	Stimulates secretion of thyroid hormones; stimulates increase in size of thyroid gland
Adrenocorticotropic hormone (ACTH)	Adrenal cortex	Stimulates secretion of adrenal cortical hormones
Gonadotropic hormones (FSH, LH)*	Gonads	Stimulate gonad function and growth
THYROID GLAND		
Thyroxine (T_4) and triiodothyronine (T_3)	General	Stimulate metabolic rate; essential to normal growth and development
Calcitonin	Bone	Lowers blood-calcium level by inhibiting Ca^{2+} release from bone
PARATHYROID GLANDS		
Parathyroid hormone (PTH)	Bone, kidneys, digestive tract	Increases blood-calcium level by stimulating Ca^{2+} release from bone; stimulates calcium reabsorption by kidneys; activates vitamin D, which increases intestinal absorption of calcium
ISLETS OF LANGERHANS OF PANCREAS		
Insulin	General	Lowers glucose concentration in the blood by facilitating glucose uptake and utilization by cells; stimulates glycogen production; stimulates fat storage and protein synthesis
Glucagon	Liver, adipose tissue	Raises glucose concentration in the blood; stimulates glycogen breakdown; mobilizes fat
ADRENAL MEDULLA		
Epinephrine and norepinephrine	Skeletal muscle; cardiac muscle; blood vessels; liver; adipose tissue	Help body cope with stress; increase heart rate, blood pressure, metabolic rate; reroute blood; mobilize fat; raise blood sugar level
ADRENAL CORTEX		
Mineralocorticoids (aldosterone)	Kidney tubules	Maintain sodium and potassium balance; increase sodium reabsorption; increase potassium excretion
Glucocorticoids (cortisol)	General	Help body cope with long-term stress; raise blood glucose level; mobilize fat
PINEAL GLAND		
Melatonin	Hypothalamus	Important in biological rhythms; influences reproductive processes in some animals; may help control onset of puberty in humans

TABLE 9-1	SOME ENDOCRINE GLANDS AND THEIR HORMONES*—cont'd	
Endocrine Gland and Hormone	**Target Tissue**	**Principal Actions**
OVARY		
Estrogens (estradiol)	General; uterus	Develop and maintain sex characteristics in female; stimulate growth of uterine lining
Progesterone	Uterus; breast	Stimulates development of uterine lining
TESTIS		
Testosterone	General; reproductive structures	Develops and maintains sex characteristics of males; promotes spermatogenesis; responsible for adolescent growth spurt
Inhibin	Anterior lobe of pituitary	Inhibits follicle-stimulating hormone (FSH) release in male

*The gonadotropic hormones (FSH and LH) and the ovaries and testes and their hormones are discussed in Chapter 17.

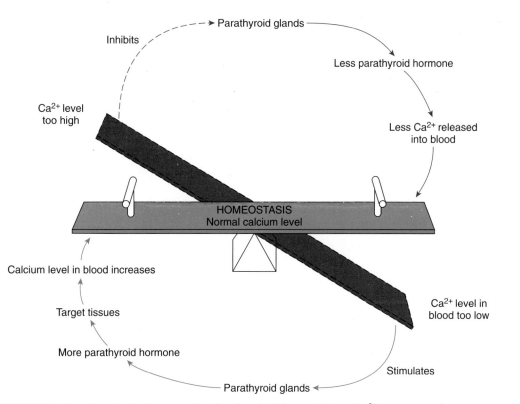

FIGURE 9-2 • Regulation by negative feedback. When calcium (Ca^{2+}) concentration exceeds its normal range in the blood, the parathyroid glands are inhibited and slow their release of parathyroid hormone (PTH). When the calcium concentration in the blood falls below its normal range, the parathyroid glands are stimulated to release more PTH. This hormone acts on target tissues that increase the calcium concentration in the blood, thus restoring homeostasis. *Green arrows,* Stimulation; *red arrows,* inhibition.

systems. Information about the amount of hormone or of some other substance in the blood or interstitial fluid is fed back to the endocrine gland, which then responds to restore homeostasis. The parathyroid glands, located in the neck, provide a good example of how negative feedback works.

The parathyroid glands regulate the calcium concentration of the blood. When the calcium concentration is not within homeostatic limits, nerves and muscles cannot function properly. For example, when insufficient amounts of calcium ions are present, neurons can fire spontaneously, causing muscle spasms. When calcium concentration varies too far from the steady state (either too high or too low), negative feedback mechanisms bring the condition back to the steady state (Figure 9-2).

A decrease in the calcium concentration in the plasma signals the parathyroid glands to release more parathyroid hormone. This hormone increases the concentration of calcium in the blood. (The details of parathyroid action are discussed later in this chapter.) When the calcium concentration rises above normal limits, the parathyroid glands slow their output of hormone. Both responses are negative feedback mechanisms. An increase in the calcium concentration results in decreased release of parathyroid hormone, whereas a decrease leads to increased hormone secretion. In each case, the response counteracts the inappropriate change, thus restoring the steady state.

When an endocrine gland is not regulated effectively, the rate of secretion becomes abnormal. In **hyposecretion,** the gland decreases its hormone output to abnormally low levels. This condition deprives target cells of needed stimulation. In **hypersecretion,** a gland increases its output to abnormally high levels, overstimulating target cells. In some endocrine disorders, an appropriate amount of hormone is secreted but the target cell receptors do not function properly. As a result, the target cells may not be able to respond to the hormone. Any of these abnormalities can lead to loss of homeostasis, resulting in predictable metabolic malfunctions and clinical symptoms (Table 9-2).

⊚ Quiz Yourself

- How do the parathyroid glands respond when the blood calcium concentration is too low?
- What is hyposecretion?

HORMONES COMBINE WITH SPECIFIC RECEPTORS ON OR IN TARGET CELLS

LEARNING OBJECTIVE

4. **Compare the mechanisms of action of hormones that work through second messengers with those of steroid hormones.**

A hormone may pass through many tissues "unnoticed" until it reaches its target cells. How do the target cells "recognize" the hormone? Specialized proteins on or in the target cell are **receptors** that bind with the hormone. This process is highly specific. The receptor is like a lock, and the hormones are like different keys. Only the hormone that fits the lock can influence the metabolic machinery of the cell. When the hormone combines with a receptor, a series of reactions is activated.

Many Hormones Activate Second Messengers

Hormones that are large molecules, such as proteins, combine with receptors on the plasma membrane of the target cell. Because the hormone turns on the system, it is referred to as the **first messenger.** The hormone relays information to a **second messenger,** which may alter the activity of the cell (Figure 9-3). Some hormones activate a series of molecular events involving several different kinds of molecules. The first molecule in the series is usually a **G protein,** a type of protein associated with the plasma membrane. Some diseases such as diabetes may be connected to malfunctioning G proteins.

TABLE 9-2	CONSEQUENCES OF ENDOCRINE MALFUNCTION	
Hormone	**Hyposecretion**	**Hypersecretion**
Growth hormone	Pituitary dwarfism	Gigantism if malfunction occurs in childhood; acromegaly in adult
Thyroid hormones	Cretinism (in children); myxedema, a condition of pronounced adult hypothyroidism (metabolic rate is reduced by about 40%; patient feels tired and may be mentally slow); dietary iodine deficiency can lead to hyposecretion and goiter (abnormal enlargement of the thyroid gland)	Hyperthyroidism; increased metabolic rate, nervousness, irritability; goiter
Parathyroid hormone	Spontaneous discharge of nerves; spasms; tetany; death	Weak, brittle bones; kidney stones
Insulin	Diabetes mellitus	Hypoglycemia
Hormones of adrenal cortex	Addison's disease (inability to cope with stress; sodium loss in urine may lead to shock)	Cushing's disease (edema gives face a full-moon appearance; fat is deposited about trunk; blood glucose level rises; immune repsonses are depressed)

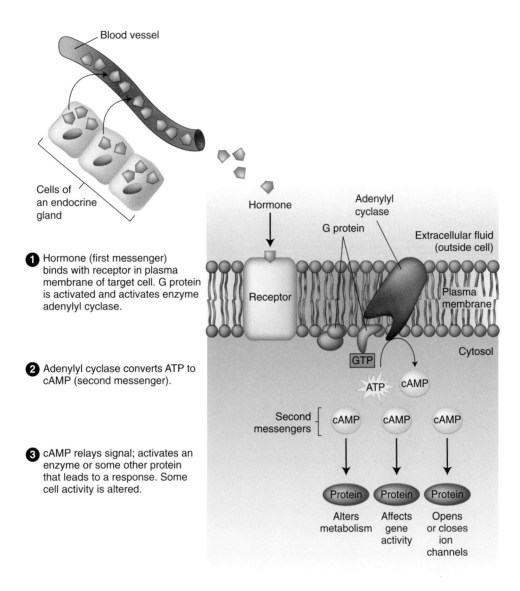

FIGURE 9-3 • Action of hormones that have membrane receptors. When a peptide hormone binds with a receptor on the plasma membrane of a target cell, the receptor converts the hormone signal to an intracellular signal. The signal may be relayed by a second messenger. Typically, a sequence of several signaling molecules relays the message. Some cell process is changed. This is the hormone action.

Cyclic AMP (cyclic adenosine monophosphate, often abbreviated as cAMP) is a common second messenger. When certain hormones bind with receptors on the extracellular surface of the plasma membrane, they activate a G protein that in turn activates an enzyme (adenylyl cyclase). This enzyme catalyzes the conversion of ATP (adenosine triphosphate) to cAMP. cAMP then activates one or more enzymes that alter specific proteins, triggering a chain of reactions that leads to a certain metabolic effect.

Calcium ions can also act as second messengers. Certain hormone receptors are linked to calcium channels. When the hormone combines with the receptor, the calcium channel opens and calcium ions move into the cell. Calcium ions bind to the protein **calmodulin.** The calmodulin molecule changes shape and can activate enzymes that regulate certain cellular processes, such as neurotransmitter release.

Steroid Hormones Activate Genes

Steroid hormones and thyroid hormones are relatively small molecules that pass easily through the plasma membrane of a target cell. They pass through the cytoplasm and into the nucleus (Figure 9-4). Specific protein receptors in the cytoplasm or in the nucleus combine with the hormone molecules. This hormone-receptor complex then interacts with the DNA (deoxyribonucleic acid) and turns specific genes on or off.

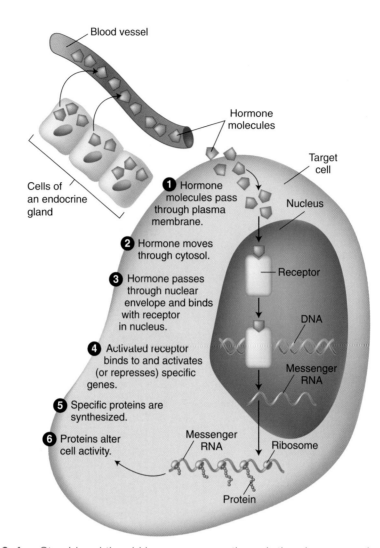

FIGURE 9-4 • Steroid and thyroid hormones pass through the plasma membrane and bind with a receptor in the cytoplasm or nucleus. The activated receptor binds with DNA in the nucleus and activates or represses specific genes. This causes changes in the protein composition of the cell. As a result, cell activity is altered. We recognize this change as the hormone's action.

When certain genes are switched on, specific proteins are synthesized. These proteins produce the changes in structure or metabolic activity responsible for the effect of the hormone.

Quiz Yourself

- What is cyclic AMP?
- What is the mechanism of action of a steroid hormone?

THE HYPOTHALAMUS REGULATES THE PITUITARY GLAND

LEARNING OBJECTIVES

5. **Justify the reputation of the hypothalamus as the link between nervous and endocrine systems.**

(**Describe the mechanisms by which the hypothalamus exerts its control.**)

6. **Compare the functions of the posterior and anterior lobes of the pituitary and describe the actions of their hormones.**

The **hypothalamus** links the nervous and endocrine systems. Directly or indirectly, the hypothalamus regulates most endocrine activity. In response to input from other areas of the brain and from hormones in the blood, the hypothalamus secretes several neurohormones. Two of these hormones—oxytocin and antidiuretic hormone—are stored in the pituitary gland. Several others are **releasing hormones** and **inhibiting hormones,** which act on the pituitary gland, regulating secretion of several pituitary hormones.

The **pituitary gland** is a remarkable organ only about the size of a pea. Connected to the hypothalamus by a stalk of tissue, the pituitary gland lies in a bony cavity (sella turcica) of the sphenoid bone. Sometimes called the *master gland of the body,* the pituitary secretes at least seven distinct hormones (Figure 9-5). These hormones control the activities of several other endocrine glands and influence many body processes. The pituitary gland consists of two main lobes—the **anterior lobe** and the **posterior lobe.**

The Posterior Lobe Releases Two Hormones Produced by the Hypothalamus

The **posterior lobe** of the pituitary gland secretes **oxytocin** (ox′-see-**tow**′-sin) and **antidiuretic** (an′-tie-die-you-**ret**′-ik) **hormone (ADH).** These hormones are actually produced in certain neurons in the hypothalamus. The hormones are enclosed within little vesicles (sacs) and pass slowly down the axons of these neurons into the posterior lobe where they are stored.

Oxytocin stimulates contraction of smooth muscle in the wall of the uterus and stimulates release of milk from the breast. Toward the end of pregnancy, the oxytocin concentration rises, stimulating the strong contractions of the uterus needed to expel a baby. Oxytocin is sometimes administered clinically (under the trade name *Pitocin*) to start or speed labor.

ADH regulates fluid balance in the body and indirectly helps control blood pressure. ADH helps the body conserve water by increasing water reabsorption from the collecting ducts in the kidney (discussed in Chapter 16). The result is a decrease in urine output and an increase in tissue fluid. Alcohol consumption increases urine output because alcohol inhibits ADH secretion. The resulting increase in urine output dehydrates the body and causes the feeling of thirst.

ADH deficiency can lead to the metabolic disorder called **diabetes insipidus,** in which enormous quantities of dilute urine may be excreted. This fluid loss must be replaced or serious dehydration rapidly develops.

The Anterior Lobe Regulates Growth and Other Endocrine Glands

The **anterior lobe** of the pituitary gland secretes growth hormone, prolactin, and several **tropic hormones**—hormones that stimulate other endocrine glands. Each of the anterior pituitary hormones is regulated in some way by a releasing hormone and in some cases also by an inhibiting hormone produced in the hypothalamus. These neurohormones enter capillaries and pass through special portal veins that connect the hypothalamus with the anterior lobe of the pituitary. (Portal veins are unusual in that they do not deliver blood to a larger vein directly but connect two sets of capillaries.) Within the anterior lobe of the pituitary, the portal veins divide into a second set of capillaries. The releasing and inhib-

iting hormones pass through the walls of these capillaries into the tissue of the anterior lobe.

During lactation (milk production), **prolactin** (pro-**lak**′-tin) stimulates the cells of the mammary glands to secrete milk. Prolactin secretion increases when the nipple is stimulated by a nursing baby.

The tropic hormones are (1) thyroid-stimulating hormone (TSH), which stimulates the thyroid gland; (2) adrenocorticotropic hormone (ACTH), which stimulates the adrenal cortex; and (3) and (4) the gonadotropic hormones, follicle-stimulating hormone (FSH) and luteinizing hormone (LH), which control the activities of the gonads (sex glands).

Growth Hormone Stimulates Protein Synthesis

Whether one will be tall or short depends on many factors, including genes, diet, hormone balance, and even emotional nurturance. **Growth hormone** (**GH,** also called *somatotropin*) stimulates body growth mainly by stimulating protein synthesis. Many of the effects of GH on skeletal growth are indirect. GH stimulates liver cells and cells of many other tissues to produce peptides called **somatomedins,** including **insulin-like growth factors (IGFs).** These growth factors promote the growth of the skeleton and stimulate general tissue growth by promoting protein synthesis.

In adults as well as in growing children, GH is secreted in pulses throughout the day. Secretion of GH is regulated by both a **growth hormone–releasing hormone (GHRH)** and a **growth hormone–inhibiting hormone (GHIH)** released by the hypothalamus. A high level of GH in the blood signals the hypothalamus to secrete the inhibiting hormone, and the pituitary release of GH slows. A low level of GH in the blood stimulates the hypothalamus to secrete the releasing hormone, which in turn stimulates the pituitary gland to release more GH. Many other factors (e.g., blood sugar level, decrease in amino acid concentration, stress) influence GH secretion.

The age-old notions that children need plenty of sleep, a proper diet, and regular exercise to grow are supported by research. Secretion of GH increases during exercise, probably because rapid metabolism by muscle cells lowers the blood sugar level. GH is secreted about 1 hour after the onset of deep sleep and in a series of pulses 2 to 4 hours after a meal.

Emotional support is also necessary for proper growth. Growth is retarded in children who are deprived of cuddling, playing, and other forms of nurture, even when their needs for food and shelter are met. In extreme cases, childhood stress can produce a form of retarded development known as *psychosocial dwarfism.*

Other hormones also influence growth. Thyroid hormones appear to be necessary for normal GH secretion and function and for normal tissue response to IGFs. Sex hormones must be present for the adolescent growth spurt to occur. However, the presence of sex hormones eventually causes the growth centers within the long bones to ossify, so further increase in height is impossible even when GH is present.

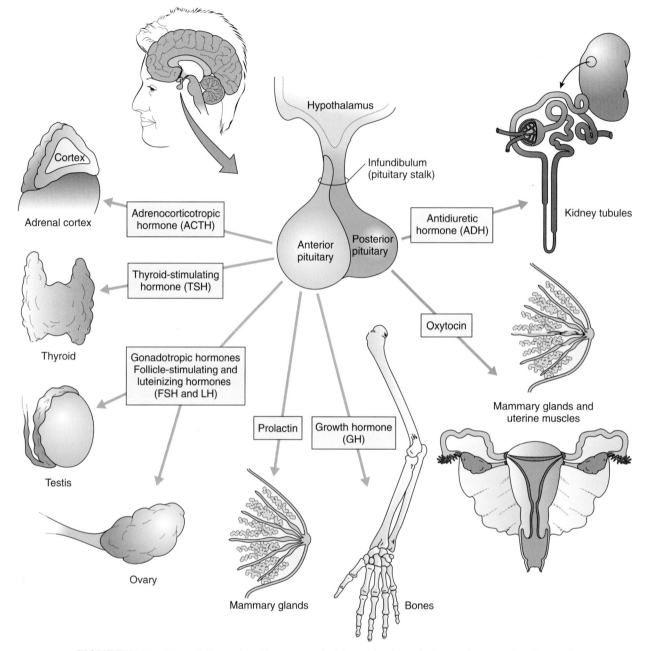

FIGURE 9-5 • The pituitary gland is suspended from the hypothalamus by a stalk of neural tissue. The hormones secreted by the anterior and posterior lobes of the pituitary gland and their target tissues are shown.

Circus midgets are **pituitary dwarfs**—individuals whose pituitary gland did not produce enough GH during childhood. Though miniature, a pituitary dwarf has normal intelligence and is usually well proportioned. If the growth centers in the long bones are still open when this condition is diagnosed, it can be treated by injection with GH.

An individual may become abnormally tall when the anterior pituitary secretes too much GH during childhood. This condition is referred to as **gigantism.** If pituitary malfunction leads to hypersecretion of GH during adulthood, the individual cannot grow taller. However, connective tissue thickens, and bones in the hands, feet, and face may increase in diameter. This condition is known as **acromegaly,** which means "large extremities."

Quiz Yourself

- What is the function of releasing hormones?
- What hormones are released by the posterior lobe of the pituitary gland? What are their actions?
- What are tropic hormones?

THYROID HORMONES INCREASE METABOLIC RATE

LEARNING OBJECTIVE

7. **Summarize the actions of the thyroid hormones and draw a diagram illustrating how they are regulated.**

Shaped somewhat like a shield, the **thyroid gland** is located in the neck. It lies anterior to the trachea and just below the larynx (see Figure 9-1). Its two lobes of dark red glandular tissue are connected by a bridge of tissue—the isthmus. The thyroid gland secretes two **thyroid hormones** and a hormone called *calcitonin* (which is discussed in connection with the parathyroid glands).

The thyroid hormones are essential for normal growth and development, and they increase metabolic rate in most tissues. The main thyroid hormone is **thyroxine** (thy-**rok'**-sin), also known as T_4 (because it has four iodine atoms in its structure). A second hormone, T_3 (triiodothyronine, pronounced tri'-i-o-doe-**thy'**-row-nene) has three iodine atoms in its structure. The protein-bound iodine, or PBI, is an index of the amount of circulating thyroid hormones and is sometimes measured clinically for that purpose.

The regulation of thyroid hormone secretion depends on a negative feedback system between the anterior pituitary and the thyroid gland (Figure 9-6). The anterior pituitary secretes **TSH,** which promotes synthesis and secretion of thyroid hormones. When the normal concentration of thyroid hormones in the blood falls, the anterior pituitary secretes more TSH.

> Low concentration of thyroid hormones → anterior pituitary secretes more TSH → thyroid gland secretes more thyroid hormones → homeostasis

When the level of thyroid hormones in the blood rises above normal, the anterior pituitary is inhibited and slows its release of TSH. Too much thyroid hormone in the blood also affects the hypothalamus, inhibiting secretion of TSH-releasing hormones.

> Concentration of thyroid hormones increases → anterior pituitary secretes less TSH → thyroid gland secretes less thyroid hormones → homeostasis

Extreme hypothyroidism during childhood results in low metabolic rate and retarded mental and physical development. This condition is called **cretinism.** (A cretin is very different from a pituitary dwarf.)

Any abnormal enlargement of the thyroid gland is termed a **goiter** and may be associated with either hyposecretion or hypersecretion. One cause is iodine deficiency. Without iodine, the gland cannot make thyroid hormones, so their concentra-

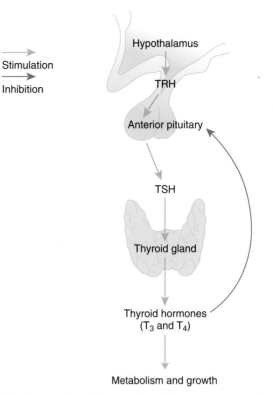

FIGURE 9-6 • Regulation of thyroid hormone secretion by negative feedback. An increase in concentration of thyroid hormones above normal levels signals the anterior pituitary to decrease production and release of TSH. Thus thyroid hormones limit their own production by negative feedback. *Green arrows,* stimulation; *red arrows,* inhibition. *TRH,* TSH-releasing hormone.

tion in the blood decreases. In response, the anterior pituitary secretes large amounts of TSH, and the thyroid gland enlarges. Thanks to iodized salt, goiter is no longer common in the United States. In other parts of the world, however, hundreds of thousands still suffer from this easily preventable disorder.

Quiz Yourself

- What are the functions of thyroid hormones?
- What is the action of TSH?

PARATHYROID GLANDS REGULATE CALCIUM CONCENTRATION

LEARNING OBJECTIVE

8. **Describe how the parathyroid and thyroid glands regulate calcium levels.**

The **parathyroid glands** are embedded in the connective tissue that surrounds the thyroid gland (see Figure 9-1).

Usually there are four glands, but the number may vary from two to ten. The parathyroid glands secrete **parathyroid hormone (PTH)**—a small protein that regulates the calcium level of the blood and tissue fluid.

Appropriate concentrations of calcium are essential for normal nerve and muscle function, bone metabolism, cell-membrane permeability, and blood clotting. PTH increases calcium levels by stimulating release of calcium from the bones and by stimulating calcium reabsorption by the kidney tubules, preventing its loss in the urine. PTH also activates vitamin D, which then increases the amount of calcium absorbed from the intestine.

The parathyroid glands are regulated by the concentration of calcium in the blood and tissue fluid (see Figure 9-2). When the calcium concentration rises above normal, the parathyroid glands slow their secretion of PTH.

> Calcium concentration too high → parathyroid glands secrete less PTH → calcium concentration decreases

When the calcium concentration becomes very high, calcitonin (kal′-sih-**tow**′-nin) is released from the thyroid gland. This hormone quickly inhibits removal of calcium from bone.

When the concentration of calcium in the tissue fluid falls even slightly, PTH secretion increases.

> Calcium concentration too low → parathyroid glands secrete more PTH → calcium concentration increases

When PTH secretion is too low, the calcium level falls. Nerve fibers become more excitable and may discharge spontaneously. This causes muscles to twitch and to go into spasms—a condition called *tetany*. Spasm of the muscles of the larynx interferes with respiration and may lead to death.

Too much PTH results in too much calcium being removed from the bones. The bones are weakened and may fracture easily. The kidneys attempt to excrete the excess calcium removed from the bones. So much calcium may be present in the urine that crystals of calcium form kidney stones.

⊚ Quiz Yourself

- What is the function of PTH? Of calcitonin?
- What happens when the calcium concentration is too low?

THE ISLETS OF LANGERHANS REGULATE GLUCOSE CONCENTRATION

LEARNING OBJECTIVE

9. **Contrast the actions of insulin and glucagon and describe the effects of diabetes mellitus.**

The pancreas, which lies in the abdomen posterior to the stomach, has both exocrine and endocrine functions. Its exocrine cells produce digestive enzymes (discussed in Chapter 15). More than a million small clusters of cells known as the **islets of Langerhans** are scattered throughout the pancreas. About 70% of the islet cells are **beta cells** that produce the hormone *insulin*. **Alpha cells** secrete the hormone *glucagon*.

Insulin (in′-suh-lin) *lowers* the concentration of glucose in the blood. It stimulates cells of many tissues, including liver, muscle, and fat cells, to take up glucose from the blood. Once glucose enters muscle cells, it is either used immediately as fuel or stored as glycogen. Insulin also inhibits liver cells from releasing glucose.

Glucagon (gloo′-kuh-gon) *raises* the blood glucose level. It does this by stimulating liver cells to convert glycogen to glucose. It also stimulates the liver cells to make glucose from noncarbohydrates. The effects of glucagon are opposite to those of insulin.

Secretion of insulin and glucagon is directly controlled by the blood glucose level. After a meal, the concentration of glucose in the blood rises. This stimulates the beta cells to increase insulin secretion. Then, as the cells remove glucose from the blood, the glucose concentration decreases. Insulin secretion decreases accordingly.

> Glucose concentration too high → beta cells secrete insulin → blood glucose concentration decreases → homeostasis

When a person has not eaten for several hours, the glucose concentration in the blood begins to fall. When it falls from its normal fasting level of about 90 mg/dl to about 70 mg/dl, the alpha cells of the islets secrete glucagon. (A dl [deciliter] equals 100 ml). Glucose is taken out of storage in the liver, and the blood glucose level returns to normal.

> Glucose concentration too low → alpha cells secrete glucagon → blood glucose concentration increases → homeostasis

Note that these are negative feedback systems and that insulin and glucagon work antagonistically to keep blood glucose concentration within normal limits (Figure 9-7). When the glucose level rises, insulin release brings it back to normal; when it falls, glucagon acts to raise it again. The insulin-glucagon system is a powerful, fast-acting mechanism for

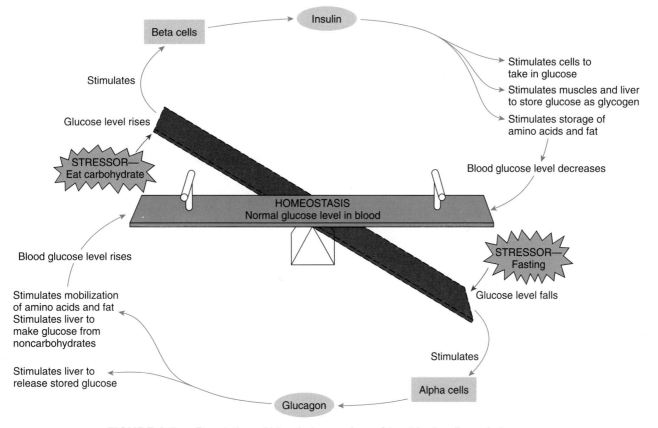

FIGURE 9-7 • Regulation of blood glucose (sugar) level by insulin and glucagon.

keeping the blood glucose level within normal limits. Why is it important to maintain a constant blood glucose level? Recall that brain cells ordinarily are unable to use other nutrients as fuel and must depend on a continuous supply of glucose.

In Diabetes Mellitus, Glucose Accumulates in the Blood

The main disorder associated with pancreatic hormones is **diabetes mellitus** (die-ah-**be′**-teez **mel′**-ih-tus). Insulin-dependent diabetes, referred to as **type 1 diabetes,** commonly develops before age 20. In this disorder there is a marked decrease in the number of beta cells in the pancreas. This loss of beta cells results in insulin deficiency. Type 1 diabetes is clinically treated with insulin injections. Researchers recently reported that injections of stem cells can be used to treat type 1 diabetes, eliminating the need for insulin injections.

About 90% of all cases of diabetes are non-insulin-dependent, or **type 2, diabetes.** This disorder develops gradually, usually in individuals who are overweight. In many cases of type 2 diabetes, sufficient insulin is released by the islets of Langerhans. The problem is that the insulin receptors on target cells are not able to bind with the insulin and use it. This condition is known as **insulin resistance.**

Similar metabolic disturbances occur in both types of diabetes mellitus. Because cells cannot take up glucose from the blood, it accumulates there and the blood glucose level rises (hyperglycemia). Instead of the normal fasting level of about 90 mg/dl, the diabetic may have from 300 to more than 500 mg/dl. Glucose does not normally appear in the urine. However, in diabetics the blood glucose concentration may be so high that glucose is excreted in the urine. Because cells cannot take up the glucose they require for fuel, they turn to fat and protein for energy. This shift leads to several problems, including an unhealthy concentration of lipids in the blood. Diabetics also have difficulty regulating their electrolytes. (Electrolytes are chemical compounds such as salts that form ions.)

Quiz Yourself

- What are the actions of insulin?
- How do insulin and glucagon work together to maintain a normal glucose level?

THE ADRENAL GLANDS FUNCTION IN METABOLISM AND STRESS

LEARNING OBJECTIVES

10. **Describe the role of the adrenal medulla in the body's responses to stress.**

11. **Identify the hormones secreted by the adrenal cortex and give the actions of glucocorticoids and mineralocorticoids.**

The paired **adrenal glands** are small yellow masses of tissue located above the kidneys (Figure 9-8). Each gland consists of a central portion, the **adrenal medulla,** and a larger outer region, the **adrenal cortex.** These regions function as distinct glands. Both secrete hormones that help regulate metabolism, and both help the body deal with stress.

The Adrenal Medulla Secretes Epinephrine and Norepinephrine

The adrenal medulla develops from nervous tissue and is sometimes considered part of the sympathetic nervous system. The adrenal medulla secretes two hormones—**epinephrine** (ep′-ih-**nef′**-rin) (also called *adrenaline*) and **norepinephrine** (nor′-ep-ih-**nef′**-rin) (also called *noradrenaline*). Norepinephrine is the same substance that is secreted as a neurotransmitter by sympathetic neurons and by some neurons in the central nervous system.

The adrenal medulla is called the *emergency gland of the body* because it prepares us to cope with threatening situations. Under normal conditions, both epinephrine and norepinephrine are secreted continuously in small amounts. Their secretion is under nervous system control. During stressful situations when anxiety is aroused, neural messages are sent through sympathetic nerves to the adrenal medulla. Hormone secretion from the adrenal medulla increases, initiating an alarm reaction. This response enables you to think quickly and then fight harder or run much faster than normal.

Anxiety affects hypothalamus → sympathetic nerves stimulate adrenal medulla → increased secretion of epinephrine and norepinephrine → physiological adjustments that help the body cope with stress

Actions of epinephrine and norepinephrine include the following:

1. Increase metabolic rate as much as 100%
2. Increase the heart rate and stimulate the heart to contract with greater strength
3. Increase blood pressure
4. Increase alertness
5. Dilate the airway so that breathing is more effective (Epinephrine and related drugs are used clinically to relieve nasal congestion and asthma.)
6. Reroute the blood so that more flows to the organs essential for emergency action. Blood vessels to the skin and most internal organs are constricted; those to the brain, muscles, and heart are dilated. Constriction of the blood vessels to the skin has the added advantage of decreasing blood loss from superficial wounds. (It also explains the sudden paleness that comes with fear or rage.)
7. Increase strength of contraction of skeletal muscles.
8. Raise glucose and fatty acid levels in the blood so that there is enough fuel to provide the extra energy needed.

The Adrenal Cortex Secretes Steroid Hormones

The **adrenal cortex** secretes three different types of steroid hormones:

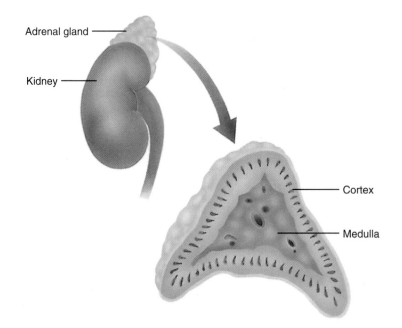

FIGURE 9-8 • The paired adrenal glands are small yellow masses of tissues that lie in contact with the upper ends of the kidneys. Each gland consists of a central medulla and an outer cortex.

1. **Glucocorticoids** (gloo'-koe-**kor'**-tih-koyds) help the body cope with stress. The main glucocorticoid is **cortisol** (also called **hydrocortisone**). The principal action of the glucocorticoids is to promote production of glucose from other nutrients. This action increases the concentration of glucose in the blood, providing glucose supplies when the body is under stress and in need of extra energy. Thus the adrenal cortex serves as an important backup system for the adrenal medulla. Glucocorticoids also reduce inflammation and are used clinically in allergic reactions, infections, arthritis, and certain other disorders. When present in large amounts over long periods, glucocorticoids can cause serious side effects. They depress the immune system and so decrease the ability to fight infections.

2. **Mineralocorticoids** (min'-er-al-o-**kor'**-tih-koyds) regulate water and salt balance. Aldosterone (al-**dos'**-ter-own) is the principal mineralocorticoid. Its main function is to maintain homeostasis of sodium and potassium ions. It does this mainly by stimulating the kidneys to conserve sodium and to excrete potassium.

3. **Sex hormones.** In both sexes, the adrenal cortex secretes small amounts of both **androgens** (hormones that have masculinizing effects) and **estrogens** (female sex hormones).

Stress stimulates the hypothalamus to secrete corticotropin-releasing factor (CRF). This hormone stimulates the anterior pituitary to secrete ACTH, which regulates both glucocorticoid and aldosterone secretion. When the body is not under

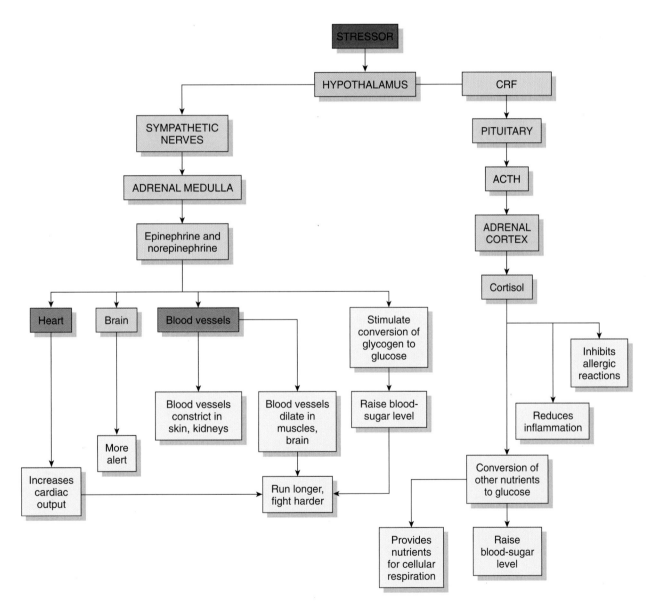

FIGURE 9-9 • The adrenal medulla and the adrenal cortex both play important roles in helping the body cope with stress. Some of the effects of their hormones are shown here.

stress, high levels of cortisol in the blood inhibit both CRF secretion by the hypothalamus and ACTH secretion by the pituitary.

Abnormally large amounts of glucocorticoids, whether resulting from disease or drugs, can result in **Cushing's disease.** In this condition, fat is mobilized from the lower part of the body and deposited about the trunk. Edema gives the patient's face a full-moon appearance. The blood glucose level rises to as much as 50% above normal, causing a type of diabetes (adrenal diabetes). The immune system is depressed, and hypertension (high blood pressure) is common.

Hyposecretion of the adrenal cortex can lead to **Addison's disease.** Reduction in cortisol prevents the body from effectively regulating the concentration of glucose in the blood because the liver cannot convert other nutrients to glucose. The cortisol-deficient patient also loses the ability to cope with stress. If cortisol levels are significantly depressed, even the stress of mild infections can cause death.

Stress Threatens Homeostasis

Good health and survival depend on maintaining homeostasis. **Stressors,** stimuli that disrupt the steady state of the body, must be dealt with swiftly and effectively. Stressors, whether in the form of infection, disease, arguments, or even the anxiety of taking a test for which one is not fully prepared, may threaten homeostasis, putting the body in a state of **stress.**

When stressed, the brain sends messages activating the sympathetic nervous system and the adrenal glands. Epinephrine and norepinephrine are released, and the body prepares for fight or flight. The hypothalamus also signals the anterior pituitary hormonally to secrete ACTH, which increases cortisol secretion, thereby adjusting metabolism to meet the increased demands of the stressful situation (Figure 9-9).

Some stressors are short lived. We react to the situation and quickly resolve it. Other stressors may be chronic, lasting for weeks or even years (e.g., a chronic disease or an unhappy marriage). Chronic stress is harmful because of the effects of long-term elevation of some hormones.

Quiz Yourself

- What are the actions of epinephrine and norepinephrine?
- What is the function of cortisol?

MANY OTHER HORMONES ARE KNOWN

LEARNING OBJECTIVE

12. **Describe the actions of hormones secreted by the pineal gland, thymus gland, and atrium of the heart.**

Many other tissues and organs of the body secrete hormones. The **pineal (pin'-ee-al) gland,** located in the brain, produces **melatonin.** This hormone facilitates the onset of sleep and influences biological rhythms and the onset of sexual maturity. Exposure to light suppresses melatonin secretion.

The digestive tract and adipose tissue secrete hormones that regulate digestive processes (discussed in Chapter 15). The **thymus gland** produces **thymosin,** a hormone that plays a role in immune responses. The atrium of the heart secretes **atrial natriuretic factor (ANF),** which promotes sodium excretion and lowers blood pressure. We discuss reproductive hormones in Chapter 17.

Quiz Yourself

- What is the action of ANF?

SUMMARY

LO 1. **Describe the sources, transport, and general functions of hormones and hormone-like substances (for example, eurohormones and prostaglandins).**

- The **endocrine system** regulates homeostasis of many metabolic processes; it consists of **endocrine glands** and tissues that release chemical messengers called **hormones.** Endocrine glands are ductless glands that secrete hormones into the tissue fluid.

LO 2. **Identify the principal endocrine glands, locate them in the body, and list the hormones secreted by each gland.**

- The principal endocrine glands are illustrated in Figure 9-1 and are described in Table 9-1.

LO 3. **Describe how endocrine glands are regulated by negative feedback systems.**

- Endocrine glands are regulated by **negative feedback systems.** Information about the concentration of the hormone is fed back to an endocrine gland, which then responds to restore homeostasis. In **hyposecretion,** the gland decreases its hormone output to abnormally low levels. In **hypersecretion,** the gland increases its output to abnormally high levels.

LO 4. **Compare the mechanisms of action of hormones that work through second messengers with those of steroid hormones.**

- Hormones are transported to **target tissues** by the blood. They stimulate the target tissue to change some metabolic activity. Protein hormones bind to **receptors** on the plasma membrane of target cells. These hormones act as **first messengers,** and they activate **second messengers,** such as calcium ions or **cyclic AMP.** The second messenger can trigger a chain of molecular events leading to the actual response.
- Steroid hormones and thyroid hormones enter target cells and combine with receptors within the cytoplasm or nucleus. The steroid-receptor complex moves into the nucleus and activates (or represses) specific genes.

LO 5. **Justify the reputation of the hypothalamus as the link between nervous and endocrine systems. (Describe the mechanisms by which the hypothalamus exerts its control.)**

- The **hypothalamus** secretes two hormones that are stored and released by the **posterior lobe** of the **pituitary gland.** The hypothalamus also secretes **releasing hormones** and **inhibiting hormones** that regulate the **anterior lobe** of the pituitary gland.

LO 6. **Compare the functions of the posterior and anterior lobes of the pituitary and describe the actions of their hormones.**

- The posterior lobe of the pituitary gland releases the hormones **oxytocin** and **ADH,** both produced by the hypothalamus. Oxytocin stimulates the uterus to contract and stimulates release of milk from the lactating breast. ADH promotes reabsorption of water by the kidney ducts.
- The anterior lobe of the pituitary gland releases growth hormone, prolactin, and several tropic hormones. **GH** stimulates growth by promoting protein synthesis. GH acts indirectly through **somatomedins.** GH is regulated by **GHRH** and **GHIH** from the hypothalamus.
- **Prolactin** stimulates milk production in the lactating breast. The **tropic hormones** include TSH, ACTH, and the gonadotropic hormones.

LO 7. **Summarize the actions of the thyroid hormones and draw a diagram illustrating how they are regulated.**

- The **thyroid hormones, T_3** and **T_4,** stimulate the rate of metabolism. A rise in thyroid hormone level in the blood inhibits secretion of **TSH** by the pituitary; a decrease stimulates TSH secretion.
- Extreme **hypothyroidism** in childhood may result in **cretinism. Goiter,** an abnormal enlargement of the thyroid gland, can result from either hyposecretion or hypersecretion of thyroid hormones.

LO = Learning Objective

LO 8. **Describe how the parathyroid and thyroid glands regulate calcium levels.**
 - The **parathyroid glands** secrete **PTH,** which increases calcium levels in the blood and tissue fluid. PTH stimulates release of calcium from bones, stimulates calcium conservation by the kidneys, and helps activate vitamin D. An increase in the calcium level inhibits PTH secretion; a decrease in the calcium level stimulates secretion.
 - When the calcium concentration is too high, the thyroid gland secretes **calcitonin,** a hormone that rapidly acts to inhibit calcium removal from bone.

LO 9. **Contrast the actions of insulin and glucagon and describe the effects of diabetes mellitus.**
 - The **islets of Langerhans** in the pancreas secrete **insulin** and **glucagon**—hormones that regulate the glucose concentration in the blood. Insulin, secreted by the **beta cells,** lowers the concentration of glucose in the blood; it stimulates cells to take in glucose and store it. Glucagon, secreted by the **alpha cells,** raises the blood glucose concentration; it stimulates the release of glucose from storage and manufacture of glucose from other nutrients.
 - **Diabetes mellitus** is the main disorder associated with pancreatic hormones. Type 2 diabetes is characterized by **insulin resistance** (insulin receptors on target cells cannot bind with insulin). In diabetes, cells cannot take up insulin from the blood. Cells turn to protein and fat for energy, and the lipid concentration increases in the blood.

LO 10. **Describe the role of the adrenal medulla in the body's responses to stress.**
 - **Stressors** are stimuli that disrupt the steady state of the body, putting the body in a state of **stress.** The **adrenal glands** consist of the adrenal medulla and the **adrenal cortex;** both glands release hormones that help the body cope with stress. The adrenal medulla releases **epinephrine** and **norepinephrine.** These hormones increase heart rate, blood pressure, metabolic rate, and strength of muscle contraction and reroute the blood to organs that need more blood in time of stress.

LO 11. **Identify the hormones secreted by the adrenal cortex and give the actions of glucocorticoids and mineralocorticoids.**
 - The adrenal cortex releases **glucocorticoids,** mainly **cortisol.** This hormone promotes glucose manufacture from other nutrients, thereby raising the blood glucose level. Cortisol provides backup to the adrenal medullary hormones.
 - The adrenal cortex also releases hormones called **mineralocorticoids.** The main one is **aldosterone,** which helps maintain sodium and potassium balance.
 - Stress stimulates the hypothalamus to secrete **CRF.** This hormone stimulates the anterior lobe of the pituitary to secrete **ACTH,** which regulates glucocorticoid and aldosterone secretion.

LO 12. **Describe the actions of hormones secreted by the pineal gland, thymus gland, and atrium of the heart.**
 - The **pineal gland** produces **melatonin,** which facilitates the onset of sleep and influences biological rhythms and the onset of sexual maturity.
 - The **thymus gland** produces **thymosin,** which plays a role in immune responses.
 - The atrium of the heart secretes **ANF,** which promotes sodium excretion and lowers blood pressure.

CHAPTER QUIZ

Fill in the Blank

1. Endocrine glands lack _____ and release _____.

2. A hormone may be defined as a _____.

3. Hormones combine with receptors on _____ cells.

4. The _____ serves as the link between nervous and endocrine systems.

5. The hormone _____ stimulates contraction of the uterus.

6. The hormone _____ stimulates milk production in the lactating breast.

7. Growth hormone is produced by the _____ _____.

8. Oxytocin is produced by the _____.

9. Oxytocin is stored and released by the _____ _____ when needed.

10. Hypersecretion of growth hormone during childhood may result in _____ _____.

11. The main function of the thyroid hormones is to stimulate _____.

12. In addition to the thyroid hormones, the thyroid gland produces a hormone called _____, which acts to _____.

13. A hormone that raises the level of sodium in the blood is _____.

14. Blood glucose concentration is lowered by the hormone _____ released from the pancreas.

15. Blood glucose concentration is raised by the hormone _____ released from the pancreas.

16. The adrenal medulla releases _____ and _____.

Multiple Choice

17. The following hormone is associated with the anterior lobe of the pituitary gland: a. oxytocin; b. glucagon; c. growth hormone; d. melatonin.

18. The following hormone is associated with the adrenal medulla: a. insulin; b. cortisol; c. aldosterone; d. norepinephrine.

19. The following hormone rapidly lowers blood calcium concentration: a. calcitonin; b. parathyroid hormone; c. aldosterone; d. cortisol.

20. The following is true about cAMP: a. it is a hormone; b. it is a neurohormone; c. it is a first messenger; d. it is a second messenger.

21. Hormones that stimulate other endocrine glands are referred to as: a. local hormones; b. tropic hormones; c. neurohormones; d. somatomedins.

22. John's physician tells him that the insulin receptors on his cells are not able to bind with insulin. The following is *not* true: a. John has insulin resistance; b. John's blood glucose level is likely to be low; c. John has type 2 diabetes; d. urinalysis would likely show glucose in the urine.

23. Which of the following pairs is *not* correct? a. cortisol/glucocorticoid; b. ACTH/tropic hormone; c. oxytocin/neurohormone; d. estrogens/mineralocorticoid.

REVIEW QUESTIONS

1. How do hormones recognize their target tissues? Compare the mode of action of a hormone such as cortisol with a larger hormone such as insulin. Draw diagrams to support your explanation.

2. List the hormones released by the anterior lobe of the pituitary gland and give their actions.

3. How is the thyroid gland regulated? Draw a diagram to illustrate your answer.

4. What are the actions of parathyroid hormone?

5. How are the parathyroid glands regulated? Draw a diagram to illustrate your answer.

6. Describe the actions of insulin and glucagon in maintaining a steady blood glucose level. Draw a diagram to illustrate your description.

7. How do the adrenal glands help the body cope with stress?

8. Label the diagram. (See Figure 9-1 to check your answers.).

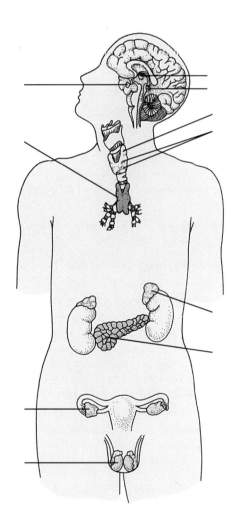

10 The Circulatory System: Blood

Chapter Outline

The **circulatory system** is the transportation system of the body. This system consists of two subsystems—the **cardiovascular** (kar′-dee-o-**vas**′-ku-lar) **system** and the **lymphatic** (lim-**fat**′-ik) **system.** In the cardiovascular system the **heart** pumps **blood** through a vast system of **blood vessels.** As it circulates, the blood transports nutrients, oxygen, hormones, and waste products. The lymphatic system helps preserve fluid balance and protects the body against disease. This chapter focuses on the blood.

THE CIRCULATORY SYSTEM PERFORMS CRITICAL FUNCTIONS

LEARNING OBJECTIVE

1. **List the functions of the circulatory system and describe the composition of blood.**

The circulatory system helps maintain homeostasis by transporting needed materials and maintaining fluid balance and acid-base balance. The circulatory system:

1. Transports nutrients from the digestive system to all of the cells
2. Transports oxygen from the lungs to all of the cells of the body
3. Transports carbon dioxide and other metabolic wastes from the cells to the excretory organs
4. Transports hormones from the endocrine glands to target tissues
5. Helps distribute metabolic heat within the body, which helps maintain a constant body temperature
6. Helps maintain fluid balance
7. Helps maintain acid-base balance
8. Protects the body against disease-causing organisms

Blood consists of red blood cells, white blood cells, and cell fragments called *platelets,* all suspended in a pale, yellowish fluid called *plasma* (Figure 10-1). In an adult weighing about 70 kg (154 lb), blood volume is normally about 5.6 L (about 6 qt). The normal pH of blood is slightly alkaline (ranging between 7.35 and 7.45).

Quiz Yourself

- What are some of the materials transported by the circulatory system?

PLASMA IS THE FLUID COMPONENT OF BLOOD

LEARNING OBJECTIVE

2. **Describe the composition of blood plasma and the functions of plasma proteins.**

Plasma (**plaz′**-muh) consists of about 92% water, about 7% protein, a sprinkling of salts, and many materials being transported, including oxygen and other dissolved gases, glucose and other nutrients, metabolic wastes, and hormones (Figure 10-2). Plasma is in dynamic equilibrium with the **interstitial fluid** (also called *tissue fluid*) bathing the cells and with the **intracellular fluid**—the fluid inside cells. As blood passes through the tiniest blood vessels (the capillaries), substances continuously move into and out of the plasma. Changes in its composition initiate responses on the part of one or more organs of the body to restore homeostasis.

Plasma contains several kinds of **plasma proteins,** each with specific properties and functions. Most of the plasma proteins are manufactured in the liver. Plasma proteins may be divided into three groups, or fractions: (1) **albumins,** (2) **globulins,** and (3) **fibrinogen** (fye-**brin′**-o-jen). Each fraction has specific properties.

Plasma proteins, especially albumins and globulins, help regulate the distribution of fluid between plasma and interstitial fluid. As blood flows through capillaries, some of the plasma seeps through the capillary walls and passes into the tissues. However, large protein molecules have difficulty passing through the capillary walls, so most of them remain in the blood. There they exert an osmotic force that helps pull plasma back into the blood. This action is important in maintaining an appropriate blood volume.

Plasma proteins (along with the hemoglobin in the red blood cells) are also important acid-base buffers. They help keep the pH of the blood within a narrow homeostatic range. **pH** is a measure of the acidity or alkalinity of a solution. pH

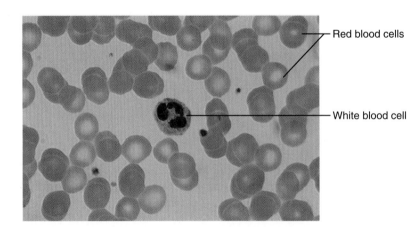

FIGURE 10-1 • Photomicrograph of blood. The cells shown are red blood cells except for one neutrophil, a type of white blood cell (magnified approximately 31,200×). (From Gartner LP, Hiatt JL: *Color textbook of histology,* ed 2, Philadelphia, 2001, WB Saunders.)

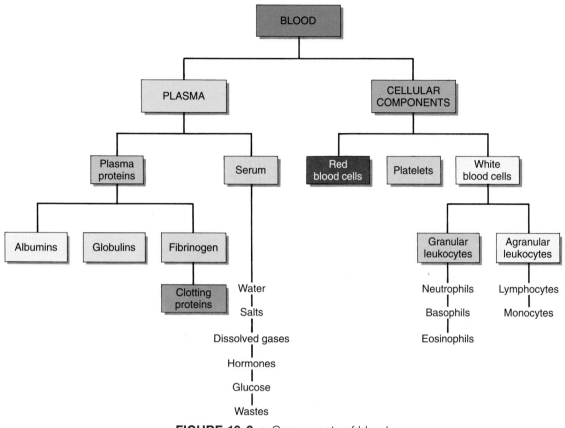

FIGURE 10-2 • Components of blood.

7 is considered neutral. A solution with a pH greater than 7 is considered alkaline (basic). A solution with a pH less than 7 is considered acidic.

Alpha globulins include certain hormones and proteins that transport hormones; *prothrombin,* a protein involved in blood clotting; and high-density *lipoproteins (HDL),* which transport fats and cholesterol. **Beta globulins** include other lipoproteins that transport fats and cholesterol, including low-density lipoproteins (LDL). Proteins that transport certain vitamins and minerals are also beta globulins.

The **gamma globulin** fraction contains antibodies that provide immunity to diseases such as measles and infectious hepatitis. Purified human gamma globulin is used to treat certain diseases or to reduce the probability of contracting a disease.

Fibrinogen and several other plasma proteins are involved in the clotting process. When the proteins involved in clotting have been removed from the plasma, the remaining liquid is called **serum.**

ⓠ Quiz Yourself

- What is the composition of plasma?
- What are the three fractions of plasma proteins?

RED BLOOD CELLS TRANSPORT OXYGEN

LEARNING OBJECTIVE

3. **Describe the structure, function, and life cycle of red blood cells.**

Red blood cells (RBCs), more formally called **erythrocytes** (eh-**rith′**-row-sites), are very small (about 7 mm in diameter and about 2 mm thick). About 3000 lined up end to end would span only about 1 inch! An adult male has about 30 trillion RBCs circulating in his blood. This amounts to more than 5 million per microliter (μL) (also expressed as cubic millimeters [mm³]). Females have slightly fewer.

RBCs are one of the most specialized cell types in the body. They are adapted for producing and packaging **hemoglobin**—the red pigment that transports oxygen. RBCs also transport carbon dioxide.

A mature RBC is a tiny, flexible, biconcave disk. (*Biconcave* means thinner in the center than around the edge.) An internal elastic framework maintains the disk shape and permits the cell to bend and twist as it passes through blood vessels even smaller than its own diameter. Its biconcave shape provides a high ratio of surface area to volume, allowing efficient diffusion of oxygen and carbon dioxide into and out of the cell.

When viewed under an ordinary light microscope, the center portion of the RBC appears relatively clear because the cytoplasm is thinnest there. A mature RBC lacks a nucleus and most other organelles.

As blood circulates through the lungs, oxygen diffuses into the blood and into the RBCs, where it combines weakly with hemoglobin to form **oxyhemoglobin.** When blood circulates through the brain or some other tissue where cells are low in oxygen, the reverse reaction occurs. The oxygen then diffuses out of the capillaries and into the cells. Oxyhemoglobin is bright red. It is responsible for the color of the oxygen-rich blood that flows through arteries. Hemoglobin that is not combined with oxygen is bluish in color and accounts for the darker appearance of venous blood.

In children, RBCs are produced in the **red bone marrow** of almost all bones. Recall that red bone marrow is a type of connective tissue found in spongy bone. In adults, red bone marrow is found only in certain bones, including the vertebrae, sternum, skull, ribs, and long bones. The red bone marrow has immature cells known as **stem cells,** which multiply, giving rise to the blood cells. (A stem cell is a relatively undifferentiated cell capable of repeated cell division. At each division, one of the daughter cells typically remains a stem cell, whereas the other cell may differentiate as a specific cell type.) After a 3- to 5-day maturation period, RBCs squeeze through the walls of capillaries within the bone marrow and enter the circulation.

The average circulating life span of a RBC is about 120 days. Without a nucleus and other organelles, it is unable to manufacture proteins. When its proteins break down, they cannot be replaced. The cell becomes fragile and may rupture as it squeezes through a tight channel in the circulation. Old or damaged cells are destroyed in the liver, spleen, or bone marrow. These RBCs are taken apart, and some of their components are recycled. Each second about 2.4 million RBCs wear out and are destroyed. New cells must be continuously manufactured to replace them. RBC production is regulated by the hormone **erythropoietin** (eh-rith′-row-**poy**′-ih-tin). This hormone is secreted by the kidneys in response to a decrease in oxygen concentration.

When production of new RBCs does not keep up with the rate of RBC destruction, the number of RBCs becomes deficient. With too few, there is a deficiency of hemoglobin. This condition is called **anemia** (ah-**nee**′-me-ah). With decreased amounts of hemoglobin, oxygen transport is reduced and cells do not receive enough oxygen.

Three general causes of anemia are (1) loss of blood as a result of hemorrhage or internal bleeding, (2) decreased production of hemoglobin or RBCs as in iron-deficiency anemia or pernicious anemia (which can be caused by vitamin B_{12} deficiency), and (3) increased rate of RBC destruction—the **hemolytic anemias,** such as sickle cell anemia. The most common cause of anemia is iron deficiency. Because iron is an essential ingredient of hemoglobin, the body cannot synthesize hemoglobin without it. That would be like trying to make a chocolate cake without chocolate.

WHITE BLOOD CELLS DEFEND THE BODY AGAINST DISEASE

LEARNING OBJECTIVE

4. **Compare the structure and functions of the main types of white blood cells.**

White blood cells (WBCs), or **leukocytes** (loo′-koe-sites), are specialized to protect the body against *pathogens*—harmful bacteria and other microorganisms that cause disease. WBCs develop from stem cells in the red bone marrow, but some types complete their maturation elsewhere in the body. Although RBCs function within the blood, many WBCs leave the circulation and perform their duties in various tissues. They move through the tissues, flowing along like amebas.

As they wander through the body, WBCs destroy bacteria and engulf dead cells and foreign matter. You may recall from Chapter 2 that **phagocytosis** (fag′-oh-sigh-**toe**′-sis) is the process by which cells engulf microorganisms, foreign particles, or other cells. Cells that are specialized to carry on phagocytosis are called **phagocytes.**

Five main types of WBCs are found in the circulating blood (Figure 10-3, Table 10-1). They can be classified as **granular leukocytes** or **agranular leukocytes.** The granular leukocytes have large, lobed nuclei and distinctive granules in their cytoplasm. The kinds of WBCs that contain granules are **neutrophils** (**noo**′-trow-fils), **basophils** (**bay**′-so-fils), and **eosinophils** (ee-o-**sin**′-o-fils).

Neutrophils are the main phagocytes in the blood (see Figure 10-1). These WBCs are adept at seeking out and ingesting bacteria. They also phagocytize dead cells—a cleanup task especially demanding after injury or infection. Most of the granules in neutrophils contain enzymes that digest ingested material.

Eosinophils have large granules that stain red with eosin, an acidic dye. The lysosomes of these WBCs contain enzymes that destroy viruses and bacteria. Some of their enzymes are especially toxic to parasitic worms. Eosinophils also play an important role in allergic reactions.

Basophils exhibit deep-blue granules when stained with basic dyes. Like eosinophils, these cells play a role in allergic reactions. Granules in their cytoplasm contain **histamine,** a substance that dilates blood vessels and makes capillaries more permeable. Basophils release histamine in injured tissues and in allergic responses. Other basophil granules contain **heparin,** an anticoagulant that helps prevent blood from clotting inappropriately within the blood vessels.

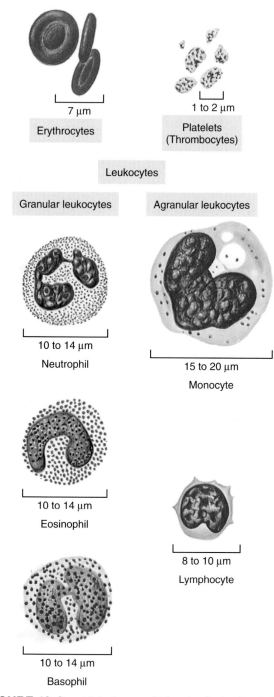

FIGURE 10-3 • Main types of blood cells in circulating blood.

Agranular WBCs have no specific granules in their cytoplasm, and their nuclei are rounded or kidney shaped. Two types of agranular leukocytes are **lymphocytes** (**lim′**-foe-sites) and **monocytes** (**mon′**-oh-sites). Some lymphocytes are specialized to produce antibodies. Others attack bacteria or viruses directly. Monocytes migrate into the connective tissues and develop into **macrophages** (**mak′**-row-faje-es)—the large scavenger cells of the body. These cells are further discussed in Chapter 13.

WBCs are far less numerous than RBCs (only about 1 WBCs to every 700 RBCs). Normally, an adult has about 7000 WBCs/mm^3 of blood. A WBC count elevated above 10,000/mm^3 may indicate the presence of bacterial infection. *Leukemia* is a form of cancer in which any one of the several types of WBCs multiply wildly within the bone marrow. They crowd out developing RBCs and platelets, leading to anemia and impaired blood clotting.

> **Quiz Yourself**
> - What are the functions of neutrophils?
> - What are agranular white blood cells?

PLATELETS FUNCTION IN BLOOD CLOTTING

LEARNING OBJECTIVE

5. **Describe the structure and function of platelets and summarize the chemical events of blood clotting.**

Platelets, also called **thrombocytes** (**throm′**-bow-sites), are not really cells. They are tiny fragments of cytoplasm that are pinched off of certain very large cells in the bone marrow. There are about 300,000 platelets/mm^3 of circulating blood! These cell fragments prevent blood loss. When a blood vessel is cut, it constricts, reducing blood loss. Platelets stick to the rough, cut edges of the blood vessel, forming a **platelet plug** that seals the hole in the blood vessel wall. A complex series of chemical reactions produces tiny fibers that reinforce the platelets, forming a strong clot.

Although the process of blood clotting is quite complex, involving more than 30 different chemical substances, we can summarize its three main steps (Figure 10-4):

1. Platelets and injured tissue release substances that activate **clotting factors** in the blood. A series of reactions takes place that result in formation of an enzyme known as **prothrombin** (pro-**throm′**-bin) **activator.**
2. Prothrombin activator catalyzes the conversion of **prothrombin** to its active form—**thrombin.** Calcium ions and clotting factors must be present for prothrombin to be converted to thrombin. Prothrombin, a globulin found in the plasma, is manufactured in the liver with the help of vitamin K.
3. In the presence of calcium ions, thrombin acts as an enzyme that converts the plasma protein fibrinogen to **fibrin**—a fibrous protein that forms long threads. These fibrin threads form the webbing of the clot. They trap blood cells, platelets, and plasma, which help to strengthen the clot.

Within a few minutes after clot formation, the clot begins to contract and squeezes out serum (plasma that contains no fibrinogen or clotting factors). As the clot contracts, the ends

TABLE 10-1 **CELLULAR COMPONENTS OF BLOOD**

Blood Component	Normal Range	Function	Pathology
Red blood cells (RBCs)	Male: 4.2–5.4 million/μL Female: 3.6–5.0 million/μL	Oxygen transport; carbon dioxide transport	Too few: anemia Too many: polycythemia
Platelets	150,000–400,000/μL	Essential for clotting	Clotting malfunctions; bleeding; easy bruising
White blood cells (WBCs)	5000–10,000/μL		
Neutrophils	About 60% of WBCs	Phagocytosis	Too many: may be the result of bacterial infection, inflammation, leukemia (myelogenous)
Eosinophils	1%–3% of WBCs	Play role in allergic reactions; destroy viruses, bacteria, and parasitic worms	Too many: may result from allergic reaction, parasitic infestation
Basophils	1% of WBCs	Play role in allergic reactions and in prevention of inappropriate clotting	
Lymphocytes	25%–35% of WBCs	Produce antibodies; destroy foreign cells	Atypical lymphocytes present in infectious mononucleosis; too many: may be the result of lymphocytic leukemia, certain viral infections
Monocytes	6% of WBCs	Differentiate to form macrophages	May increase in monocytic leukemia and fungal infections

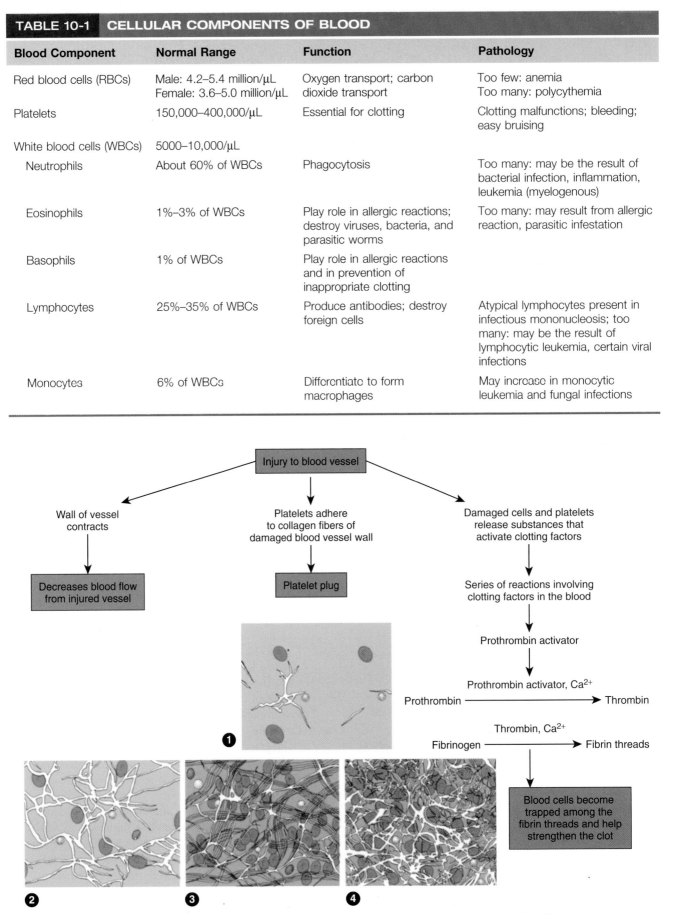

FIGURE 10-4 • Overview of blood clotting. Fibrin threads form the webbing of the clot. Blood cells, platelets, and plasma become trapped among the fibrin threads and help strengthen the clot.

of the damaged blood vessel are pulled closer together and the clot itself becomes smaller and harder.

Quiz Yourself

- What are platelets? What is their function?
- What are three main steps in blood clotting?

SUCCESSFUL BLOOD TRANSFUSIONS DEPEND ON BLOOD GROUPS

LEARNING OBJECTIVES

6. **Identify the antigen and antibody associated with each ABO blood type and explain why blood types must be carefully matched in transfusion therapy.**
7. **Identify the cause and importance of Rh incompatibility.**

Blood transfusions, the transfer of blood cells, platelets, or plasma from healthy **donors** to **recipients** in need of blood, are routine, lifesaving procedures. Whole blood or blood components can be stored in blood banks and withdrawn as needed. When blood loss occurs, whole blood can be transfused to restore an adequate volume of circulating blood. Blood components can be separated by centrifuging (spinning the blood at high speed so that the heavier components settle at the bottom of a tube). Then, platelets and other specific components of blood can be transfused. Plasma can be used to expand blood volume in patients who are in circulatory shock (discussed in Chapter 12).

Before transfusing blood, the blood of the donor and recipient must be carefully matched. If the blood is not compatible, a *transfusion reaction* will occur. This is a serious allergic reaction in which antibodies in the recipient's blood attack the foreign RBCs in the transfused blood, causing them to **agglutinate** (clump). RBCs may rupture, releasing hemoglobin into the plasma—a process known as **hemolysis** (he-**mol′**-ih-sis).

The ABO Blood Groups Are Based on Antigens A and B

Although several blood groups are known, the most important clinically are the ABO and Rh groups. Blood types are inherited. Each of us has either type A, B, AB, or O blood (Table 10-2). RBCs have specific proteins called **antigens** (**an′**-tih-jens) on their surfaces. (These antigens are also called *agglutinogens*.) The antigens are different in persons with different blood types (Figure 10-5).

The RBCs of individuals with type A blood have type A antigen. Individuals with type B blood have type B antigen, and those with type AB blood have both kinds of antigen—A and B. Individuals with type O blood have neither type of

TABLE 10-2	**ABO BLOOD TYPES**	
Blood Type	Antigen on RBC	Antibodies in Plasma
O	—	Anti-A, anti-B
A	A	Anti-B
B	B	Anti-A
AB	A, B	—

antigen on their RBCs. They are referred to as **universal donors** because, theoretically, they can donate blood to patients with any blood type.

Certain **antibodies** (also called *agglutinins*) are found in the plasma. Antibodies are specific proteins that recognize and bind to specific antigens. Individuals with type A blood have anti-B antibodies circulating in their blood. Those with type B blood have anti-A antibodies. Persons with type AB blood have neither type of antibody, and those with type O blood have both types.

Each type of antibody recognizes a specific type of antigen. For example, if a patient with type A blood is accidentally given type B blood, his anti-B antibodies will combine with the type B antigens on the surfaces of the donated RBCs. This causes the donated cells to agglutinate, resulting in hemolysis. Such mismatching can be fatal, especially if the mistake is ever repeated.

Blood typing is routinely carried out by mixing a sample of a person's blood with serum containing different types of antibodies to determine whether agglutination occurs. Because individuals with type AB blood do not have antibodies to either type A or type B blood, they are referred to as **universal recipients.** Theoretically, they can safely receive blood of any ABO type. In practice, however, whenever possible, recipients are transfused with donor blood that matches their blood type.

The Rh System Consists of Several Rh Antigens

The Rh system consists of more than 40 kinds of Rh antigens, each referred to as an **Rh factor.** By far the most important of these factors is **antigen D.** Most persons of Western European descent are Rh positive, which means that they have antigen D on the surfaces of their RBCs (as well as the antigens of the ABO system appropriate to their blood type). The 15% or so of the population who are Rh negative have no antigen D on their RBC surfaces. Unlike the antibodies of the ABO system, antibody D does not occur in the blood of Rh-negative persons unless they have been exposed to antigen D. However, once antibodies to Rh blood have been produced, they remain in the blood.

Although several kinds of maternal-fetal blood-type incompatibilities are known, *Rh incompatibility* is the most serious.

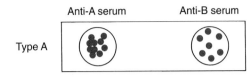

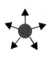
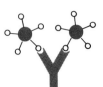

Anti-A serum   Anti-B serum

Type A

Type A RBC

Antibody in
anti-A serum

Agglutination

(A) Type A blood has type A antigen; it agglutinates when mixed
with anti-A serum (serum containing antibodies to type A blood).

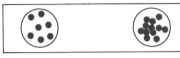

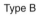
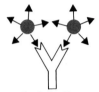

Type B

Type B RBC

Antibody in
anti-B serum

Agglutination

(B) Type B blood has type B antigen; it agglutinates when mixed
with anti-B serum (serum containing antibodies to type B blood).

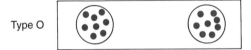

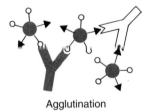

Type AB

Type AB RBC

Agglutination

(C) Type AB blood has both type A and type B antigens; it agglutinates
when mixed with serum containing antibodies to type A or type B blood.

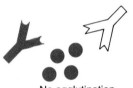

Type O

Type O RBC

No agglutination

(D) Type O blood has neither type A nor type B antigens; it does not agglutinate
when mixed with serum containing antibodies to type A or type B blood.

FIGURE 10-5 • Typing blood. Each blood type has a different combination of antigen and
antibody. In typing blood, serum containing antibody to type A blood is placed on one area
of a slide and serum containing antibody to type B is placed on another area of the slide.
A drop of blood is mixed with each type of serum. If the blood contains A antigen, it will
agglutinate with the anti-A serum. If the blood contains B antigen, it will agglutinate with the
anti-B serum.

When an Rh-negative woman and an Rh-positive man produce
an Rh-positive baby, the mother may be exposed to antigen
D. Although the baby's and the mother's blood do not ordinarily mix during fetal development, during the birth process
a small amount of the baby's blood may mix with the mother's
blood. This contact stimulates the mother to produce antibodies against the Rh-positive blood.

If the mother carries an Rh-positive child in a subsequent
pregnancy, her antibodies can cross the placenta (the organ of
exchange between mother and developing baby) and cause
hemolysis of the baby's RBCs, causing hemolytic anemia
(Figure 10-6). The baby's ability to transport oxygen is reduced,

and breakdown products of the hemoglobin released into the
circulation can damage organs, including the brain. Severe
cases of this condition are called *erythroblastosis fetalis* (ee-rith-
row-blas-**tow'**-sis fee-**tal'**-is).

🌀 *Quiz Yourself*

- A student has type AB blood. What type of antigens does she have on her RBCs. What type of
  antibodies in her blood serum?
- What causes Rh incompatibility?

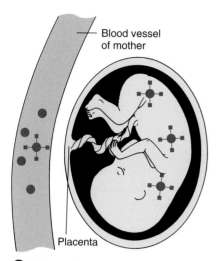
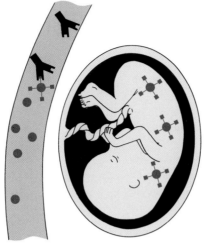
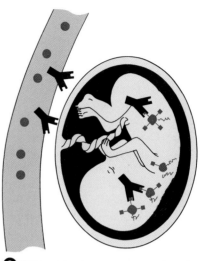

Blood vessel of mother

Placenta

❶ A few Rh⁺ RBCs leak across the placenta from the fetus into the mother's blood

❷ The mother produces anti-Rh antibodies in response to Rh antigen on Rh⁺ RBCs

❸ If the woman becomes pregnant again with an Rh⁺ fetus, serious problems can develop. Some of the mother's anti-Rh antibodies cross the placenta and enter the blood of the fetus, causing hemolysis. This Rh incompatibility can cause hemolytic anemia and erythroblastosis fetalis.

● Rh⁻ RBC of mother

✛ Rh⁺ RBC of fetus with Rh antigen on surface

➤ Anti-Rh antibody made against Rh⁺ RBC

✻ Hemolysis of Rh⁺ RBC

FIGURE 10-6 • Rh incompatibility can cause serious problems when an Rh-negative woman and an Rh-positive man produce Rh-positive offspring.

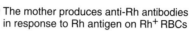

SUMMARY

LO 1. List the functions of the circulatory system and describe the composition of blood.
- The circulatory system transports nutrients, oxygen, wastes, and hormones; helps maintain body temperature, fluid balance, and acid-base balance; and protects the body against pathogens.
- Blood consists of red blood cells, white blood cells, and platelets suspended in plasma.

LO 2. Describe the composition of blood plasma and the functions of plasma proteins.
- Blood **plasma** consists of water, plasma proteins, salts, nutrients, oxygen and other gases, hormones, and wastes. Plasma is in dynamic equilibrium with the **interstitial fluid** that bathes the cells and with the **intracellular fluid** inside cells. Three fractions of **plasma proteins** are **albumins, globulins,** and **fibrinogen.**

LO = Learning Objective

- Plasma proteins exert an osmotic force that helps maintain appropriate blood volume. They also help maintain appropriate pH.
- **Alpha globulins** and **beta globulins** include lipoproteins that transport fats and cholesterol.
- **Gamma globulins** are **antibodies** that provide immunity to disease.

LO 3. Describe the structure, function, and life cycle of red blood cells.
- **Red blood cells (RBCs),** or **erythrocytes,** are tiny, biconcave disks that contain **hemoglobin**—the red pigment that transports oxygen and carbon dioxide. Oxygen combines weakly with hemoglobin to form **oxyhemoglobin.**
- RBCs develop from **stem cells** in the **red bone marrow.** RBCs lack a nucleus and other organelles; their life span is only about 120 days.
- The hormone **erythropoietin,** produced by the kidneys, regulates RBC production.

- **Anemia,** a deficiency in hemoglobin, can be caused by loss of blood, decreased hemoglobin or RBC production (e.g., iron-deficiency anemia), or increased RBC destruction (**hemolytic anemia**).

LO 4. **Compare the structure and functions of the main types of white blood cells.**
- **White blood cells (WBCs),** or **leukocytes,** defend the body against pathogens and other foreign substances. **Granular leukocytes** include the neutrophils, eosinophils, and basophils.
- **Neutrophils** are the main **phagocytes** in the blood. They engulf bacteria, foreign matter, and dead cells. **Eosinophils** destroy pathogens, especially parasitic worms. Eosinophils and **basophils** are important during allergic reactions. Basophils release **histamine,** a substance that dilates blood vessels and makes capillaries more permeable. They also release **heparin,** an anticoagulant.
- **Agranular leukocytes** include the lymphocytes and monocytes.
- Some **lymphocytes** produce antibodies. Others attack viruses or bacteria directly. **Monocytes** develop into **macrophages**—large phagocytic cells.

LO 5. **Describe the structure and function of platelets and summarize the chemical events of blood clotting.**
- **Platelets** are cell fragments that pinch off from large cells in the bone marrow; they function in blood clotting. Platelets patch tears in blood vessel walls by forming a **platelet plug.**
- Platelets also release **clotting factors** that activate **prothrombin activator.** This enzyme converts **prothrombin** to **thrombin.** Prothrombin is produced in the liver with the help of vitamin K.
- Thrombin converts **fibrinogen** to **fibrin.**

LO 6. **Identify the antigen and antibody associated with each ABO blood type and explain why blood types must be carefully matched in transfusion therapy.**
- A **blood transfusion** is the transfer of blood from a **donor** to a **recipient.**
- Blood is typed on the basis of specific **antigens** (specific proteins) on the surfaces of RBCs. When blood is not carefully matched, antibodies in the recipient's blood attack RBCs in the transfused blood, causing them to **agglutinate,** or clump. This can result in **hemolysis**—in which RBCs rupture, releasing hemoglobin.
- Each type of antibody recognizes a specific antigen. Individuals with type A blood have type A antigen and anti-B antibodies. Individuals with type B blood have type B antigen and anti-A antibodies. People with type AB blood have both types of antigens and no antibodies to A or B blood. They are referred to as **universal recipients** because they can receive blood of any ABO type. Individuals with type O blood have neither type of antigen but both types of antibodies. They are **universal donors.**

LO 7. **Identify the cause and importance of Rh incompatibility.**
- People with Rh-positive blood have antigen D, the most important Rh factor, on the surface of their RBCs. Rh-negative individuals may produce antibodies to antigen D when exposed to Rh-positive blood. When an Rh-negative woman gives birth to an Rh-positive baby, anti-D antibodies may develop. Rh incompatibility can then occur in future pregnancies.

CHAPTER QUIZ

Fill in the Blank

1. The function of red blood cells is to transport _____.

2. The liquid portion of the blood is called _____.

3. Some of the gamma globulins serve as _____.

4. Fibrinogen functions in blood _____.

5. Red blood cells are produced in the _____ _____ _____.

6. A deficiency of hemoglobin is called _____.

7. The function of neutrophils is to _____.

8. _____ patch damaged blood vessels.

9. Fibrinogen is converted to _____ by an enzyme called _____.

10. A person with type B blood has type _____ antigens on the surfaces of his red blood cells and _____ antibodies in his plasma.

11. Hemolytic anemia in the newborn may occur when there is _____ incompatibility. This may occur when a woman with _____ blood produces a baby with _____ blood.

Multiple Choice

12. Which of the following produce antibodies? a. basophils; b. neutrophils; c. monocytes; d. lymphocytes.

13. Prothrombin: a. is produced in the bone marrow; b. production requires vitamin K; c. is a clotting factor; d. is released by platelets.

14. An individual with type B blood: a. has anti-A antibodies; b. has anti-B antibodies; c. has type A antigen and type B antigen; d. will have hemolysis if transfused with Rh blood.

15. The following is *least* likely to cause a problem: a. a woman with type AB blood who is transfused with type O blood; b. a man with type B blood who is transfused with type AB blood; c. a woman with Rh-negative blood who gives birth to her second child with Rh-positive blood; d. a man with Rh-negative blood who is transfused with blood that has antigen D.

REVIEW QUESTIONS

1. List six functions of the circulatory system and identify which specific blood components carry out each job.

2. What are the functions of the plasma proteins as a group? Of globulins specifically?

3. In what ways are mature red blood cells adapted to perform their function?

4. What are the functions of platelets? Explain.

5. Imagine that a patient with type AB blood is accidentally given type A blood in a transfusion. What, if any, ill effects may occur? What if a patient with type O blood is given type A blood?

6. What happens when an Rh-negative woman has Rh-positive children?

11 The Circulatory System: The Heart

Chapter Outline

The heart is a hollow, muscular organ not much bigger than a fist. It weighs less than a pound. In an average lifetime, the heart pumps about 300 million liters (80 million gallons) of blood through the complex of blood vessels that bring oxygen and nutrients to the cells of the body. Depending on the body's needs, the heart can vary its output from 5 to 35 liters of blood per minute.

THE HEART WALL CONSISTS OF THREE LAYERS

LEARNING OBJECTIVE

1. **Locate the heart and describe the structure of its wall.**

The **heart** is located in the thorax between the lungs. About two thirds of this cone-shaped organ lies to the left of the body's midline. When you place your fingers on the left side of the chest between the fifth and sixth ribs, you can feel the heart pulsate each time it beats.

The wall of the heart is richly supplied with nerves, blood vessels, and lymph vessels. From the inside out, the layers of the heart are the endocardium, myocardium, and pericardium.

1. The **endocardium** (en′-doe-**kar**′-dee-um) consists of a smooth endothelial lining resting on connective tissue.
2. By far the greatest bulk of the heart wall consists of **myocardium** (my′-oh-**kar**′-dee-um), the cardiac muscle that contracts to pump the blood.
3. The outer layer of the heart is the **epicardium** (ep-ih-**kar**′-dee-um), also referred to as the **visceral pericardium** (per-ih-**kar**′-dee-um). The visceral pericardium is the inner layer of the two-layered **pericardium.** The two layers are separated by a potential space, the **pericardial cavity.** The outer layer, the **parietal pericardium,** forms a strong sac for the heart and helps to anchor it within the thorax.

Quiz Yourself

- Which layer of the heart wall is thickest?
- Which is the outer layer of the heart?

THE HEART HAS FOUR CHAMBERS

LEARNING OBJECTIVE

2. **Identify the chambers of the heart and compare their functions.**

The heart is a double pump. The right and left sides of the heart are completely separated by a wall or **septum.** The heart has four chambers: a **right atrium** and **right ventricle** and a **left atrium** and **left ventricle** (Figures 11-1 through 11-3). The atria receive blood returning to the heart from the veins and act as reservoirs between contractions of the heart. The ventricles pump blood into the great arteries leaving the heart.

The right atrium receives oxygen-poor blood (blood somewhat depleted of its oxygen supply) returning from the tissues,

and the right ventricle pumps it into the **pulmonary circulation**—the system of blood vessels that connect the heart and lungs. Pulmonary arteries carry blood to the lungs, where gases are exchanged. Pulmonary veins then return oxygen-rich blood to the left atrium. The left ventricle pumps oxygen-rich blood into the **aorta**—a large artery of the **systemic circulation,** the network of blood vessels that delivers blood to all the body systems. The sequence of blood flow through the heart is as follows:

> Right atrium → right ventricle → through pulmonary circulation → left atrium → left ventricle → through systemic circulation

The wall between the atria is the **interatrial septum.** The wall between the ventricles is the **interventricular septum.** A small, muscular pouch called the **auricle** (**aw**′-reh-kle) increases the surface area of each atrium. It can be seen at the upper surface of each atrium in Figure 11-1. Irregular muscle columns project from the inner surface of both ventricles.

Quiz Yourself

- What is the function of the atria? Of the ventricles?
- What is the interventricular septum?

VALVES PREVENT BACKFLOW OF BLOOD

LEARNING OBJECTIVE

3. **Locate the atrioventricular and semilunar valves and compare their structure.**

When blood is pumped from either atrium into the corresponding ventricle, pressure in the ventricle becomes greater than in the atrium. When the atrium relaxes, blood must be prevented from flowing backward into it. To prevent such backflow of blood, an **atrioventricular** (a′-tree-o-ven-**trik**′-u-lar) **(AV) valve** guards the passageway between each atrium and ventricle (Figures 11-3 and 11-4). The AV valves consist of flaps, or cusps, of fibrous tissues that project from the heart wall. The AV valves are held in place by connective tissue cords called *chordae tendineae*, popularly referred to as the "heart strings." The chordeae tendineae attach the valves to the **papillary** (**pap**′-il-ler-ee) **muscles,** which project from the walls of the ventricles.

The AV valve between the right atrium and the right ventricle has three cusps and is called the **tricuspid** (try-**kus**′-pid) **valve.** The left AV valve, with only two cusps, is the **bicuspid** (bi-**kus**′-pid) **valve,** but it is commonly known as the **mitral** (**my**′-tril) **valve.** *Mitral stenosis,* a narrowing of the opening of

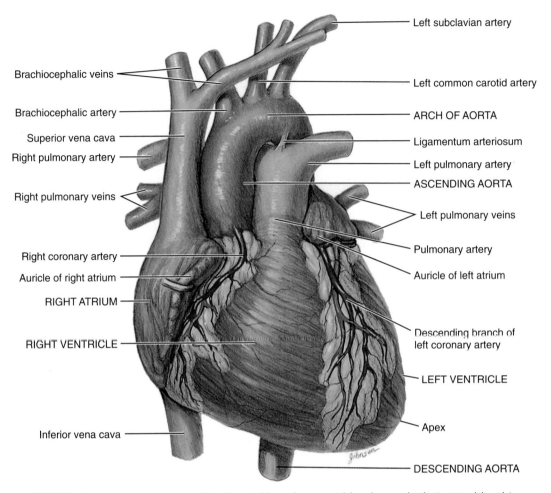

Left subclavian artery

Brachiocephalic veins

Brachiocephalic artery

Superior vena cava

Right pulmonary artery

Right pulmonary veins

Right coronary artery

Auricle of right atrium

RIGHT ATRIUM

RIGHT VENTRICLE

Inferior vena cava

Left common carotid artery

ARCH OF AORTA

Ligamentum arteriosum

Left pulmonary artery

ASCENDING AORTA

Left pulmonary veins

Pulmonary artery

Auricle of left atrium

Descending branch of left coronary artery

LEFT VENTRICLE

Apex

DESCENDING AORTA

FIGURE 11-1 • Anterior view of the heart. Note the great blood vessels that carry blood to and from the heart. (From Guyton AC: *Anatomy and physiology,* Philadelphia, 1985, Saunders College Publishing.)

the mitral valve, is a common valve deformity. In this condition, the valve is thickened and slows the flow of blood from the left atrium into the left ventricle. The heart must work harder to pump blood through the narrow opening. The most common cause of mitral stenosis is rheumatic fever inflammation. Diseased valves can be surgically removed and replaced with artificial valves.

Valves also guard the exits from the ventricles. The three cusps of each **semilunar** (sem-ee-loo′-nar) **valve** are shaped like half-moons. The semilunar valve between the left ventricle and the aorta is known as the **aortic** (ay-or′-tik) **semilunar valve,** and the one between the right ventricle and the pulmonary artery is the **pulmonary semilunar valve.**

THE HEART HAS ITS OWN BLOOD VESSELS

LEARNING OBJECTIVE

4. **Identify the principal blood vessels that serve the heart wall.**

Although the heart is filled with blood, its wall is so thick that oxygen and nutrients cannot effectively diffuse to all of its cells. Blood vessels must deliver oxygen and nutrients to the hard-working cardiac muscle in the heart wall. The right and left **coronary arteries** branch off from the aorta (the large artery that receives blood from the left ventricle) as it leaves the heart (see Figure 11-1). Branches of the two coronary arteries bring blood to all the tissue of the heart. After passing through capillaries in the heart wall, blood flows through **coronary veins.** These veins join to form a large vein, the **coronary sinus,** which empties into the right atrium.

Coronary artery disease (CAD), a leading cause of death in the United States, develops when the coronary arteries or

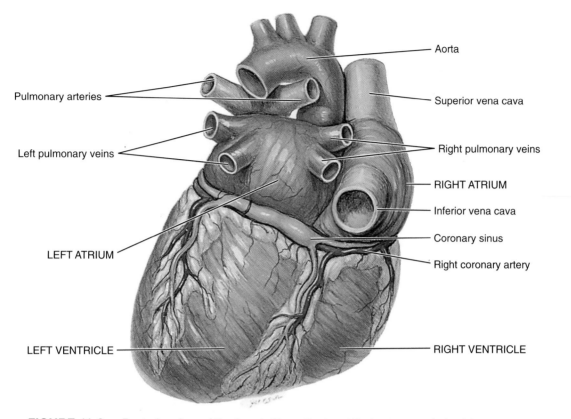

FIGURE 11-2 • Posterior view of the heart. (From Guyton AC: *Anatomy and physiology,* Philadelphia, 1985, Saunders College Publishing.)

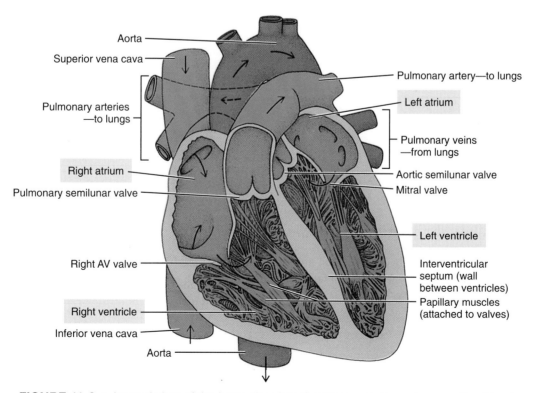

FIGURE 11-3 • Internal view of the heart showing chambers, valves, and connecting blood vessels. *Arrows* indicate the direction of blood flow.

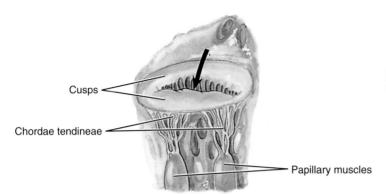

Cusps

Chordae tendineae

Papillary muscles

(A) Mitral valve open. When the atria contract, the mitral valve opens and blood flows from the left atrium into the left ventricle.

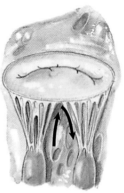

(B) Mitral valve closed. When the ventricles contract, blood is forced against the valve cusps, closing the valve. The papillary muscles contract, tightening the chordae tendineae. This prevents the cusps of the AV valve from opening backward into the atrium when blood pushes against them.

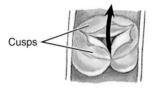

Cusps

(C) Semilunar valve open. When the pressure in the ventricle is higher than the pressure in the aorta (or pulmonary artery), the semilunar valve opens, allowing blood to flow from the ventricle into the artery.

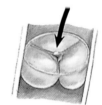

(D) Semilunar valve closed. The semilunar valves close when the ventricles relax and their pressure falls below that of the artery. The backflow of blood fills the cusps and closes them. Their upper edges fit tightly together preventing blood from flowing backward into the ventricle.

FIGURE 11-4 • How the valves of the heart work.

their branches become thickened or blocked, reducing blood flow. There are many causes of CAD. When a branch of a coronary artery becomes blocked, blood flow to part of the cardiac muscle is decreased or even halted. The affected cardiac muscle becomes **ischemic,** or lacking in blood supply. The tissue is deprived of an adequate supply of oxygen and nutrients. This condition can lead to a **myocardial infarction (MI),** commonly known as a heart attack.

Quiz Yourself

- Which arteries deliver blood to the heart wall?
- What is the function of the coronary sinus?

THE CONDUCTION SYSTEM CONSISTS OF SPECIALIZED CARDIAC MUSCLE

LEARNING OBJECTIVE

5. Trace the path of an electrical impulse through the conduction system of the heart.

You may have viewed horror films in which a heart beats spookily after being separated from the body of its owner. Some scriptwriters may have rooted their fantasies in a knowledge of cardiac physiology. When removed from the body, the heart can continue to beat for many hours if it is provided with appropriate nutrients and salts. This is possible because the heart has its own specialized **conduction system** and can beat independently of its nerve supply.

The heart's conduction system includes the sinoatrial node, the atrioventricular node, and the atrioventricular bundle (Figure 11-5). Each heartbeat is initiated by the **sinoatrial (SA) node** (sie-no-**ay**′-tree-al), or **pacemaker**—a small mass of specialized muscle in the posterior wall of the right atrium. The SA node generates electrical impulses (action potentials) 70 to 80 times each minute.

The ends of the fibers of the SA node fuse with surrounding ordinary muscle fibers of the atrium, so the muscle impulse spreads through the atria, producing atrial contraction. One group of atrial muscle fibers conducts the electrical impulse directly to the **atrioventricular (AV) node,** located in the right atrium along the lower part of the septum. Here, transmission of the impulse is delayed briefly. This delay allows the atria to complete their contraction before the ventricles begin to contract.

From the AV node the impulse spreads into specialized muscle fibers that form the **atrioventricular (AV) bundle** (also called the *bundle of His*). These large fibers conduct impulses about six times faster than ordinary cardiac muscle fibers. The AV bundle divides into right and left bundle branches, which extend into the right and left ventricles. Fibers of the bundle branches divide into smaller branches ending in terminal fibers known as **Purkinje** (per-**kin**′-jee) **fibers.** The Purkinje fibers end on fibers of ordinary cardiac muscle within the myocardium, and the impulse spreads through the ventricles.

Cardiac muscle fibers are joined at their ends by dense bands called **intercalated disks.** These tight junctions between the muscle cells allow the impulse to pass rapidly from cell to cell. The entire atrium or ventricle contracts as if it were one giant cell.

In summary, the pathway taken by an electrical impulse through the heart is as follows:

> SA node → cardiac muscle of atria (atria contract) → AV node → AV bundle → right and left branches → Purkinje fibers → ordinary muscle fibers of ventricles (ventricles contract)

THE CARDIAC CYCLE INCLUDES CONTRACTION AND RELAXATION PHASES

LEARNING OBJECTIVE

6. **Describe the events of the cardiac cycle and correlate them with normal heart sounds.**

The events that occur during one complete heartbeat make up the **cardiac cycle.** Each complete cycle lasts for about 0.8 second and occurs about 72 times per minute. It consists of a contraction in which blood is forced out of the heart and then a relaxation in which the heart fills with blood. The period of

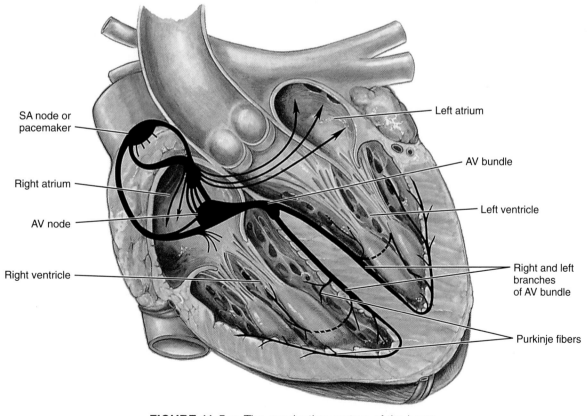

FIGURE 11-5 • The conduction system of the heart.

contraction is known as **systole** (sis'-tow-lee); the period of relaxation is **diastole** (dye-**as'**-tow'-lee).

Each cardiac cycle begins with an electrical impulse that spreads from the SA node throughout the atria, resulting in the contraction of the atria. As the atria contract, the AV valves are open and blood is forced from the atria into the ventricles. As this happens, the semilunar valves are closed (Figure 11-6).

As the atria relax, they are filled with blood from the veins. During this time, the AV valves are closed and the ventricles are contracting, forcing blood through the semilunar valves into the arteries. Then, as the ventricles begin to relax, the semilunar valves close and the AV valves open. Blood flows into the ventricles, and the cycle begins again.

While the atria are contracting, the ventricles are relaxed. Then the atria relax while the ventricles contract. The atria remain relaxed during the first part of ventricular relaxation.

As each wave of contraction spreads through the heart, electrical currents flow into the tissues surrounding the heart and onto the body surface. By placing electrodes on the body surface on opposite sides of the heart, the electrical activity can be amplified and recorded either by an oscilloscope or an electrocardiograph. The written record produced is called an **electrocardiogram** (**ECG** or **EKG**). Abnormalities in the ECG indicate disorders in the heart or its rhythm.

When you listen to the heart through a stethoscope, you can hear certain characteristic sounds, usually described as a "lub-dup." These sounds are produced each time the valves

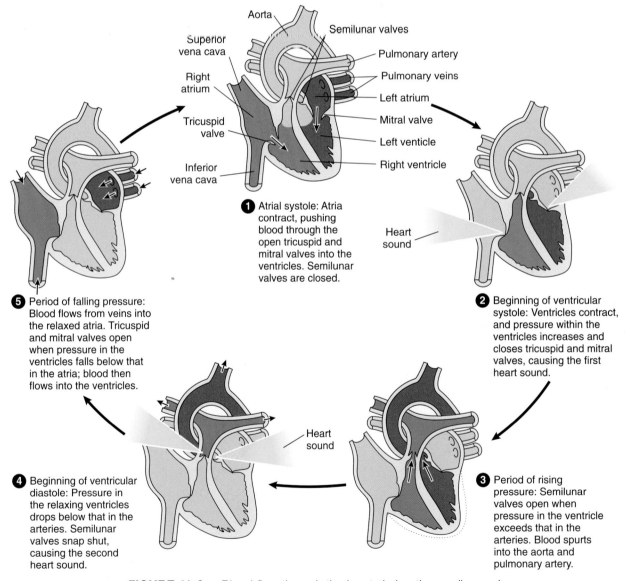

1 Atrial systole: Atria contract, pushing blood through the open tricuspid and mitral valves into the ventricles. Semilunar valves are closed.

2 Beginning of ventricular systole: Ventricles contract, and pressure within the ventricles increases and closes tricuspid and mitral valves, causing the first heart sound.

3 Period of rising pressure: Semilunar valves open when pressure in the ventricle exceeds that in the arteries. Blood spurts into the aorta and pulmonary artery.

4 Beginning of ventricular diastole: Pressure in the relaxing ventricles drops below that in the arteries. Semilunar valves snap shut, causing the second heart sound.

5 Period of falling pressure: Blood flows from veins into the relaxed atria. Tricuspid and mitral valves open when pressure in the ventricles falls below that in the atria; blood then flows into the ventricles.

FIGURE 11-6 • Blood flow through the heart during the cardiac cycle.

close. The first sound, the "lub," marks the beginning of ventricular systole (contraction). Heard as a low-pitched, relatively long sound, it is caused by the closure of the AV valves as the ventricles begin to contract.

The second sound, which marks the beginning of ventricular diastole, is caused by the closing of the semilunar valves. Because these valves close very rapidly, the "dup" sound is heard as a quick snap. Diastole is longer than systole, so when the heart is beating at a normal rate, there is a slight pause after the second sound. Thus one hears "lub-dup," pause, "lub-dup," pause.

Abnormal heart sounds called **heart murmurs** indicate the possibility of valve disorders. When a valve does not close properly, some blood may flow backward. This can result in a hissing sound. Murmurs can also be detected when a valve becomes narrowed (stenosis) and rough.

Quiz Yourself

- An electrical impulse passes through the cardiac muscle of the atria. Where does it go next?
- What causes the first heart sound?

CARDIAC OUTPUT DEPENDS ON STROKE VOLUME AND HEART RATE

LEARNING OBJECTIVE

7. **Define cardiac output and identify factors that affect it.**

The **cardiac output** is the volume of blood pumped by the left ventricle into the aorta in one minute. The volume of blood pumped by one ventricle during one beat is called the **stroke volume.** By multiplying the stroke volume by the number of times the left ventricle beats per minute, the cardiac output can be computed. For example, in a resting adult the heart may beat about 72 times per minute and pump about 70 ml of blood with each contraction.

$$\text{Cardiac output} = \text{Stroke volume} \times \text{Heart rate (number of}$$
$$\text{ventricular contractions/min)}$$
$$= 70 \text{ ml/Stroke} \times 72 \text{ Strokes/min}$$
$$= 5040 \text{ ml/min (about 5 L/min)}$$

Note that cardiac output varies with changes in either stroke volume or heart rate. Stroke volume depends mainly on venous return—the amount of blood delivered to the heart by the veins. According to **Starling's law of the heart,** the greater the amount of blood delivered to the heart by the veins, the more blood the heart pumps (within physiological limits). When extra amounts of blood fill the heart chambers, the cardiac

muscle fibers are stretched to a greater extent. This stretching causes the cardiac muscle to contract with greater force, and as a result the heart pumps a larger volume of blood into the arteries. This increase in stroke volume increases the cardiac output (Figure 11-7).

Quiz Yourself

- What is cardiac output?
- How does stroke volume affect cardiac output?

THE HEART IS REGULATED BY THE NERVOUS AND ENDOCRINE SYSTEMS

LEARNING OBJECTIVE

8. **Describe how the nervous and endocrine systems regulate the heart.**

The normal heart rate is about 72 beats per minute. The heart rate and cardiac output can vary dramatically with the changing needs of the body. Although the heart is capable of beating rhythmically on its own, it cannot by itself change the strength and rate of contraction to meet the changing needs of the body. Such changes are regulated by the nervous and endocrine systems.

Sensory receptors in the walls of certain blood vessels and heart chambers are sensitive to changes in blood pressure. When stimulated, they send messages to **cardiac centers** in the medulla of the brain. The cardiac centers maintain control over two sets of autonomic nerves (parasympathetic and sympathetic nerves) that signal the SA node.

Parasympathetic and sympathetic nerves have opposite effects on heart rate. Parasympathetic nerves release the neurotransmitter acetylcholine, which slows the heart. Sympathetic nerves release norepinephrine, which speeds the heart rate and increases the strength of contraction. When the force of contraction increases, the heart pumps more blood per stroke. This increase in stroke volume increases cardiac output. (Both norepinephrine and acetylcholine act indirectly on ion channels in the plasma membrane.) Norepinephrine binds to receptors known as beta-adrenergic receptors. These receptors are targeted by beta blockers—drugs used clinically in the treatment of hypertension and other types of heart disease. The balance between sympathetic and parasympathetic nerve stimulation determines the heart rate.

In response to physical stressors (e.g., exercise) and emotional stressors, the adrenal glands release norepinephrine and epinephrine, which increase heart rate. These hormones also increase the force of contraction of the cardiac muscle fibers. During vigorous exercise, the normal heart can beat as many

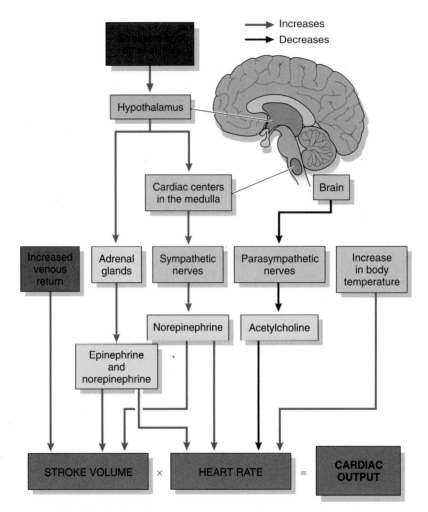

FIGURE 11-7 • Some factors that influence cardiac output.

as 200 times per minute and increase its output four to five times, so that up to 35 liters of blood can be pumped per minute. In a trained athlete, the heart enlarges and is capable of pumping a greater quantity of blood per beat. An athlete's heart is thus very efficient.

Increased body temperature, whether it results from strenuous exercise or fever, increases heart rate. A fast heart rate—more than 100 beats per minute—is called **tachycardia** (tak'-ee-**kar**'-dee-ah). A slow heart rate—less than 60 beats per minute—is referred to as **bradycardia** (brad'-ee-**kar**'-dee-ah).

Heart rate decreases when the body temperature is lowered. This is why a patient's temperature is sometimes deliberately lowered during heart surgery.

Quiz Yourself

- How does acetylcholine affect the heart?
- How does norepinephrine affect the heart?

SUMMARY

LO 1. Locate the heart and describe the structure of its wall.

- The **heart** is a hollow, muscular organ that lies in the thorax between the lungs.
- The bulk of the heart wall consists of **myocardium**—the middle layer, which is made up of cardiac muscle. The inner layer of the heart wall is the **endocardium.**
- The outer layer of the heart wall is the **epicardium, or visceral pericardium.**
- The visceral pericardium is the inner layer of the **pericardium.** The outer layer of the pericardium is the **parietal pericardium,** which forms a protective sac around the heart. The potential space between the two layers of the pericardium is the **pericardial cavity.**

LO 2. Identify the chambers of the heart and compare their functions.

- The heart has four chambers—the right and left **atria,** which receive blood returning to the heart; and the right and left **ventricles,** which pump blood out into the great arteries. The left ventricle pumps oxygen-rich blood into the **systemic circulation.** The right ventricle pumps oxygen-poor blood into the **pulmonary circulation.**
- The **interatrial septum** is the wall between the atria. The **auricle** increases the surface area of each atrium. The **interventricular septum** is the wall between the ventricles. The **papillary muscles** project from the inner wall of both ventricles.

LO 3. Locate the atrioventricular and semilunar valves and compare their functions.

- The entrance and exit of each ventricle is guarded by a valve that prevents backflow of blood. The entrance of each ventricle has an **atrioventricular valve:** the **tricuspid valve** between the right atrium and ventricle and the **mitral valve (bicuspid valve)** between the left atrium and ventricle.
- The **semilunar valves** are located between each ventricle and the artery into which it pumps blood. The semilunar valve between the left

ventricle and aorta is the **aortic semilunar valve.** The semilunar valve between the right ventricle and pulmonary artery is the **pulmonary semilunar valve.**

LO 4. Identify the principal blood vessels that serve the heart wall.

- The **coronary arteries** deliver blood to the heart wall. The **coronary veins** return blood to the **coronary sinus,** which empties into the right atrium.

LO 5. Trace the path of an electrical impulse through the conduction system of the heart.

- The heart has its own **conduction system** and can beat independently of its nerve supply. Each heartbeat begins in the **sinoatrial node**—the **pacemaker** of the heart. The electrical impulse spreads through the atria, causing atrial contraction. One group of fibers conducts the impulse to the **atrioventricular node.**
- From the atrioventricular node the impulse spreads through the **atrioventricular bundle,** which divides into right and left bundle branches that extend into the ventricles. The impulse spreads into **Purkinje fibers** that end on ordinary cardiac muscle fibers of the ventricles. The ventricles contract.

LO 6. Describe the events of the cardiac cycle and correlate them with normal heart sounds.

- The sequence of events that occurs during one complete heartbeat is a **cardiac cycle.** The contraction phase is **systole;** the relaxation phase is **diastole.**
- Each cardiac cycle begins with the generation of an impulse in the sinoatrial node that produces atrial systole (contraction). As the atria contract, additional blood is forced into the ventricles. Ventricular systole occurs next, forcing blood through the semilunar valves into the systemic and pulmonary circulations. At the same time, the atria have returned to diastole and are again filling with blood.
- When listening to the heart through a stethoscope, one can hear a "lub" sound when the atrioventricular valves close, followed by a "dup" sound when the semilunar valves snap shut. **Heart murmurs** are abnormal heart sounds that may be caused by valve disorders.

LO = Learning Objective

LO 7. Define cardiac output and identify factors that affect it.

- **Cardiac output** is the amount of blood pumped by the left ventricle into the aorta in 1 minute. Cardiac output equals stroke volume times heart rate.
- The **stroke volume** is the amount of blood pumped by one ventricle during one beat. According to **Starling's law of the heart,** the more blood returned to the heart by the veins, the greater the volume of blood that will be pumped during the next systole.
- Stroke volume depends mainly on venous return—the amount of blood delivered to the heart by the veins. Stroke volume is also influenced by neural messages and hormones, especially epinephrine and norepinephrine.

LO 8. Describe how the nervous and endocrine systems regulate the heart.

- The nervous and endocrine systems regulate the heartbeat so that its rate and strength of contraction adjusts to the changing needs of the body. **Cardiac centers** in the medulla regulate the heart by way of autonomic nerves.
- Parasympathetic nerves release **acetylcholine,** which slows the heart rate. Sympathetic nerves release **norepinephrine,** which speeds the heart rate.
- In response to stress, the adrenal glands release epinephrine and norepinephrine, hormones that increase heart rate and stroke volume.

CHAPTER QUIZ

Fill in the Blank

1. The outer layer of the heart is the visceral _____.

2. The bulk of the heart wall consists of _____.

3. The wall separating the ventricles of the heart is called the _____ _____.

4. The left AV valve is often called the _____ valve.

5. Aortic and pulmonary valves are _____ valves.

6. Blood is delivered to the heart wall by the _____ arteries.

7. The _____ _____ is called the pacemaker of the heart.

8. From the AV node, the electrical impulse spreads into specialized muscle fibers that form the AV _____.

9. In the cardiac cycle, the period of contraction is called _____ and the period of relaxation is called _____.

10. At the time the atria are contracting, the ventricles are in _____.

11. The volume of blood pumped by one ventricle in 1 minute is the _____ _____.

12. The amount of blood pumped by one ventricle during one beat is the _____ _____.

13. Heart rate is slowed by _____ nerves and speeded by _____ nerves.

Multiple Choice

14. The left ventricle: a. receives blood from the systemic circulation; b. receives blood from the pulmonary circulation; c. pumps blood into the systemic circulation; d. pumps blood into the pulmonary circulation.

15. When the atrium relaxes, blood is prevented from flowing backward into it by the: a. atrioventricular valve; b. semilunar valve; c. aortic valve; d. pulmonary valve.

16. From the sinoatrial node, impulses pass into ordinary muscle fibers of the: a. atrioventricular bundle; b. atrium; c. ventricle; d. atrioventricular node.

17. Delay of impulse transmission in the atrioventricular node: a. allows the atria to relax while the ventricles are relaxing; b. allows blood to pass through the semilunar valves; c. allows the electrical activity of the heart to cease momentarily; d. allows the atria to complete systole before the ventricles contract.

18. Increased venous return: a. increases stroke volume; b. decreases cardiac output; c. decreases epinephrine release; d. decreases heart rate.

REVIEW QUESTIONS

1. Relate the structure of the heart wall to the heart's function.

2. Trace a drop of blood through the heart, listing each structure through which it passes in sequence.

3. Name and locate the four valves of the heart and give the function of each.

4. Why does the heart wall require its own blood supply? Name the blood vessels that bring blood to and from the heart wall.

5. Why is the sinoatrial node called the pacemaker of the heart?

6. Trace an electrical impulse through the heart.

7. Define systole and diastole and describe the cardiac cycle.

8. What causes each of the heart sounds?

9. Define cardiac output and explain how it is influenced by venous return.

10. Describe the regulation of the heart by sympathetic and parasympathetic nerves.

11. Label the diagram. (See Figure 11-3 to check your answers.)

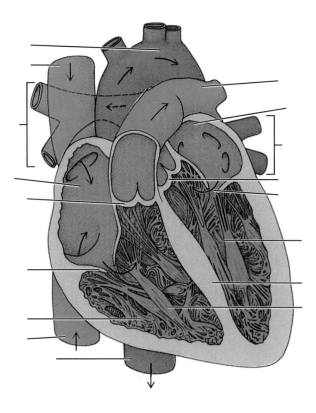

12 Circulation of Blood and Lymph

Chapter Outline

Blood vessels are the tubes that deliver blood to the tissues. The smaller types of blood vessels are quite leaky. As blood circulates through blood vessels in the tissues, some of the plasma is forced out of the blood vessels. The plasma contains nutrients, oxygen, and other materials needed by the cells. When plasma enters the tissues, it is called **interstitial fluid,** or **tissue fluid.** Interstitial fluid nourishes the cells and keeps them moist.

   In this chapter we first examine the various types of blood vessels and some of their pathways through the body. Then we look at the physiology of blood circulation. Finally, we examine how the lymphatic system returns fluid to the blood.

THREE MAIN TYPES OF BLOOD VESSELS CIRCULATE BLOOD

LEARNING OBJECTIVE

1. **Compare the structure and functions of arteries, capillaries, and veins.**

The main types of blood vessels—the arteries, capillaries, and veins—vary with respect to their structure and functions (Figure 12-1).

Arteries Carry Blood Away From the Heart

Arteries carry blood from the ventricles of the heart to the organs of the body. Arteries carry blood rich in oxygen.

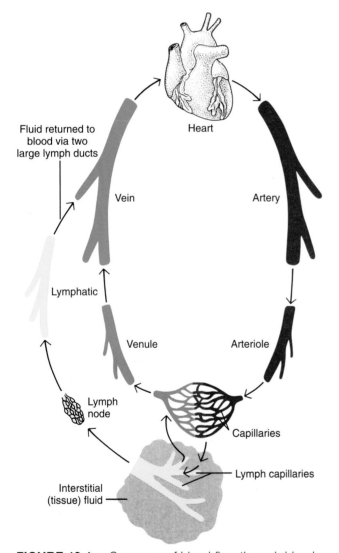

FIGURE 12-1 • Sequence of blood flow through blood vessels and lymphatic vessels. As blood circulates through capillaries, some plasma leaves the circulation and becomes interstitial fluid. Some of this fluid is returned to the blood by way of the lymph system.

As we will learn, the pulmonary arteries are an important exception. Arteries are strong vessels adapted to carry blood under high pressure. The smallest branches of an artery, called **arterioles** (ar-**teer'**-ee-olz), are important in regulating blood pressure.

The wall of an artery or vein has three layers, or **tunics** (Figure 12-2). The inner layer, called **tunica intima,** consists of **endothelium** (en'-doe-**thee'**-lee-um) (similar to simple squamous epithelium) that forms a smooth surface for the blood. The middle layer, or **tunica media,** consists of connective tissue and smooth muscle. In large arteries, this is the thickest layer and contains several layers of elastic fibers. The outer layer, the **tunica adventitia,** is a relatively thin layer in arteries. It consists of connective tissue rich in elastic and collagen fibers.

Smooth muscle in its wall allows an arteriole to constrict (**vasoconstriction**) or relax (**vasodilation),** changing the radius of the arteriole. Such changes help maintain appropriate blood pressure and can help control the volume of blood passing to a particular tissue. Changes in blood flow are regulated by the nervous system in response to the metabolic needs of the tissue and by the demands of the body as a whole. For example, when a tissue is metabolizing rapidly, it needs a greater supply of nutrients and oxygen. During exercise, arterioles within the muscles dilate, increasing by more than tenfold the amount of blood flowing to the muscle cells.

Capillaries Are Exchange Vessels

From the arterioles blood flows through **capillaries** (kap'-ih-lar-ees), tiny vessels that form extensive networks within each tissue. Capillaries are located close to almost every cell in the body. The total length of all capillaries in the body has been estimated to be more than 60,000 miles! Capillary walls are thin and somewhat porous, permitting plasma to pass through them into the tissues. Capillaries permit oxygen, nutrients, and other materials to be exchanged between the blood and tissues.

The capillary wall consists mainly of endothelium. At the point where a capillary branches from an arteriole, a smooth muscle cell surrounds the vessel. By contracting or relaxing, this muscle regulates the flow of blood into the capillaries.

Metarterioles are small vessels that directly link arterioles with venules (small veins). The so-called *true capillaries* branch off from the metarterioles and then rejoin them (see Figure 12-2). True capillaries also interconnect with one another. Wherever a capillary branches from a metarteriole, a smooth muscle cell called a **precapillary sphincter** is present. Precapillary sphincters open and close continuously, directing blood first to one and then to another section of tissue. These sphincters also (along with the smooth muscle in the walls of arteries and arterioles) regulate the blood supply to each organ and its subdivisions.

If all the blood vessels were dilated at the same time, there would not be sufficient blood to fill them completely.

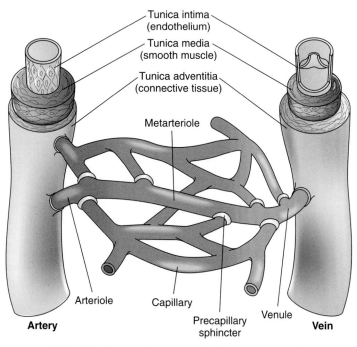

Tunica intima (endothelium)
Tunica media (smooth muscle)
Tunica adventitia (connective tissue)
Metarteriole
Arteriole
Capillary
Precapillary sphincter
Venule
Artery
Vein

FIGURE 12-2 • Structure of blood vessel walls.

Normally the liver, kidneys, and brain receive the lion's share of blood. However, when an emergency occurs requiring rapid action, the blood is rerouted quickly in favor of the heart and muscles. This enables rapid, effective action. At such a time, the digestive system and kidneys can do with less blood because they are not critical in responding to the crisis.

In the liver, spleen, and bone marrow, arterioles and venules are connected by capillary-like vessels called **sinusoids** rather than by typical capillaries. The endothelial cells lining a sinusoid do not all come into contact with one another, leaving gaps in the wall. For this reason, sinusoids are very leaky. White blood cells can move in and out of the circulation through their walls. Macrophages lie along the outer walls of sinusoids. They reach into the vessels to remove worn-out blood cells and foreign matter from the circulation.

Veins Carry Blood Back to the Heart

Blood passes from capillaries into **veins,** the vessels that conduct blood back toward the heart. The smallest veins are called **venules.** All veins except the pulmonary veins carry blood that is poor in oxygen. In general, veins have thinner walls than arteries have. The outer layer, the tunica adventitia, is the thickest layer in the walls of large veins.

Most large veins have valves that permit the vein to conduct blood toward the heart, even against the force of gravity. A vein valve usually consists of two cusps formed by inward extensions of the endothelium. These cusps prevent blood from flowing backward.

Quiz Yourself

• What is the function of arteries? Of capillaries?
• How does the capillary wall differ from the wall of a vein?

BLOOD CIRCULATES THROUGH TWO CIRCUITS

LEARNING OBJECTIVES

2. **Trace a drop of blood through the pulmonary and systemic circulations, listing the principal vessels and heart chambers through which it must pass on its journey from one part of the body to another. (For example, trace a drop of blood from the inferior vena cava to an organ such as the brain and then back to the heart.)**
3. **Identify the main divisions of the aorta and its principal branches.**
4. **Trace a drop of blood through the brain.**
5. **Trace a drop of blood through the hepatic portal system.**

Blood flows through a continuous network of blood vessels that forms a double circuit: (1) the **pulmonary circulation** connects heart and lungs and (2) the **systemic circulation** connects the heart and all the organs and tissues. The left ventricle pumps blood into the systemic circulation, which brings oxygen-rich blood to all the different organs and tissues. Blood that is poor in oxygen but loaded with carbon dioxide wastes returns to the right atrium of the heart. Then the blood is pumped by the right ventricle into the pulmonary circulation, where gases are exchanged.

From the pulmonary circulation, blood is returned to the left atrium. It is pumped into the left ventricle, which pumps it back out into the systemic circulation. This general pattern of circulation is shown in Figure 12-3. A more detailed view is shown in Figure 12-4.

The Pulmonary Circulation Carries Blood to and From the Lungs

The right atrium receives blood returning to the heart from the systemic circulation. This blood, which is poor in oxygen, is pumped into the right ventricle and then into the **pulmonary arteries.** These blood vessels deliver blood to the lungs, where they give rise to an extensive network of capillaries. As

blood flows through the pulmonary capillaries, carbon dioxide diffuses out of the blood and oxygen diffuses into it.

The **pulmonary veins** return blood, rich in oxygen once more, to the left atrium. Blood then passes into the left ventricle and is pumped into the systemic circulation again. Note that the pulmonary veins are the only veins that carry oxygen-rich blood, and the pulmonary arteries are the only arteries that transport blood that is poor in oxygen. In summary, blood flows through the pulmonary circulation in the following sequence:

> Right atrium → right ventricle → pulmonary arteries → pulmonary capillaries → pulmonary veins → left atrium

The Systemic Circulation Carries Blood to and From the Tissues

Blood returning from the pulmonary circulation enters the left atrium and is pumped into the left ventricle. The left ventricle pumps the blood into the largest artery in the body—the **aorta** (ay-**or**′-tah). Branches of the aorta deliver blood to all the organs and tissues of the body.

The Aorta Has Four Main Regions

We can identify four regions of the aorta (Figure 12-5):

1. The **ascending aorta,** the first part of the aorta, travels upward (superiorly).
2. The **aortic arch** curves from the ascending aorta and makes a U-turn.
3. The **thoracic** (thow-**ras**′-ik) **aorta** descends from the aortic arch, passing through the thorax. It lies posterior to the heart.
4. The **abdominal aorta,** the region of the aorta below the diaphragm, is the longest region of the aorta. The abdominal aorta descends downward through the abdominal cavity. The thoracic aorta and abdominal aorta together make up the **descending aorta.**

The principal branches of each region of the aorta are listed in Table 12-1.

The Superior and Inferior Venae Cavae Return Blood to the Heart

As blood circulates through capillaries in the tissues, it delivers nutrients and oxygen to the cells and picks up carbon dioxide. Capillaries deliver blood to venules, and these small veins merge to form larger veins. Veins bringing blood back from the tissues drain into two very large veins. The **superior vena cava** (**vee**′-nah **kay**′-vah) receives blood from the upper portions of the body (Table 12-2). The **inferior vena cava** receives blood returning from below the level of the diaphragm. The superior and inferior venae cavae return blood to the right atrium of the heart.

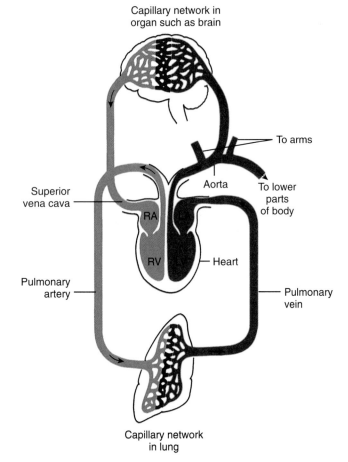

Capillary network in organ such as brain

To arms

Superior vena cava

Aorta

To lower parts of body

RA

RV

Heart

Pulmonary artery

Pulmonary vein

Capillary network in lung

FIGURE 12-3 • Simplified diagram of circulation through the systemic and pulmonary circuits. *Red* represents oxygen-rich blood; *blue* represents oxygen-poor blood. *RA,* Right atrium; *LA,* left atrium; *RV,* right ventricle; *LV,* left ventricle.

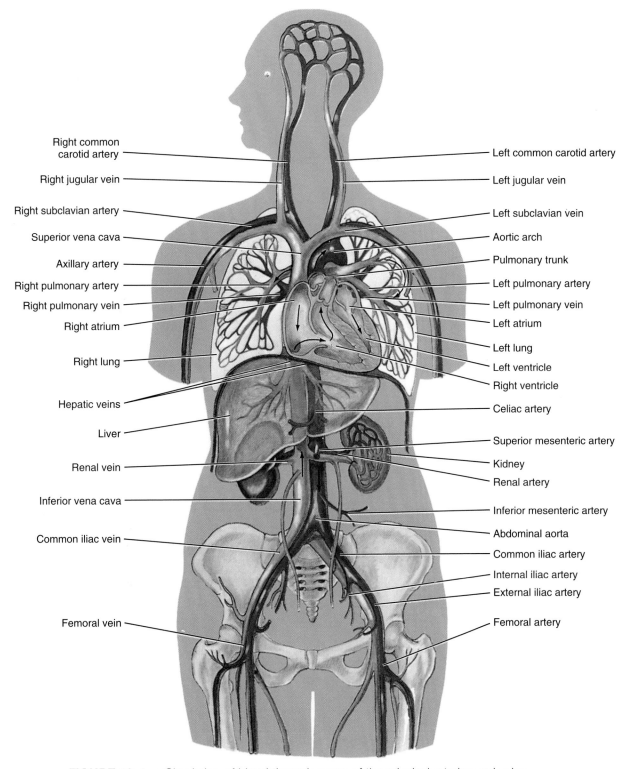

Right common carotid artery

Right jugular vein

Right subclavian artery

Superior vena cava

Axillary artery

Right pulmonary artery

Right pulmonary vein

Right atrium

Right lung

Hepatic veins

Liver

Renal vein

Inferior vena cava

Common iliac vein

Femoral vein

Left common carotid artery

Left jugular vein

Left subclavian vein

Aortic arch

Pulmonary trunk

Left pulmonary artery

Left pulmonary vein

Left atrium

Left lung

Left ventricle

Right ventricle

Celiac artery

Superior mesenteric artery

Kidney

Renal artery

Inferior mesenteric artery

Abdominal aorta

Common iliac artery

Internal iliac artery

External iliac artery

Femoral artery

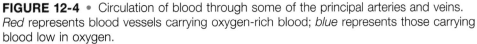

FIGURE 12-4 • Circulation of blood through some of the principal arteries and veins. *Red* represents blood vessels carrying oxygen-rich blood; *blue* represents those carrying blood low in oxygen.

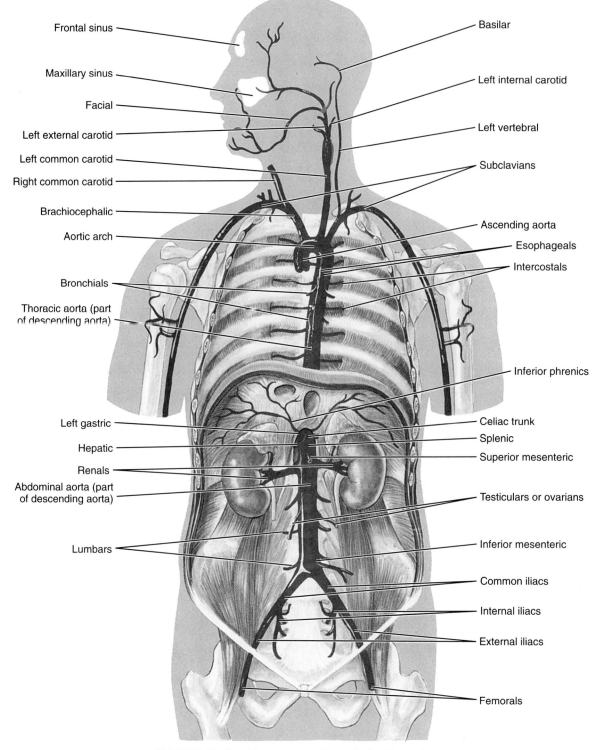

FIGURE 12-5 • The aorta and its principal branches.

TABLE 12-1	THE AORTA AND ITS PRINCIPAL BRANCHES	
Division of Aorta	**Arterial Branch**	**Region Supplied**
Ascending aorta	Coronary arteries	Wall of heart
Aortic arch	Brachiocephalic (innominate)	
	Right common carotid	Branches into external carotid (supplying head and neck) and internal carotid (supplying brain and head)
	Right subclavian	Sends branches to neck and right upper limb
	Left common carotid	Branches into external carotid (supplying head and neck) and internal carotid (supplying brain and head)
	Left subclavian	Sends branches to neck and left upper limb
Thoracic aorta	*Visceral branches*	
	Bronchial	Bronchi of lungs
	Esophageal	Esophagus
	Parietal branches	
	Several pairs of posterior intercostal arteries	Intercostal and other chest muscles and pleurae; join with other arteries that serve chest wall
	Subcostal	Last pair of arteries to branch from thoracic aorta; serve chest wall
Abdominal aorta	*Visceral branches*	
	Celiac	Branches to supply the liver (hepatic artery), stomach (gastric artery), and spleen, pancreas, and stomach (splenic artery)
	Superior mesenteric	Small intestine and first part of large intestine
	Suprarenal	Adrenal glands
	Renal	Kidneys
	Ovarian (in female)	Ovaries
	Testicular (in male)	Testes
	Inferior mesenteric	Colon, rectum
	Common iliac	
	External	Lower limbs
	Internal	Branches supply gluteal muscles, urinary bladder, uterus, vagina
	Parietal branches	
	Inferior phrenic	Diaphragm
	Lumbar	Spinal cord and lumbar region of back
	Middle sacral	Sacrum, coccyx, gluteus maximus, and rectum

TABLE 12-2	VEINS DRAINING INTO THE VENAE CAVAE	
Vein	**Formed From**	**Area(s) Drained**
INTO SUPERIOR VENA CAVA		
Internal jugular	Sinuses of dura matter	Brain, skull
External jugular	Veins of face	Muscles and skin of face and scalp
Subclavian	Axillary, cephalic, basilic and their tributaries, scapular, and thoracic veins	Upper limb, chest, mammary glands
Brachiocephalic (innominate)	Internal jugular, external jugular, and subclavian	Brain, face, neck
Azygos	Lumbar and intercostal veins	Posterior aspect of thorax and abdominal cavities
INTO INFERIOR VENA CAVA		
Hepatics	Sinusoids of liver	Liver
Renals	Veins of kidneys	Kidneys
Ovarians or testiculars	Veins of gonads	Ovaries or testes
Common iliac	External iliac (extension of the femoral vein)	Lower limbs
	Internal iliac	Organs of lower abdomen

Four Arteries Supply the Brain

Four arteries bring blood to the brain. The two **internal carotid arteries** enter the cranial cavity in the midregion of the cranial floor. The two **vertebral arteries** (branches of the subclavian arteries) pass through the foramen magnum (the opening in the occipital bone through which the spinal cord passes) and join on the ventral surface of the brainstem. Together they form the **basilar artery** (Figure 12-6).

Branches of the internal carotid arteries and basilar artery form a circle of arteries at the base of the brain. This circuit is called the **circle of Willis.** The joining of two or more arteries is called an arterial **anastomosis** (ah′-nas-tow-**mow**′-sis). If one of the arteries serving the brain becomes blocked or damaged in some way, this arterial circuit helps ensure that the brain cells will continue to receive an adequate blood supply through other vessels.

From the brain capillaries, blood drains into large **venous sinuses** located in the folds of the dura mater (the outer covering of the brain) (Figure 12-7). A venous sinus is a specialized vein that has no smooth muscle in its wall. Blood from the venous sinuses empties into the **internal jugular veins** at either side of the neck. From there, blood passes through the **brachiocephalic** (bray′-kee-o-seh-**fal**′-ik) **veins** and into the superior vena cava, which returns it to the heart.

A simplified summary of blood flow to and from the brain follows:

Aorta → common carotid artery → internal carotid artery (with branches of basilar artery) → circle of Willis → capillaries in brain → venous sinus → internal jugular vein → brachiocephalic vein → superior vena cava

The Liver Has an Unusual Circulation

As you have seen, blood typically flows from arteries to capillaries and then to veins. The veins conduct the blood back toward the heart. However, the body has a few veins that carry blood to a second set of exchange vessels (capillaries or sinusoids). Such veins are called **portal veins.** The **hepatic portal vein** delivers blood from the organs of the digestive system to the liver.

Blood is delivered to the intestines by the **mesenteric** (mez-en-**ter**′-ik) **arteries** and enters capillaries in the intestinal wall. Nutrients are absorbed into these capillaries. Then the blood, rich in nutrients, flows into the **superior mesenteric vein.** This vein empties into the hepatic portal vein, which also receives blood returning from the lower portion of the intestine and from the spleen (Figure 12-8).

The hepatic portal vein conducts blood to the liver, where it gives rise to an extensive network of hepatic sinusoids—exchange vessels somewhat like capillaries. As blood flows through the sinusoids, liver cells remove and store nutrients whose concentrations are above homeostatic levels. Liver cells

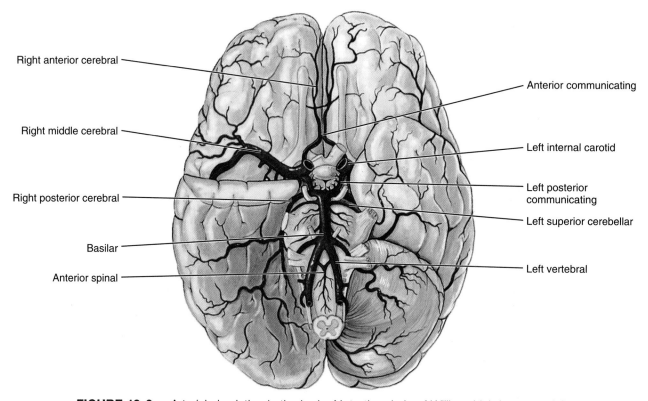

FIGURE 12-6 • Arterial circulation in the brain. Note the circle of Willis, which is an arterial anastomosis formed from branches of the internal carotid arteries and basilar artery. It provides alternative circulatory pathways to ensure an adequate blood supply to the brain cells. Inferior view of brain.

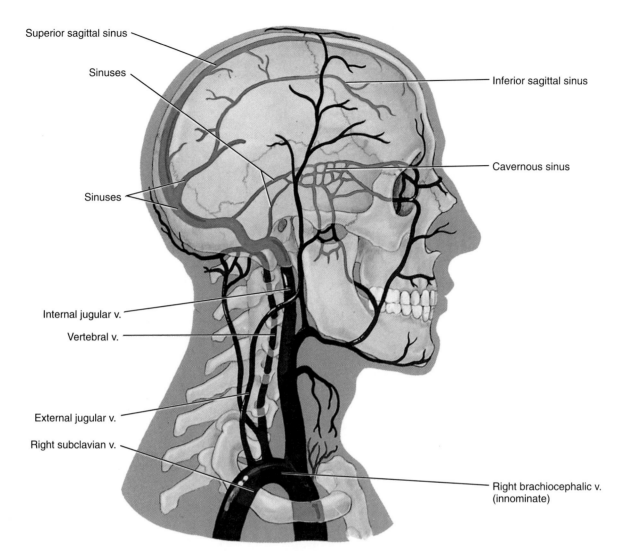

Superior sagittal sinus

Sinuses

Inferior sagittal sinus

Cavernous sinus

Sinuses

Internal jugular v.

Vertebral v.

External jugular v.

Right subclavian v.

Right brachiocephalic v. (innominate)

FIGURE 12-7 • Venous circulation in the brain. Large sinuses receive blood from brain capillaries and deliver it to veins that leave the brain and return blood to the heart. *v.,* Vein.

also remove toxic substances from the blood. The hepatic sinusoids deliver blood to the hepatic veins, which leave the liver and empty into the inferior vena cava.

Quiz Yourself

- What are the four divisions of the aorta?
- What are the four main arteries that supply the brain?
- What are portal veins?

SEVERAL FACTORS INFLUENCE BLOOD FLOW

LEARNING OBJECTIVES

6. State the physiological basis for arterial pulse and describe how pulse is measured.

7. State the relationship among blood pressure, blood flow, and resistance, and describe how blood pressure is measured.
8. Compare blood pressure in the different types of blood vessels of the systemic circulation.
9. Describe the mechanisms by which the nervous and endocrine systems regulate blood pressure.

In Chapter 11 we discussed some of the factors that influence cardiac output. Here we focus on the physiology of circulation through the blood vessels.

The Alternate Expansion and Recoil of an Artery Is Its Pulse

Each time the left ventricle pumps blood into the aorta, the elastic wall of the aorta stretches. This expansion moves down the aorta and its branches in a wave that is faster than the flow of the blood itself. As soon as the wave has passed, the elastic

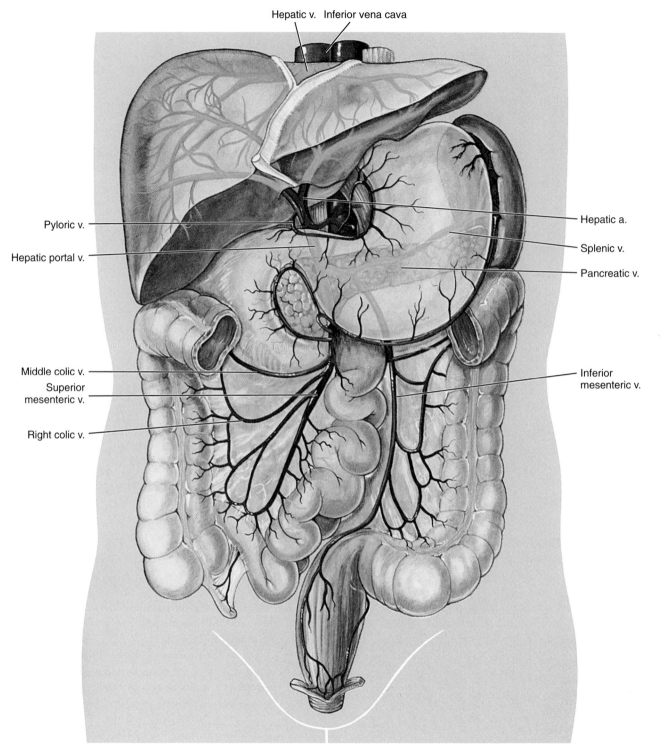

FIGURE 12-8 • The hepatic portal system. Blood circulating through the hepatic portal vein has passed through capillaries in the intestine and is partly depleted of its oxygen supply. Oxygen-rich blood is delivered to the hepatic sinuses of the liver by branches of the hepatic arteries. The oxygen-rich blood mixes with the venous blood from the hepatic portal vein. *v.*, Vein; *a.*, artery.

wall of the artery snaps back to its normal size. This alternate expansion and recoil of an artery is the **arterial pulse.**

The ability of the large arteries to expand and then snap back to their original diameter is important in maintaining a continuous flow of blood. As the left ventricle forces a large volume of blood into the aorta during systole, the aorta expands to accommodate it. During diastole, as the walls of the aorta recoil to normal size, the blood is kept flowing into the capillaries. Without this mechanism, blood would rush through the arteries and into the arterioles and capillaries in enormous gushes each time the ventricle contracted. This would damage the delicate walls of the capillaries.

When you place your finger over an artery near the skin surface, you can feel the pulse. The **radial artery** in the wrist is used most frequently to measure pulse. However, the *common carotid artery* in the neck region or any other superficial artery that lies over a bone or other firm structure may be used (Figure 12-9). These locations are sometimes referred to as *pressure points* because pressure applied directly on the vessel at these points may stop arterial bleeding if a wound is distal to the pressure point.

The number of pulsations counted per minute indicates the number of heartbeats per minute. This is because every time the heart contracts, a pulse wave is initiated. Because it takes time for the pulse wave to pass from the ventricle to the artery, the pulse is felt just after the ventricles contract.

Blood Pressure Depends on Blood Flow and Resistance to Blood Flow

Blood pressure is the force exerted by the blood against the inner walls of the blood vessels. It is determined by (1) the flow of blood and (2) the resistance to that flow. The flow of blood depends directly on the pumping action of the heart.

When cardiac output increases, blood flow increases, causing a rise in blood pressure (Figure 12-10). When cardiac output decreases, blood flow decreases, causing a fall in blood pressure.

Blood flow is directly affected by blood volume. The normal volume of blood in the body is about 5 liters. If blood volume is reduced by hemorrhage or by chronic bleeding, the blood pressure drops. On the other hand, an increase in blood volume causes an increase in blood pressure. For example, a high dietary intake of salt causes water to be retained in the body.

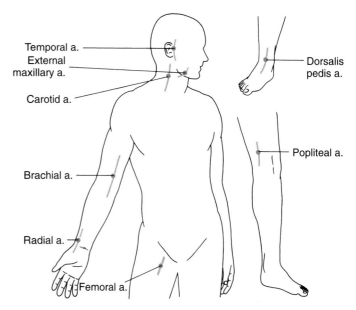

FIGURE 12-9 • The pulse may be felt at any of the locations indicated in the diagram. All the arteries indicated lie near the body surface over a bone or other firm structure. *a.,* Artery.

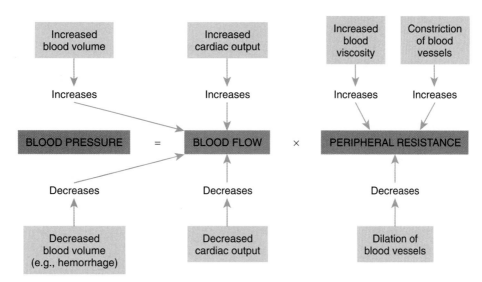

FIGURE 12-10 • Some factors that influence blood pressure. Any factor that increases either blood flow or peripheral resistance increases blood pressure. Any factor that decreases either blood flow or peripheral resistance decreases blood pressure.

This may result in an increase in blood volume and may lead to an increase in blood pressure.

Blood flow is slowed by resistance. **Peripheral resistance** is the opposing force to blood flow caused by viscosity of the blood and by the friction between the blood and the wall of the blood vessel. When the peripheral resistance increases, blood pressure increases. Viscosity remains fairly constant in a healthy person and is only a minor factor influencing changes in blood pressure. More important is the friction between the blood and the wall of the blood vessel.

The length and diameter of a blood vessel determine the amount of surface area in contact with the blood. The length of a blood vessel does not change, but the diameter, especially of an arteriole, does. A small change in the diameter of a blood vessel causes a big change in blood pressure.

Pressure Changes as Blood Flows Through the Systemic Circulation

Because arteries are large, their walls do not present much resistance to blood flow. Arterioles, however, have a much smaller diameter, so they offer a great deal of resistance to blood flow. This permits relatively high pressures to build up in the blood behind them. More important, arterioles can constrict and dilate by increasing or decreasing the extent of contraction of the muscle in their walls. **Vasoconstriction,** a decrease in blood vessel diameter, increases resistance to blood flow. **Vasodilation,** an increase in blood vessel diameter, decreases resistance to blood flow. Changes in resistance affect the blood pressure and the rate of blood flow. In fact, the blood pressure within the arteries is regulated mainly by the degree of constriction or dilation of the arterioles.

The diameter of a capillary is very small, so individual capillaries offer great resistance to blood flow. However, blood has so many capillaries through which to pass that the *total* resistance, when all the capillaries are considered together, is far less than that of the arterioles.

As blood flows through capillaries, most of the pressure caused by the action of the heart is spent. By the time the blood passes into the veins, its pressure is very low. However, even this small pressure is usually sufficient to push blood through the veins to the heart.

Very little pressure is needed to force the blood through the veins because veins offer little resistance to blood flow. Their diameters are large, and vein walls are thin and can easily be stretched. As a result, they can hold large volumes of blood. Indeed, at any moment more than 60% of all the blood in the circulation can be found within the veins. Thus veins serve as a kind of blood reservoir.

When the body is in an upright position, gravity offers a great deal of resistance to venous blood flow. It is really quite remarkable that blood in the feet manages to make its way back to the heart. How is this accomplished? Blood is pushed along by the pressure of blood behind it and by compression of veins when skeletal muscle contracts. Vein valves, especially those in the legs, prevent backflow that would occur because of the force of gravity.

During exercise, increased muscle contraction results in increased flow of blood through the veins and into the heart. Cardiac output increases. On the other hand, when one stands still for a long period (e.g., when a soldier stands at attention or a store clerk stands at a cash register), blood pools in the veins. When fully distended, veins can accept no more blood from the capillaries. Pressure in the capillaries increases, and large amounts of plasma may be forced out of the circulation through capillary walls. Within just a few minutes, as much as 20% of the blood volume can be lost from the circulation—with drastic effect. Arterial blood pressure falls dramatically, reducing blood flow to the brain. The resulting lack of oxygen in the brain can cause fainting, which is a protective response. Lying in a prone position increases blood supply to the brain. In fact, lifting a person who has fainted to an upright position can result in *circulatory shock.* In this condition, the blood pressure may fall drastically so that blood flow to the tissues is not adequate, leading to death.

Blood Pressure Is Expressed as Systolic Pressure Over Diastolic Pressure

In arteries, blood pressure rises during systole and falls during diastole. A blood pressure reading is expressed as **systolic pressure** over **diastolic pressure.** The National Institutes of Health defines normal blood pressure as systolic pressure less than 120 and diastolic pressure less than 80. An example of a normal blood pressure for a young adult is 112/72. The numbers refer to *millimeters of mercury,* abbreviated *mm Hg.* Systolic pressure is represented by the numerator and diastolic by the denominator. Blood pressure may vary greatly with physical exertion and emotional stress.

Clinically, blood pressure can be measured with a *sphygmomanometer* (sfig'-mow-mah-**nom'**-eh-ter) and stethoscope. The sphygmomanometer consists of a column of mercury connected by a rubber tube to an inflatable rubber cuff. An air pump with a valve is attached to the cuff. To measure the pressure, the cuff is wrapped around a patient's arm over the brachial artery. Air is pumped into the cuff until the air pressure is great enough to compress the artery so that no pulse is heard on the anterior surface of the elbow joint (with the stethoscope). Then the valve is opened slightly so that the pressure in the cuff begins to fall. Soon, a distinct sound is heard as blood spurts into the artery again. The pressure at that instant is read as the systolic pressure. The sound gets louder, then changes in quality, and finally becomes inaudible. Pressure at the instant the sound is no longer heard is read as the diastolic pressure.

When the systolic pressure consistently measures 140 mm Hg or higher or diastolic pressure consistently measures 90 mm Hg or higher, a person has high blood pressure, or **hypertension.** This condition is a risk factor for cardiovascular disease. In hypertension, there is usually increased vascular resistance, especially in the arterioles and small arteries. The heart's workload increases because it must pump against this greater resistance. If this condition persists, the left ventricle enlarges and may begin to deteriorate in function. Heredity, aging, ethnicity, and lifestyle are factors in the development of hypertension.

If your systolic blood pressure is between 120 and 139 and your diastolic pressure is 80 to 89, you are *prehypertensive*. To prevent cardiovascular disease, you need to modify your lifestyle. Changes that reduce risk include exercising, losing excess weight, following a heart-healthy diet, reducing salt intake, not smoking, and limiting alcohol intake.

Blood Pressure Must Be Carefully Regulated

Whenever you change position, blood pressure fluctuates. It is kept within normal limits by the interaction of several complex homeostatic mechanisms. When blood pressure falls, sympathetic nerves signal arterioles to constrict. Vasoconstriction results in an increase in blood pressure.

Baroreceptors (bar′-o-re-**sep**′-tors) are specialized receptors present in the walls of certain arteries and in the heart wall. These receptors are sensitive to changes in blood pressure. Some baroreceptors respond to high blood pressure, while others respond to low blood pressure. When blood pressure increases, certain baroreceptors are stretched. They send messages to cardiac centers in the medulla. Then parasympathetic nerves signal the heart to slow—an action that lowers blood pressure. The cardiac centers also inhibit sympathetic nerves that constrict arterioles; this action causes vasodilation, which lowers blood pressure. These neural reflexes continuously work in this complementary way to maintain blood pressure within normal limits.

Hormones are also important in regulating blood pressure. In response to low blood pressure, the kidneys release **renin.** This enzyme acts on a plasma protein (angiotensinogen), initiating a series of reactions that produces **angiotensin II,** a hormone that acts as a powerful vasoconstrictor. Angiotensin II also acts indirectly to maintain blood pressure by signaling the adrenal glands to increase its output of **aldosterone.** This hormone increases the retention of sodium ions by the kidneys, resulting in greater fluid retention and increased blood volume. As a result, blood pressure increases.

When blood is lost during hemorrhage, arterial pressure may fall drastically. Baroreceptors respond, causing the veins to constrict. Large amounts of blood leave the veins and enter the heart. This response prevents the heart from failing and may keep the circulation going even when large amounts of blood are lost. In severe hemorrhage, *circulatory shock* may occur. In this condition, blood pressure may fall so drastically that blood flow to the tissues is not adequate and tissue damage and death may occur.

Quiz Yourself

- What is peripheral resistance?
- What are some of the factors that affect blood pressure?
- What is the function of baroreceptors?

THE LYMPHATIC SYSTEM IS AN ACCESSORY CIRCULATORY SYSTEM

LEARNING OBJECTIVES

10. Describe the functions, tissues, and organs of the lymphatic system.
11. Trace the flow of lymph from a lymph capillary to the left or right subclavian vein.

The **lymphatic system** has three principal functions:

1. Collects and returns interstitial fluid (tissue fluid) to the blood and thus helps maintain fluid balance
2. Defends the body against disease by launching immune responses
3. Absorbs lipids from the intestine and transports them to the blood

The lymphatic system consists of the clear, watery **lymph** that is formed from interstitial fluid, the lymphatic vessels that conduct the lymph, and **lymph tissue.** The lymph tissue is a type of connective tissue with large numbers of lymphocytes. It is organized into small masses of tissue called **lymph nodules** and **lymph nodes.** The tonsils, spleen, and thymus gland are also part of the lymph system (Figure 12-11).

The Lymph Circulation Is a Drainage System

The lymph circulation collects excess interstitial fluid and returns it to the blood. The lymph system has neither a heart nor arteries. It has three types of lymphatic vessels: lymph capillaries, lymphatics, and lymph ducts. The microscopic dead-end **lymph capillaries** extend into most tissues, alongside the blood capillaries. Lymph capillaries conduct lymph to larger vessels called **lymphatics** (lim-**fat**′-iks). At strategic locations, lymphatics enter lymph nodes. As the lymph flows slowly through lymph sinuses (very small, irregular channels) within the tissue of the lymph node, it is filtered.

Lymphatics that leave the lymph nodes conduct lymph toward the shoulder region. Lymphatic vessels from all over the body except the upper right quadrant drain into the **thoracic duct.** This duct delivers the lymph into the base of the left subclavian vein. Lymph from the lymphatic vessels in the upper right quadrant of the body drains into the **right**

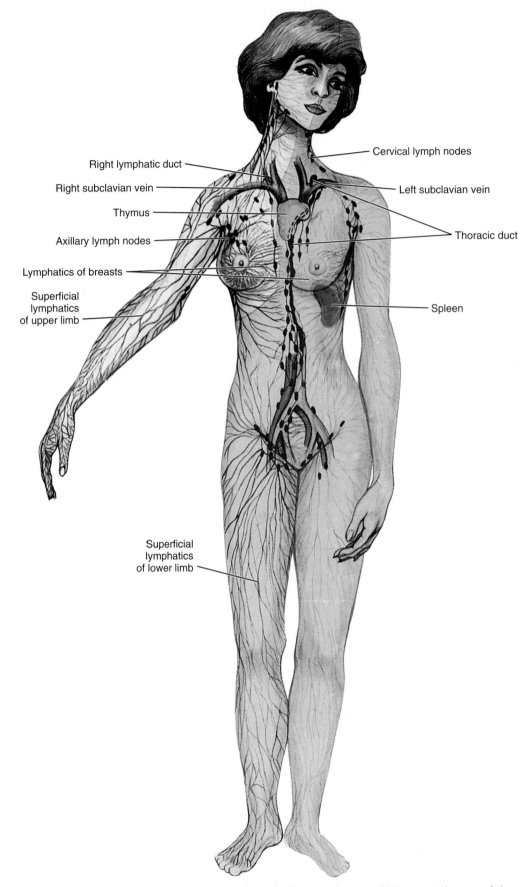

Cervical lymph nodes

Right lymphatic duct

Right subclavian vein

Left subclavian vein

Thymus

Axillary lymph nodes

Thoracic duct

Lymphatics of breasts

Superficial lymphatics of upper limb

Spleen

Superficial lymphatics of lower limb

FIGURE 12-11 • The lymphatic system. Lymphatic vessels extend into most tissues of the body, but lymph nodes are clustered in certain regions. The right lymphatic duct drains lymph from the upper right quadrant of the body. The thoracic duct drains lymph from other regions of the body.

lymphatic duct, which empties lymph into the base of the right subclavian vein. In this way, lymph continuously empties into the blood, where it mixes with the plasma. Thus interstitial fluid from the tissues is returned to the blood. Here is the general pattern of lymph circulation:

> Lymph capillaries → lymphatic → lymph sinuses in lymph node → lymphatic → thoracic duct (or right lymphatic duct) → subclavian vein

Lymph Nodes Filter Lymph

Lymph nodes, sometimes called *lymph glands,* are masses of lymph tissue surrounded by a connective tissue capsule. Their main function is to filter the lymph. Lymph nodes are distributed along the main lymphatic routes. As illustrated in Figure 12-11, they are most numerous in the axillary and groin regions and many are located in the thorax and abdomen.

As lymph passes through lymph sinuses in lymph nodes, macrophages and other phagocytic cells remove bacteria and other foreign matter, as well as damaged cells and cellular debris. By filtering and destroying bacteria from the lymph, the lymph nodes help prevent the spread of infection. When bacteria are present, lymph nodes may increase in size and become tender. For example, you may have experienced the swollen cervical lymph nodes that often accompany a sore throat. An infection in almost any part of the body may result in swelling and tenderness of the lymph nodes that drain that area.

Tonsils Filter Interstitial Fluid

Tonsils are masses of lymph tissue located under the epithelial lining of the oral cavity and pharynx. Their major function is to filter interstitial fluid. The **lingual (ling′-gwal) tonsils** are located at the base of the tongue. The **pharyngeal tonsil** is located in the posterior wall of the nasal portion of the pharynx above the soft palate. When enlarged (usually as a result of infection or allergy), the pharyngeal tonsil is called the *adenoids.*

Most prominent are the paired **palatine tonsils** on each side of the throat. These oval masses of lymphatic tissue are thickenings in the mucous membrane of the throat. The stratified epithelium of the throat that overlies the tonsils dips down to form 10 to 20 pits, or crypts, in each tonsil. Bacteria often accumulate in these crypts and may invade the lymphatic tissue of the tonsil. This may cause an increase in the mass of the tonsil. Sometimes bacterial invasion of the tonsils becomes a chronic problem and the tonsils are surgically removed by the well-known procedure called *tonsillectomy.* After a child is about 7 years old, the lymphatic tissue of the tonsils begins to shrink in size.

The Spleen Filters Blood

The **spleen** is the largest organ of the lymphatic system (see Figure 12-11). It lies in the abdominal cavity posterior and lateral to the stomach and is protected by the ribs. Because it holds a great deal of blood, the spleen has a distinctive rich purple color.

One of the main functions of the spleen is to filter blood. As blood flows slowly through the spleen, macrophages remove bacteria and other disease organisms. Macrophages also remove worn-out red blood cells and platelets. The spleen stores platelets, and a large percentage of the body's platelets are normally found there.

Although the spleen performs these important functions, it is not vital to life. This is fortunate because the spleen is the most easily and most frequently injured of all of the abdominal organs. A severe blow or crushing injury to the upper abdomen or lower left chest may fracture the ribs that protect the spleen and cause rupture of the spleen itself. When the spleen is ruptured, extensive, sometimes massive, hemorrhage occurs. Prompt surgical removal of the spleen *(splenectomy)* prevents the loss of blood and the circulatory shock that could cause death. When the spleen is surgically removed, some of its functions are taken over by the bone marrow and liver; other functions are simply absent, and the body manages without them.

The Thymus Gland Plays a Role in Immune Function

The **thymus gland** is a pinkish gray lymphatic organ located in the upper thorax posterior to the sternum and anterior to the great vessels as they emerge from the heart (see Figure 12-11). During fetal life and childhood, it is quite large. It reaches its largest size at puberty and then begins to become smaller with age. The thymus gland plays a key role in the body's immune processes (see Chapter 13). It produces several hormones collectively called *thymosin.* The thymus prepares one type of lymphocyte (T lymphocytes) for action.

Quiz Yourself

- What are three main functions of the lymphatic system?
- Through what structures does lymph pass as it moves from a lymph capillary back to the blood circulation?

SUMMARY

LO 1. Compare the structure and functions of arteries, capillaries, and veins.

- Blood vessels are tubes that circulate blood through the body. Three main types of blood vessels are arteries, capillaries, and veins.
- An **artery** conducts blood away from the heart and toward some organ. An **arteriole** is a small artery that can constrict or dilate, thereby changing the flow of blood into a tissue and affecting blood pressure. **Metarterioles** are small vessels that link arterioles and venules.
- **Capillaries** are microscopic blood vessels with very thin walls. Plasma leaks through the walls into the tissues, taking with it oxygen, nutrients, and other materials. A capillary that branches from a metarteriole has a **precapillary sphincter** that regulates the flow of blood into the capillary. In the liver, spleen, and bone marrow, small, leaky vessels called **sinusoids** connect arterioles and venules.
- A **vein** conducts blood away from an organ and back toward the heart.
- The walls of arteries and veins consist of three layers: an endothelium lining, the **tunica intima;** a middle layer, **tunica media,** consisting of connective tissue and smooth muscle; and an outer connective tissue layer, **tunica adventitia.**

LO 2. Trace a drop of blood through the pulmonary and systemic circulations, listing the principal vessels and heart chambers through which it must pass on its journey from one part of the body to another. (For example, trace a drop of blood from the inferior vena cava to an organ such as the brain and then back to the heart.)

- Blood is circulated through two circuits: the **pulmonary circulation** and the **systemic circulation.** The sequence of blood flow through the pulmonary circulation is as follows: The right ventricle pumps oxygen-poor blood into the pulmonary arteries, which transport it to the lungs. As blood flows through pulmonary capillaries, carbon dioxide diffuses out of the blood and oxygen diffuses into the blood. Blood rich in oxygen enters the pulmonary veins and is transported to the left atrium. Blood then passes into the left ventricle.

- The left ventricle pumps oxygen-rich blood into the systemic circulation. The **aorta,** the largest artery in the body, receives blood from the left ventricle. Branches of the aorta deliver blood to all parts of the body. Blood flows through capillaries and then passes into veins that conduct blood toward the heart. The **superior vena cava** receives blood from the upper portions of the body and returns it to the right atrium. The **inferior vena cava** receives blood from below the diaphragm and returns it to the right atrium.

LO 3. Identify the main divisions of the aorta and its principal branches.

- The main divisions of the aorta are the **ascending aorta, aortic arch, thoracic aorta,** and **abdominal aorta.** The **descending aorta** is made up of the thoracic aorta and the abdominal aorta. The main branches of each division of the aorta are listed in Table 12-1.

LO 4. Trace a drop of blood through the brain.

- Blood is conducted to the brain by the **internal carotid arteries** and the **vertebral arteries.** The vertebral arteries form the **basilar artery.** Branches of these arteries join to form the **circle of Willis.** From the brain capillaries, blood passes into venous sinuses and then into the **internal jugular veins** (see Table 12-2).

LO 5. Trace a drop of blood through the hepatic portal system.

- Blood from the intestine drains into the **superior mesenteric vein.** Blood then passes into the **hepatic portal vein,** which conducts it to the liver. Within the liver, blood flows into an extensive network of sinusoids. Blood from the hepatic sinusoids passes into **hepatic veins,** which empty into the inferior vena cava. Note that instead of conducting blood into another vein, the hepatic portal vein empties into an extra set of exchange vessels (sinusoids).

LO 6. State the physiological basis for arterial pulse and describe how pulse is measured.

- **Arterial pulse** is caused by the elastic expansion and recoil of arteries as they fill with blood. This ability of large arteries to expand and then snap back to their original diameter helps maintain a continuous flow of blood. Pulse can be measured by placing a finger over an artery near the skin surface—for example, the **radial artery.**

LO = Learning Objective

LO 7. **State the relationship among blood pressure, blood flow, and resistance, and describe how blood pressure is measured.**

- Blood pressure is the force exerted by the blood against the inner walls of the blood vessels. Blood pressure equals blood flow times the resistance to that flow.
- Blood flow depends on cardiac output. When cardiac output increases, blood flow increases, causing a rise in blood pressure. When cardiac output decreases, blood flow decreases, causing a fall in blood pressure.
- **Peripheral resistance** is the resistance to blood flow caused by the viscosity of blood and by the friction between the blood and the wall of the blood vessel. A small change in the diameter of a blood vessel causes a big change in blood pressure. The blood pressure is regulated mainly by **vasoconstriction,** narrowing of the diameter of the arterioles, or **vasodilation,** expansion of the diameter of the arterioles.
- In severe hemorrhage, circulatory shock may occur. The blood pressure may fall drastically so that blood flow to the tissues is not adequate and death may result.
- A blood pressure reading is expressed as **systolic pressure** over **diastolic pressure.** Blood pressure can be measured with a sphygmomanometer and a stethoscope. In **hypertension** (systolic pressure consistently measures 140 mm Hg or higher or diastolic pressure consistently measures 90 mm Hg or higher), there is typically increased vascular resistance, especially in the arterioles and small arteries.

LO 8. **Compare blood pressure in the different types of blood vessels of the systemic circulation.**

- Blood pressure is greatest in the arteries, decreases in the arterioles, and continues to decrease as blood flows through capillaries, and finally veins.

LO 9. **Describe the mechanisms by which the nervous and endocrine systems regulate blood pressure.**

- When blood pressure *decreases,* sympathetic nerves signal vasoconstriction in blood vessels so that pressure rises again. When blood pressure *increases,* specialized receptors, called **baroreceptors,** present in the walls of certain arteries and in the heart wall, send messages to cardiac

centers in the medulla. Then, parasympathetic nerves signal the heart to slow—an action that lowers blood pressure. The cardiac centers also inhibit sympathetic nerves that constrict arterioles. Inhibiting these nerves lowers blood pressure.

- When blood pressure decreases, the kidneys secrete **renin.** This enzyme acts on a plasma protein, initiating a series of reactions that produces **angiotensin II**—a hormone that is a powerful vasoconstrictor. Angiotensin II also stimulates the adrenal glands to secrete **aldosterone.** This hormone increases blood pressure by increasing reabsorption of sodium ions by the kidneys. As a result, more fluid is retained. Blood volume increases, which raises blood pressure.

LO 10. **Describe the functions, tissues, and organs of the lymphatic system.**

- The **lymphatic system** collects and returns interstitial (tissue) fluid to the blood, defends the body against disease, and absorbs lipids from the intestine.
- The **lymph** is formed from interstitial fluid. The lymph circulates through a system of **lymph capillaries** and **lymphatics;** as it passes through **lymph nodes,** it is filtered.
- The lymphatic system includes the tonsils, spleen, and thymus gland. The main **tonsils** are the palatine tonsils on each side of the throat. Tonsils filter interstitial fluid. The **spleen** filters blood and stores platelets. The **thymus gland** produces hormones and prepares one type of lymphocyte for its function in immunity.

LO 11. **Trace the flow of lymph from a lymph capillary to the left or right subclavian vein.**

- A drop of lymph flows from lymph capillaries to a lymphatic vessel and then through the lymph sinuses in a lymph node, where it is filtered. The lymph then flows into another lymphatic.
- Lymphatic vessels from all over the body, except the upper right quadrant, drain into the **thoracic duct,** which delivers lymph into the left subclavian vein. Lymph from the lymphatic vessels in the upper right quadrant of the body drains into the **right lymphatic duct,** which empties lymph into the right subclavian vein.

CHAPTER QUIZ

Fill in the Blank

1. Blood vessels that transport blood away from the heart and toward some organ or tissue are called _____.

2. Materials are exchanged between blood and tissues through the thin walls of _____.

3. By constricting and dilating, arterioles help regulate blood _____.

4. The left ventricle pumps blood into the _____ circulation.

5. Blood from the right ventricle is pumped into the _____ artery.

6. The pulmonary vein carries _____ (oxygen-rich or oxygen-poor) blood.

7. The _____ aorta is the region of the aorta that descends from the aortic arch.

8. Blood returning to the heart from the tissues, above the level of the diaphragm, drains into a large vein, the _____ _____ _____.

9. An important arterial circuit at the base of the brain is the _____ of _____.

10. Blood is delivered to the brain by the _____ and the _____ arteries.

11. Blood from the digestive tract passes from the superior mesenteric vein into the _____ vein, which takes it to the _____

12. The alternate expansion and recoil of an artery is called _____.

13. The force exerted by the blood against the inner walls of the blood vessels is called _____ _____.

14. The _____ system returns interstitial fluid to the blood.

15. Tonsils are masses of _____ tissue.

16. Vessels that conduct lymph into a lymph node are called _____.

Multiple Choice

17. When plasma enters the tissues, it is called: a. interstitial fluid; b. blood; c. lymph; d. capillary fluid.

18. Arterioles: a. conduct blood to arteries; b. are important in regulating blood pressure; c. have very leaky walls; d. are characterized by the baroreceptors in their walls.

19. Endothelium: a. is found mainly in the outer layer of arterial walls; b. is found mainly in the middle layer of vein walls; c. lines blood vessels; d. makes up the middle layer of the heart.

20. Metarterioles: a. are large arterioles that regulate blood pressure; b. link the aorta with smaller arteries; c. are leaky vessels found mainly in the liver and spleen; d. are small vessels that directly link arterioles and venules.

21. Blood flowing through the brachiocephalic vein next flows into the: a. internal jugular vein; b. superior vena cava; c. inferior vena cava; d. descending aorta.

22. A large organ in the abdominal cavity that filters blood is the: a. lymph nodes; b. palatine tonsils; c. spleen; d. thymus gland.

REVIEW QUESTIONS

1. Compare the wall of an artery with that of a capillary.

2. Why is the ability of arterioles to dilate and constrict important?

3. What is the function of the valves found in some veins?

4. Why are capillaries referred to as exchange vessels?

5. Name the divisions of the aorta and list the main arteries that branch from each division.

6. Trace a drop of blood from the inferior vena cava to the thoracic aorta by listing (in order) each blood vessel and each part of the heart through which it must pass.

7. What blood vessels bring blood to the brain? What is the significance of the circle of Willis?

8. Trace a drop of blood from the: (a) subclavian vein to the left ventricle; (b) right atrium to the renal vein; (c) inferior vena cava to the superior vena cava; (d) hepatic portal vein to the right common carotid artery.

9. Trace a drop of blood from the: (a) coronary vein to a pulmonary capillary; (b) iliac vein to the brain; (c) kidney to the liver; (d) inferior vena cava to the arm.

10. What factors determine blood pressure? How does the nervous system regulate blood pressure? How does the endocrine system help regulate blood pressure?

11. Trace a drop of lymph from a lymph capillary to the thoracic duct.

12. Label the diagram of the circulatory system. (See Figure 12-4 to check your answers.)

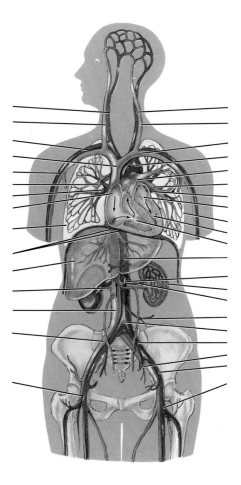

13

Internal Defense: Immune Responses

Chapter Outline

The body has remarkable defense mechanisms that protect against disease-causing organisms that enter the body with air, food, and water; during copulation; and through wounds in the skin. Disease-causing organisms, or **pathogens** (**path'**-o-jens), include certain bacteria, viruses, fungi, and protozoa. The body also protects itself against other kinds of foreign agents, including foreign cells that enter the body. Some immune responses target cancer cells.

Immunology, the study of internal defense mechanisms, is one of the most rapidly changing and exciting fields of biomedical research today. (The term *immune* is derived from a Latin word meaning "safe.") Among the greatest accomplishments of immunologists have been the development of vaccines that prevent disease and techniques for transplanting tissues and organs.

In this chapter we discuss nonspecific and specific immune responses. We describe the processes of cell-mediated and antibody-mediated immunity. We then briefly discuss immune responses that can cause problems, such as allergic reactions and autoimmune disease.

IMMUNE RESPONSES CAN BE NONSPECIFIC OR SPECIFIC

LEARNING OBJECTIVE

1. **Contrast nonspecific and specific immune responses.**

An **immune response** involves recognition of foreign or harmful molecules and an action aimed at eliminating them. Immune responses depend on communication among cells, or **cell signaling.** Cells of the immune system communicate directly with their surface molecules and indirectly by releasing signaling (messenger) molecules.

Two main types of immune responses are nonspecific and specific immune responses. **Nonspecific immune responses** provide general protection against pathogens. These responses prevent most pathogens from entering the body (e.g., the skin is a barrier) and rapidly destroy those pathogens that do penetrate the outer defenses.

Specific immune responses are precise responses against specific foreign molecules that have gained entrance to the body. Any molecule that can be specifically recognized as foreign by cells of the immune system is called an **antigen.** Typically, antigens are large molecules, such as proteins and polysaccharides (large carbohydrates). An important specific defense mechanism is the production of **antibodies**—highly specific proteins that recognize and bind to specific antigens.

Immune responses depend largely on the body's ability to distinguish *self* from *nonself,* that is, to distinguish between itself and pathogens that infect it. A single bacterium may have 10 to more than 1000 distinct proteins on its surface. When a bacterium invades, the body recognizes these surface proteins as foreign and launches an attack. Each type of organism and, indeed, each individual human are biochemically unique. In humans, this uniqueness depends largely on a group of inherited cell surface proteins known as **MHC (major histocompatibility complex) antigens.** The body "knows" its own molecules and "recognizes" those of other organisms (including other humans) as foreign. Before tissues or organs are transplanted from a donor to a patient, the tissues must be carefully matched. Cell typing is somewhat similar to blood typing but depends on matching MHC antigens as closely as possible. Only identical twins have exact matches.

Quiz Yourself

- What is the function of nonspecific immunity?
- What are antibodies?

NONSPECIFIC DEFENSE MECHANISMS ARE RAPID

LEARNING OBJECTIVE

2. **Describe several nonspecific immune responses, including barriers, proteins such as cytokines and complement, phagocytosis, and inflammation.**

Our first line of defense is our skin, the outer covering of the body. Skin and other barriers stop most pathogens from entering the body. When pathogens do succeed in penetrating the body, the immune system responds quickly to destroy them. Among the major nonspecific defenses are (1) mechanical and chemical barriers, (2) proteins that mediate immune responses, (3) cells that destroy pathogens, and (4) inflammation (Figure 13-1).

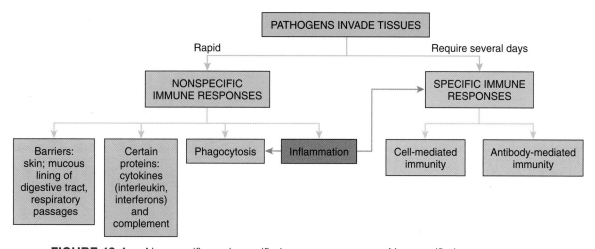

FIGURE 13-1 • Nonspecific and specific immune responses. Nonspecific immune responses prevent entry of many pathogens and act to destroy those that do manage to cross the barriers. Cytokines released by cells during inflammation signal the immune system to launch specific immune responses. Specific immune responses take longer to mobilize but are highly effective in destroying invaders.

Mechanical and Chemical Barriers Prevent Entry of Most Pathogens

The skin and the mucous membranes that line passageways into the body are the first line of defense against pathogens and other harmful substances. The skin is more than just a mechanical barrier. It is populated by large numbers of harmless bacteria. These bacteria inhibit the multiplication of harmful bacteria that happen to land on it. Sweat and other secretions on the surface of the skin contain chemicals that destroy certain types of bacteria.

Pathogens that enter the body with inhaled air may be filtered out by hairs in the nose or trapped in the sticky mucous lining of the respiratory passageway. Once trapped, pathogens may be destroyed by phagocytes. Bacteria that enter with food are usually destroyed by the acid and enzymes of the stomach.

Several Types of Proteins Mediate Immune Responses

Cytokines and complement are two major groups of proteins that are important in nonspecific immune responses.

Cytokines Are Important Signaling Molecules

Cytokines (**sigh′**-tow-kines) are a large group of peptides and proteins that cells use to signal one another. Some cytokines, like many hormones, circulate in the blood and affect distant tissues. The functions of nonspecific and specific immune responses overlap, and some cytokines have roles in both of these subsystems. We discuss two groups of cytokines: interferons and interleukins.

When infected by viruses or other intracellular parasites (some types of bacteria, fungi, and protozoa), cells respond by secreting cytokines called **interferons** (in′-ter-**feer′**-ons). When viruses infect a cell, they take over the cellular machinery and use it to make more viruses. Eventually, the infected host cell bursts, releasing many new viruses, which can then infect surrounding cells. Interferons do not protect the cells that produce them. They signal neighboring cells and stimulate them to produce antiviral proteins. Viruses produced in cells exposed to interferon are less effective at infecting new cells.

Since their discovery in 1957, interferons have been the focus of much research, and they are now being used to treat several diseases, including hepatitis B and hepatitis C, a type of leukemia, and a type of multiple sclerosis. Researchers are testing interferons in clinical trials for treatment of **human immunodeficiency virus (HIV)** infection and several types of cancer.

Interleukins are a diverse group of proteins secreted mainly by macrophages and lymphocytes. They regulate interactions between lymphocytes and other cells of the body, and some interleukins have widespread effects. For example, during infection, an interleukin resets the body's thermostat in the hypothalamus, resulting in fever and its symptoms.

Complement Leads to Pathogen Destruction

Complement, so named because it *complements* the action of other immune responses, consists of more than 20 proteins present in plasma and other body fluids. Normally, complement proteins are inactive until the body is exposed to an antigen. Certain pathogens activate the complement system directly. (In other cases, the binding of an antigen and antibody stimulates activation.) Complement activation involves a series of reactions, with each protein acting on the next in the series. Once activated, proteins of the complement system work to destroy pathogens. Some complement proteins can rupture the cell wall of the pathogen. Others promote phagocytosis and inflammation.

Phagocytes and Natural Killer Cells Destroy Pathogens

Recall that **phagocytes** (**fag′**-o-sites) are cells that ingest bacteria and other foreign matter. In **phagocytosis,** a cell flows around a bacterium and engulfs it (Figure 13-2). As a bacterium is ingested, it is packaged within a vesicle formed by membrane pinched off from the plasma membrane. Lysosomes adhere to the vesicle and release enzymes into it that kill the bacterium. **Neutrophils** (the most common type of white blood cell, see Chapter 10) and **macrophages** are the phagocytes of the immune system. A neutrophil can phagocytize 20 or so bacteria before it becomes inactivated and dies. A macrophage can phagocytize about 100 bacteria during its life span.

Natural killer (NK) cells are large, granular lymphocytes that originate in the bone marrow. When they were first identified, immunologists thought that NK cells functioned only against tumor cells. However, studies have demonstrated that these cells recognize and are active against a wide variety of targets, including cells infected with viruses, some bacteria, and some fungi. NK cells release cytokines and enzymes that destroy target cells. These killer cells also destroy target cells by specific (antibody-requiring) processes.

Inflammation Is a Protective Response

When pathogens invade tissues, **inflammation** develops within a few hours. The clinical characteristics of inflammation are *heat, redness, edema,* and *pain* (Figure 13-3). Inflammation is regulated by proteins in the plasma, by cytokines, and by **mast cells**—large connective tissue cells filled with distinctive granules.

Platelets, basophils, and mast cells release **histamine** and **serotonin**—compounds that dilate blood vessels in the affected area and increase capillary permeability. Vasodilation allows increased blood flow to the infected region, bringing great numbers of neutrophils and other phagocytic cells. The increased blood flow makes the skin feel warm and makes skin that contains little pigment appear red.

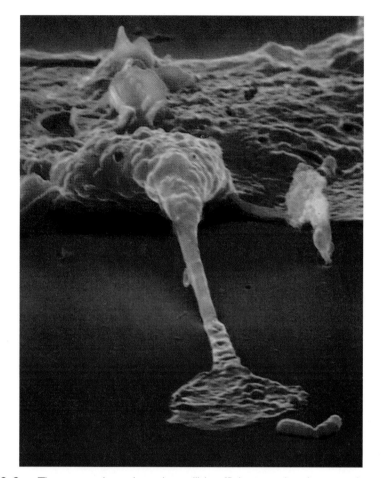

FIGURE 13-2 • The macrophage is an incredibly efficient warrior. A macrophage *(gray)* extends a pseudopod toward an invading *Escherichia coli* bacterium *(green)* that is already multiplying. The macrophage will trap the bacterium and take it into the macrophage cell. The macrophage's plasma membrane will seal over the bacterium, and powerful lysosomal enzymes will destroy it. (Copyright Boehringer Ingelheim Pharma KG, photograph Lennart Nilsson/Albert Bonniers Forlag AB.)

Increased capillary permeability also occurs during the inflammatory response. Fluid carries antibodies out of the circulation and into the tissues. As the volume of interstitial fluid increases, **edema** (swelling) occurs. The edema (and also certain enzymes in the plasma) causes the pain characteristic of inflammation. Phagocytes easily migrate out of the permeable capillaries and into the infected tissues. Increased phagocytosis appears to be one of the main functions of inflammation. Cytokines released by cells during inflammation signal other cells that function in specific immune responses.

Although inflammation is often a local response, sometimes the entire body is involved. **Fever** is a common clinical sign of widespread inflammatory response. Fever helps the body fight infection. For example, the increased body temperature interferes with the growth and replication of some microorganisms and may kill some pathogens. A short-term low fever helps speed recovery.

Quiz Yourself

- What is the function of interferons?
- What is the function of natural killer cells?
- Blood flow to the infected area increases during inflammation. How is that helpful?

SPECIFIC DEFENSE MECHANISMS INCLUDE CELL-MEDIATED IMMUNITY AND ANTIBODY-MEDIATED IMMUNITY

LEARNING OBJECTIVES

3. Identify and give the functions of the principal cells of the immune system.

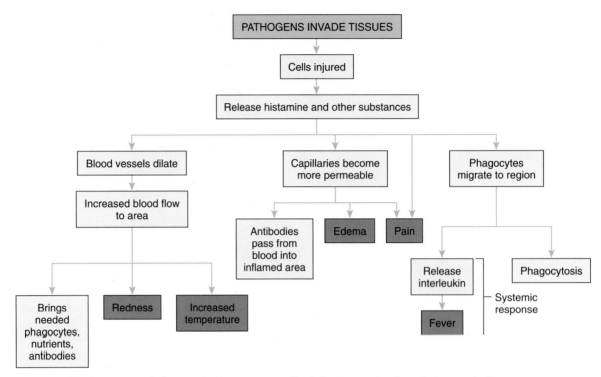

FIGURE 13-3 • Inflammation is a nonspecific defense mechanism that speeds the passage of phagocytic cells, antibodies, and other needed compounds into infected tissues.

4. **Describe cell-mediated immunity, including development of memory cells.**
5. **Describe antibody-mediated immunity, including the effects of antigen-antibody complex on pathogens both directly and through the complement system.**
6. **Compare primary and secondary immune responses.**
7. **Contrast active and passive immunity and give examples of each.**

While nonspecific immune responses rapidly destroy pathogens and prevent the spread of infection, specific immune mechanisms are being mobilized. Several days are required to activate specific immune responses, but once in gear, these mechanisms are extremely effective. Specific immunity is the job of the lymphatic system. This system can mobilize armies of highly specialized cellular soldiers and can wage sophisticated chemical warfare. Two main types of specific immunity are **antibody-mediated immunity** and **cell-mediated immunity.**

Many Types of Cells Participate in Specific Immune Responses

The principal warriors in specific immune responses are the trillion or so lymphocytes stationed strategically in the lymph tissue throughout the body. Many other types of cells participate in specific immune responses, including neutrophils, macrophages, and dendritic cells (Figure 13-4). Note that some types of cells are involved in both nonspecific and specific immune responses.

Lymphocytes Are the Principal Warriors in Specific Immune Responses

Three main types of lymphocytes are **T lymphocytes,** or **T cells; B lymphocytes,** or **B cells;** and NK cells. As already discussed, NK cells kill virus-infected cells and tumor cells.

T cells are responsible for **cell-mediated immunity.** They attack body cells infected by invading pathogens, foreign cells (e.g., those introduced in tissue grafts or organ transplants), and cells altered by mutation (cancer cells). T cells originate from stem cells in the bone marrow. On their way to the lymph tissues, T cells stop off in the **thymus gland,** where they mature. (The "T" in T cells stands for *thymus-derived.*) The thymus makes T cells *competent,* that is, capable of making immune responses. As T cells move through the thymus, they divide many times and develop specific surface receptors, called **T-cell receptors.**

B cells, which are responsible for **antibody-mediated immunity,** mature into *plasma cells* that produce specific antibodies. Millions of B cells are produced in the bone marrow daily. B cells mature in the fetal liver and in the adult bone marrow. Each B cell is genetically programmed to produce and display a specific type of receptor that binds with a specific type of antigen. After they leave the bone marrow and thymus gland, B cells and T cells reside in the spleen, lymph nodes, tonsils, and other lymphatic tissues strategically positioned throughout the body.

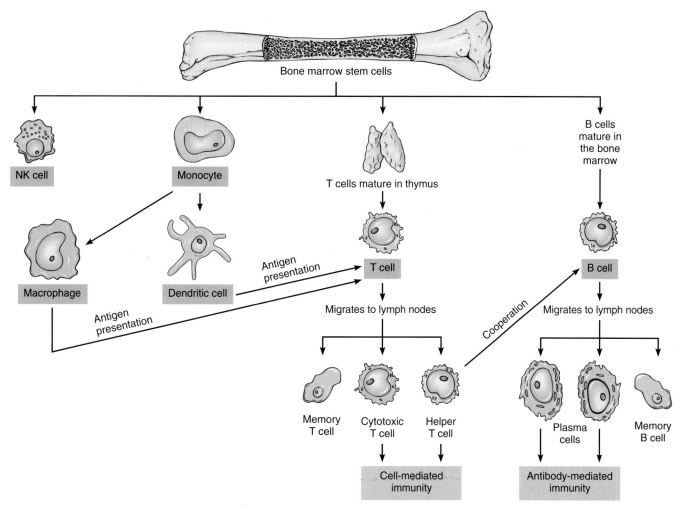

Bone marrow stem cells

NK cell

Monocyte

T cells mature in thymus

B cells mature in the bone marrow

Macrophage

Dendritic cell

Antigen presentation

T cell

B cell

Antigen presentation

Migrates to lymph nodes

Cooperation

Migrates to lymph nodes

Memory T cell

Cytotoxic T cell

Helper T cell

Plasma cells

Memory B cell

Cell-mediated immunity

Antibody-mediated immunity

FIGURE 13-4 • Some cells of the immune system. These cells interact by complex signaling.

Macrophages and Dendritic Cells Present Antigens

Macrophages and **dendritic cells** both develop from monocytes (a type of white blood cell). Macrophages secrete about 100 different compounds, including interferons and enzymes that destroy bacteria. When a macrophage ingests a bacterium, most but not all of the bacterial antigens are degraded by lysosomal enzymes. Fragments of the foreign antigens are then displayed on the surface of the macrophage. These foreign antigens are displayed in association with MHC—the cell's own self-molecules.

Dendritic cells are strategically stationed in the skin and in the linings of the digestive, respiratory, urinary, and vaginal passageways into the body. Like macrophages, dendritic cells capture foreign antigens and break them down. They display fragments of the foreign antigens on their cell surface. Dendritic cells also instruct T cells to locate to specific regions of the body.

Macrophages, dendritic cells, and B cells function as **antigen-presenting cells (APCs).** They display fragments of foreign antigens as well as their own surface proteins. APCs present the displayed antigens to T cells.

T Cells Are Responsible for Cell-Mediated Immunity

In cell-mediated immunity, T cells attack invading pathogens directly. There are thousands of different T cells, each distinguished by a specific T-cell receptor and each capable of responding to a specific type of antigen.

Several types of T cells have been identified. One group, known as **killer T cells,** or **cytotoxic T cells,** recognizes and destroys cells with foreign antigens on their surfaces. Killer T cells are also called *CD8 cells* because they have a protein known as CD8 on the surface of the plasma membrane. Among their target cells are virus-infected cells, cancer cells, and foreign tissue grafts. Killer T cells kill their target cells by releasing a variety of cytokines and enzymes that destroy cells. **Helper T cells**, also known as *CD4 cells,* secrete cytokines that activate B cells and enhance immune responses. **Regulatory T cells** suppress immune responses after pathogens have been destroyed.

After a virus enters the body and infects cells, some of the viral antigen is displayed on the cell surface of APCs. The types of T cells able to react to the foreign antigen become activated. Once stimulated, a T cell multiplies by mitosis, giving rise to a sizable clone of cells identical to itself (Figure 13-5). These differentiated (specialized) T cells then make their way to the site of infection. Killer T cells release powerful enzymes and cytokines that kill the infected cells directly and also increase inflammation.

> Virus infects body → antigen-presenting cells display foreign antigen → certain T cells are activated → activated T cells multiply, forming clones of activated T cells → killer T cells migrate to infected area → release enzymes that destroy the pathogens

Some differentiated T cells remain in the lymph tissue as **memory T cells** for years or even decades. If the same type of pathogen ever attacks again, the memory cells quickly go into action, destroying the invaders so rapidly that they usually do not have time to cause symptoms of the disease.

B Cells Are Responsible for Antibody-Mediated Immunity

As with T cells, thousands of different kinds of B cells exist, each specialized to respond to a specific type of antigen. However, B cells respond differently. Instead of going out to meet the invader, B cells produce specific antibodies and send them out to do the job. Recall that antibodies, also known as **immunoglobulins,** are highly specific proteins that serve as cell surface receptors that combine with antigens. Only a B cell displaying a matching receptor on its surface can bind a particular antigen.

In most cases, activation of B cells is a complex process that involves APCs and helper T cells. Macrophages or dendritic cells capture the foreign antigen in the infected tissues and migrate to the lymph tissues. There, they present the foreign antigen to helper T cells and B cells that have receptors matching the foreign antigen. The helper T cells secrete cytokines that help activate the B cells.

The activated B cells multiply. Within a few days an activated B cell produces a large clone of identical B cells (Figure 13-6). Most of these cells mature and become **plasma cells.** Plasma cells secrete antibodies, a form of their specific receptor molecule that can be secreted. Antibodies are carried by the lymph to the blood and are then transported to the infected region.

> Pathogen infects body → APCs present foreign antigen to helper T cells → activated helper T cells activate B cells with receptors that match the antigen → activated B cells multiply → clones of activated B cells → develop into plasma cells → plasma cells secrete antibodies → antibodies are transported to infected area

Some of the activated B cells become **memory B cells** and continue for years to produce small amounts of antibody. Should the pathogen ever enter the body again, this circulating antibody (part of the *gamma globulin fraction* of the plasma) immediately binds with it. At the same time, the memory cells respond by quickly multiplying to produce new clones of the needed type of plasma cells.

Antibodies are grouped into five classes according to their structure. With the abbreviation **Ig** used for immunoglobulin, the classes are designated *IgG, IgM, IgA, IgD,* and *IgE.* Each class has different functions. Normally, about 75% of the antibodies in the body belong in the IgG group, part of the gamma globulin fraction of the blood.

The principal job of an antibody is to identify a pathogen as foreign. It does this by combining with one or more antigens on the surface of the pathogen. An antibody usually combines with several antigens, creating a mass of clumped **antigen-antibody complex.** The antigen-antibody complex activates several defense mechanisms:

1. The antigen-antibody complex may inactivate the pathogen or its toxin. For example, once an antibody has attached to the surface of a virus, the virus may lose its ability to infect a new cell.
2. The antigen-antibody complex stimulates phagocytes to destroy the pathogen.
3. Antibodies of the IgG and IgM groups work by activating the complement system.

Long-Term Immunity Depends on Memory Cells

Memory B and memory T cells are responsible for long-term immunity. They enable the body to launch more effective immune responses, thus providing protection against disease. The first time we are exposed to a particular antigen, the body launches a **primary response** (Figure 13-7, *A*). Approximately 3 to 14 days are required to mobilize specific T cells and antibodies. After an immune response, memory cells group strategically in many nonlymphatic tissues, including the lung, liver, kidney, and digestive tract. Many infections occur in these organs, and T cells already stationed there can respond quickly.

A second exposure to the same antigen, even years later, results in a **secondary response,** which is much more rapid (Figure 13-7, *B*). Memory T cells quickly become killer T cells and produce interferon and other substances that kill invading cells before we develop the disease. Memory B cells multiply

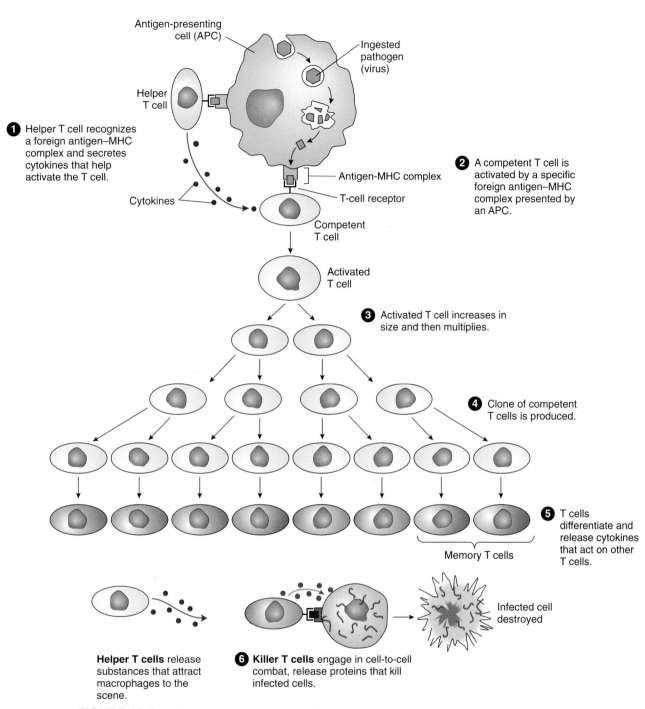

Antigen-presenting cell (APC)

Ingested pathogen (virus)

Helper T cell

❶ Helper T cell recognizes a foreign antigen–MHC complex and secretes cytokines that help activate the T cell.

Cytokines

Antigen-MHC complex

T-cell receptor

Competent T cell

❷ A competent T cell is activated by a specific foreign antigen–MHC complex presented by an APC.

Activated T cell

❸ Activated T cell increases in size and then multiplies.

❹ Clone of competent T cells is produced.

Memory T cells

❺ T cells differentiate and release cytokines that act on other T cells.

Infected cell destroyed

Helper T cells release substances that attract macrophages to the scene.

❻ **Killer T cells** engage in cell-to-cell combat, release proteins that kill infected cells.

FIGURE 13-5 • Cell-mediated immunity. When activated by a foreign antigen presented by an APC, a competent T cell gives rise to a large clone of cells. Many of these differentiate to become killer T cells, which migrate to the site of infection. There they release proteins that destroy invading pathogens. They also release cytokines that stimulate macrophages and other lymphocytes. Some of the T cells remain in the lymph nodes as memory cells. (Other T cells produce clones of helper T cells in a similar way.)

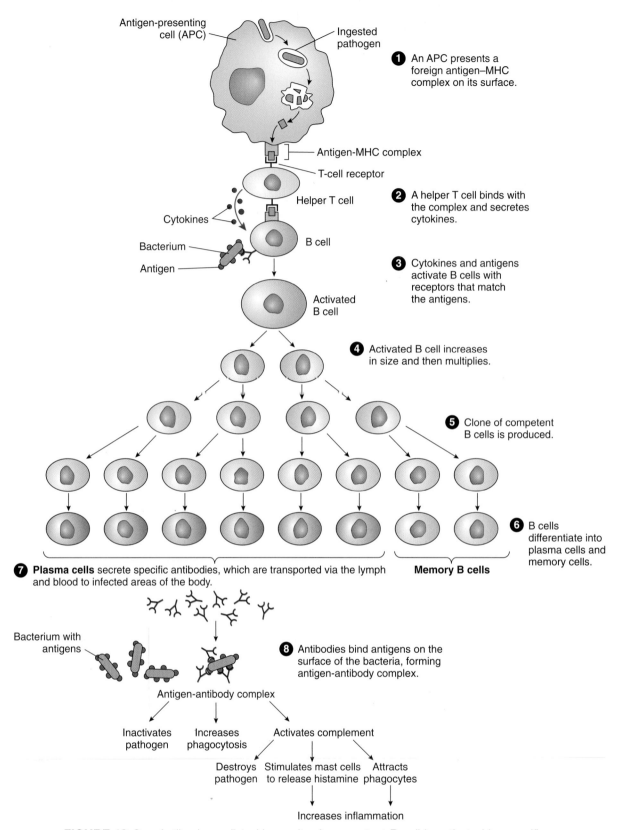

① An APC presents a foreign antigen–MHC complex on its surface.

Antigen-presenting cell (APC)

Ingested pathogen

Antigen-MHC complex

T-cell receptor

Helper T cell

② A helper T cell binds with the complex and secretes cytokines.

Cytokines

Bacterium

Antigen

B cell

③ Cytokines and antigens activate B cells with receptors that match the antigens.

Activated B cell

④ Activated B cell increases in size and then multiplies.

⑤ Clone of competent B cells is produced.

⑥ B cells differentiate into plasma cells and memory cells.

Memory B cells

⑦ **Plasma cells** secrete specific antibodies, which are transported via the lymph and blood to infected areas of the body.

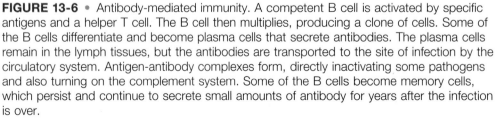

Bacterium with antigens

Antigen-antibody complex

⑧ Antibodies bind antigens on the surface of the bacteria, forming antigen-antibody complex.

Inactivates pathogen

Increases phagocytosis

Activates complement

Destroys pathogen

Stimulates mast cells to release histamine

Attracts phagocytes

Increases inflammation

FIGURE 13-6 • Antibody-mediated immunity. A competent B cell is activated by specific antigens and a helper T cell. The B cell then multiplies, producing a clone of cells. Some of the B cells differentiate and become plasma cells that secrete antibodies. The plasma cells remain in the lymph tissues, but the antibodies are transported to the site of infection by the circulatory system. Antigen-antibody complexes form, directly inactivating some pathogens and also turning on the complement system. Some of the B cells become memory cells, which persist and continue to secrete small amounts of antibody for years after the infection is over.

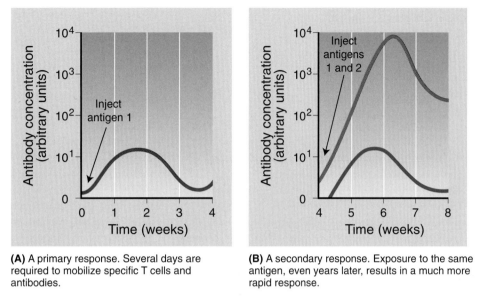

(A) A primary response. Several days are required to mobilize specific T cells and antibodies.

(B) A secondary response. Exposure to the same antigen, even years later, results in a much more rapid response.

— Antibodies to antigen 1—primary response
— Antibodies to antigen 1—secondary response
— Antibodies to antigen 2—primary response

FIGURE 13-7 • Immunological memory.

and rapidly increase antibody production. Because of memory cells, we do not usually become ill from the same type of infection more than once.

You may wonder, then, how someone can get a cold or influenza (the "flu") more than once. The answer is that these infections have many varieties, each caused by a slightly different virus. Furthermore, viruses frequently mutate (i.e., their gene structure changes) and develop slightly different surface antigens. Even a slight change in an antigen can prevent memory cells from recognizing the pathogen; the body must treat each different antigen as a new immunological challenge. A familiar example is the situation with the influenza virus. New strains of the influenza virus evolve each year, challenging microbiologists and public health officials to develop and distribute new vaccines.

Active Immunity Can Be Induced by Immunization

Active immunity typically develops naturally from exposure to antigens and production of memory cells. Active immunity can also be artificially induced by **immunization,** that is, by injection of a vaccine. For example, if you are immunized against measles, your body reacts just as though it had been exposed to someone with measles. The body launches an immune response against the antigens in the measles vaccine and develops memory cells. Vaccines are prepared in a variety of ways. Many consist of the entire pathogen that has been weakened or killed; others consist of an antigen from the pathogen.

Passive Immunity Is Borrowed Immunity

In **passive immunity,** an individual is given antibodies actively produced by other humans or by animals. Passive immunity is borrowed immunity, so its effects do not last. Antibodies produced by pregnant women can cross the placenta and enter the blood of the fetus. This gives the baby some protection for a few months after birth. Babies who are breast-fed receive antibodies in their milk. These antibodies provide immunity to the pathogens responsible for gastrointestinal infection and perhaps to other pathogens.

Passive immunity can be used clinically to boost defenses against a particular disease. For example, when individuals are exposed to a disease such as viral hepatitis or anthrax, they can be injected with gamma globulin (containing antibody to the pathogen) to help protect them from the disease. Unfortunately, these injected antibodies last only a few months. Do you know why? It is because the body has not actively launched an immune response. No memory cells have been developed, so the body cannot produce antibodies to the pathogen. Once the injected antibodies wear out, the immunity disappears.

Quiz Yourself

- Which types of cells function as antigen-presenting cells? What is their function?
- What is the function of killer T cells?
- How do B cells become plasma cells?
- Why is passive immunity temporary?

IMMUNE RESPONSES ARE SOMETIMES INADEQUATE OR HARMFUL

LEARNING OBJECTIVE

8. **Describe several examples of unwanted immune responses.**

Sometimes pathogens outmaneuver the immune defenses and cause disease. Some diseases, as well as certain genetic mutations, prevent or reduce immune function. **HIV,** the virus that causes **acquired immunodeficiency syndrome (AIDS),** infects helper T cells. Destruction of these cells seriously impairs immune function and puts the patient at risk for other infections.

Cancer cells are cells that have been transformed in a way that changes their growth-regulating mechanisms. They multiply in an uncontrolled way, invading tissues and may metastasize (spread) to other tissues. Cancer cells have abnormal surface proteins that the immune system targets as foreign antigens. However, cancer cells often evade the immune system and multiply unchecked.

At times, the immune system overfunctions, as in **allergic reactions.** The body produces antibodies against mild antigens (e.g., pollen, household dust) that normally do not stimulate an immune response. Mast cells release histamine and other substances that cause inflammation and other symptoms of allergy.

In about 8% of adults (mainly women), immune responses are directed against the body's own cells, resulting in **autoimmune diseases.** Examples are rheumatoid arthritis, multiple sclerosis, and insulin-dependent diabetes. Both genetic susceptibility and environmental factors, such as certain infections, contribute to the development of these disorders.

The immune system sometimes responds in ways that are clinically inconvenient as in Rh incompatibility (discussed in Chapter 10) or in destruction of tissue and organ transplants. Transplanted organs have foreign antigens that stimulate **graft rejection,** an immune response in which T cells destroy the cells of the transplant. To prevent graft rejection, physicians use antirejection drugs to suppress the immune system.

Quiz Yourself

- What are autoimmune diseases?
- What is graft rejection?

SUMMARY

LO 1. Contrast nonspecific and specific immune responses.
- In an **immune response,** the body recognizes foreign molecules and responds to eliminate them. Immunity depends on the body's ability to distinguish between self and nonself (e.g., pathogens). **Nonspecific immune responses** are rapid responses directed against foreign agents in general.
- **Specific immune responses** are directed against particular pathogens. In specific immune responses, the body produces **antibodies** that recognize and bind specific **antigens**—large molecules that can be recognized as foreign.

LO 2. Describe several nonspecific immune responses, including barriers, proteins such as cytokines and complement, phagocytosis, and inflammation.
- Barriers to pathogen entry include the skin, the mucous lining of the respiratory passageways, and acid secretions in the stomach.

LO = Learning Objective

- **Cytokines** are signaling molecules that regulate interactions between cells in both nonspecific and specific immune responses. **Interferons** are cytokines produced by cells infected by viruses; they signal other cells to produce antiviral proteins. **Interleukins** regulate interactions between lymphocytes and other cells.
- **Complement** is a group of proteins in plasma and other body fluids that destroy pathogens both directly and indirectly.
- **Phagocytes,** including **neutrophils** and **macrophages,** ingest bacteria and other foreign matter by phagocytosis. Lysosomes release enzymes that kill the bacteria. **Natural killer cells** destroy cancer cells and cells infected with viruses or other pathogens.
- The clinical characteristics of **inflammation** are heat, redness, **edema** (swelling), and pain. During inflammation, vasodilation brings more blood to the infected area. Increased capillary permeability results in antibodies leaving the circulation. Phagocytes move into the infected area, increasing phagocytosis. **Fever** is a clinical sign of widespread inflammation.

LO 3. Identify and give the functions of the principal cells of the immune system.

- **Lymphocytes** are the main warriors in specific immune responses. Three main types of lymphocytes are **T lymphocytes, or T cells; B lymphocytes, or B cells;** and natural killer (NK) cells. NK cells kill virus-infected cells and tumor cells. T cells are responsible for **cell-mediated immunity.** B cells, which are responsible for **antibody-mediated immunity,** mature into *plasma cells* that produce specific antibodies.
- Macrophages and **dendritic cells** are **antigen-presenting cells (APCs)** that break down foreign antigens and display antigen fragments on their cell surface.

LO 4. Describe cell-mediated immunity, including development of memory cells.

- Specific immune responses include cell-mediated immunity and antibody-mediated immunity. In cell-mediated immunity, specific T cells are activated when they come into contact with specific antigens. Activated T cells multiply, giving rise to a clone of identical cells.
- Some T cells differentiate to become **killer T cells** (also known as **cytotoxic T cells**) that migrate to the site of infection and kill pathogens. **Helper T cells** secrete cytokines that activate B cells and promote immune responses. Some activated T cells remain in the lymph nodes as **memory T cells.**

LO 5. Describe antibody-mediated immunity, including the effects of antigen-antibody complex on pathogens both directly and through the complement system.

- In antibody-mediated immunity, specific **B cells** are activated by the presence of specific antigens. Activated B cells multiply and give rise

to **plasma cells** that secrete specific antibodies. **Memory B cells** are also produced.
- Antibodies are transported by the circulatory system to the site of infection. Their main job is to identify an antigen as foreign. Antibodies combine with specific antigens to form **antigen-antibody complex.** This may inactivate the pathogen, stimulate phagocytes, or activate the complement system.

LO 6. Compare primary and secondary immune responses.

- Long-term immunity depends on memory cells. A **primary response,** launched at first exposure to a particular antigen, requires up to 2 weeks. A **secondary response** occurs when the body is exposed to the same antigen a second time; it is much faster because memory cells are already present.

LO 7. Contrast active and passive immunity and give examples of each.

- **Active immunity,** whether natural or by immunization, involves exposure to an antigen and an active immune response. Memory cells are produced and provide long-term protection.
- In **passive immunity,** antibodies are borrowed from another person or animal that has produced them. Passive immunity is temporary.

LO 8. Describe several examples of unwanted immune responses.

- The immune system sometimes responds in ways that are inconvenient, as in allergic reactions, autoimmune disease, or when an immune response destroys the cells of tissue and organ transplants. Transplanted tissues have foreign antigens that stimulate **graft rejection**—an immune response in which T cells destroy the transplant.

CHAPTER QUIZ

Fill in the Blank

1. Disease-causing organisms such as bacteria and viruses are called _____.

2. The body's first line of defense against pathogens is the _____.

3. The increased blood flow characteristic of inflammation brings _____ cells to the infected area.

4. When certain types of cells are infected by viruses, they release proteins called _____.

5. Molecules, such as certain proteins, that stimulate immune responses are called _____.

6. Plasma cells produce proteins called _____, which help destroy antigens.

7. B cells are responsible for _____-mediated immunity.

8. T cells are responsible for _____-mediated immunity.

9. Activated B or T cells that remain in the lymph nodes for many years after an infection are called _____ cells.

10. The main job of an antibody is to identify a pathogen as foreign by combining with _____ on its surface.

Multiple Choice

11. The group of more than 20 proteins found in plasma that are activated by certain pathogens is called:
a. complement; b. interferon; c. cytokine; d. interleukin.

12. Which of the following cells are antigen-presenting cells? a. plasma cells; b. memory T cells; c. basophils; d. dendritic cells.

13. An activated T cell has just formed a clone of cells. What happens next is: a. antibodies are released; b. antigen must be displayed on an APC; c. killer T cells migrate to the infected area; d. plasma cells differentiate.

14. The temporary immunity gained when one is injected with gamma globulin: a. is called active immunity; b. is called passive immunity; c. is similar to the immunity developed from vaccines; d. depends on development of memory cells.

15. An autoimmune disease may develop when: a. complement proteins are overactive; b. the immune system attacks self molecules; c. the body produces antibodies against mild foreign antigens; d. HIV infects helper T cells.

REVIEW QUESTIONS

1. Contrast nonspecific and specific immune responses.

2. How does the inflammatory response help restore homeostasis?

3. What is fever? Why is it considered a defense mechanism?

4. What are cytokines? How does interferon work?

5. Define: (a) antigen; (b) antibody.

6. Contrast the origins and actions of T and B cells.

7. Contrast cell-mediated immunity with antibody-mediated immunity, giving their principal differences.

8. Compare (a) the immune response that occurs when someone with measles sneezes on someone who has not had measles and has not been immunized against measles; (b) the response stimulated when you are immunized against measles; and (c) the immune response that might occur if you were injected with gamma globulin containing antibodies against measles.

9. What is the function of antibodies? How do they work?

10. What is the basic difference between a primary and a secondary immune response?

14

The Respiratory System

Chapter Outline

I. The respiratory system consists of the airway and lungs

    A. The nasal cavities are lined with a mucous membrane

    B. The pharynx is divided into three regions

    C. The larynx contains the vocal cords

    D. The trachea is supported by rings of cartilage

    E. The primary bronchi enter the lungs

    F. The lungs provide a large surface area for gas exchange

II. Ventilation moves air into and out of the lungs

III. Gas exchange occurs by diffusion

IV. Gases are transported by the circulatory system

V. Respiration is regulated by the brain

VI. The respiratory system defends itself against polluted air

Respiration, which means to "breathe again," is the exchange of gases between the body and its environment. Respiration supplies the cells of the body with oxygen and rids them of carbon dioxide. The process of respiration includes breathing, gas exchange between the lungs and the blood, transport of gases through the body by the blood, gas exchange between the blood and the cells, and cellular respiration. **Cellular respiration** is the process by which cells capture energy from nutrients that serve as fuel molecules. Oxygen is required for cellular respiration, and carbon dioxide is produced as a waste product.

THE RESPIRATORY SYSTEM CONSISTS OF THE AIRWAY AND LUNGS

LEARNING OBJECTIVES

1. Trace a breath of air through the respiratory system from nose to alveoli.
2. Describe the structure and functions of the respiratory organs, including the lungs.

The **respiratory system** consists of the lungs and the airway, a series of tubes through which air flows to and from the air sacs of the lungs (Figure 14-1). A breath of air enters the body through the **nostrils,** the openings into the **nose;** flows through the **nasal cavities** to the **pharynx** (**far′**-inks); through the **larynx** (**lar′**-inks), popularly known as the voice box; and into the **trachea** (**tray′**-kee-ah), or windpipe. Air then enters the right or left **primary bronchus** (**brong′**-kus) (plural—*bronchi*). One bronchus enters each lung. After passing through smaller branches of the bronchi, air flows into the **bronchioles** (**brong′**-kee-oles). These divide again and again until the air

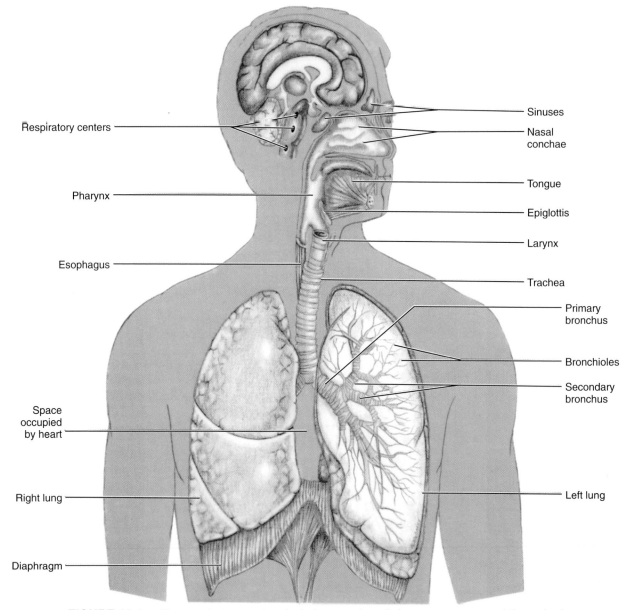

FIGURE 14-1 • The respiratory system includes a series of air passageways and the paired lungs. The lungs are located in the thoracic cavity. The muscular diaphragm forms the floor of the thoracic cavity, separating it from the abdominal cavity below. An internal view of one lung illustrates its extensive system of air passageways. The microscopic alveoli (air sacs) are shown in Figure 14-2. Note the respiratory centers in the medulla and pons.

reaches the microscopic **air sacs,** called **alveoli** (al-**vee′**-o-lee). Oxygen diffuses from the air sacs into the blood.

> Nasal cavities → pharynx → larynx → trachea → primary bronchus (enters lung) → bronchioles (in lung) → alveoli (air sacs in lung)

The Nasal Cavities Are Lined With a Mucous Membrane

Air passes into the nose through its two openings, the nostrils, also called *nares* (**nay′**-reez). Coarse hairs in the nostrils prevent large particles from entering the nose. The nostrils open into the two nasal cavities, which are separated by a partition, the **nasal septum.** The nasal septum and walls of the nose consist of bone covered with a mucous membrane. Three bony projections, the **nasal conchae** (**kong′**-kee), project from the lateral walls of the nose. The conchae increase the surface area over which air must pass as it moves through the nose.

The mucous membrane lining the nose has a rich blood supply that heats and moistens the lining and the air that comes in contact with it. Thus as air passes through the nose, it is filtered, moistened, and brought to body temperature. The nasal cavity contains the receptors for the sense of smell.

Mucous cells within the lining produce more than a pint of mucus a day and even more during infections or allergic reactions. Inhaled dirt and other foreign particles are trapped in the layer of mucus that forms along the surface of the mucous membrane. Ciliated epithelial cells of the membrane push a steady stream of mucus along with its trapped particles toward the throat. The mucus is swallowed with the saliva. In this way foreign particles are delivered to the digestive system, which is far more capable of disposing of them than are the delicate lungs.

Several **paranasal sinuses** (small cavities) in the bones of the skull communicate with the nasal cavities by small channels. They are lined with mucous membrane that sometimes becomes inflamed and infected (sinusitis).

The Pharynx Is Divided Into Three Regions

Whether you breathe through your nose or your mouth, air finds its way into the pharynx or throat because posteriorly, the nasal cavities are continuous with the pharynx. Air enters the **nasopharynx** (nay′-zo-**far′**-inks)—the superior part of the pharynx. Air then moves down into the **oropharynx** (oh′-row-**far′**-inks) behind the mouth. The oropharynx also receives food from the mouth. Finally, air passes through the **laryngopharynx** (lah-ring′-oh-**far′**-inks) and enters the larynx. Posterior to the opening into the larynx, a second opening in the laryngopharynx leads into the esophagus (part of the digestive tract).

The Larynx Contains the Vocal Cords

The opening into the larynx is the **glottis.** The wall of the larynx is supported by cartilage that protrudes from the midline of the neck and is sometimes referred to as the *Adam's apple.* The Adam's apple is more prominent in males than in females. Inflammation of the larynx, called *laryngitis,* is most often caused by a respiratory infection or by irritating substances such as cigarette smoke. The **vocal cords** are muscular folds of tissue that project into the larynx from its lateral walls. (The larynx is often referred to as the *voice box*). The vocal cords vibrate as air from the lungs rushes past them during expiration (breathing out).

During swallowing, a flap of tissue, the **epiglottis** (ep-ih-**glot′**-is), automatically closes off the larynx so food and water cannot enter the lower airway. When this mechanism fails, foreign matter comes into contact with the sensitive larynx. A cough reflex is stimulated to expel the material from the respiratory system.

The Trachea Is Supported by Rings of Cartilage

The trachea, or windpipe, is located anterior to the esophagus. It extends from the larynx to the middle of the chest. Like the larynx, the trachea is kept from collapsing by rings of cartilage in its wall. The open parts of these **C**-shaped rings of cartilage face posteriorly, toward the esophagus.

The larynx, trachea, and bronchi are lined by a mucous membrane that traps dirt and other foreign matter. Ciliated cells in this lining continuously beat a stream of mucus upward to the pharynx, where the mucus is swallowed. This *cilia-propelled mucus elevator* keeps foreign material out of the lungs.

The Primary Bronchi Enter the Lungs

The trachea divides into right and left primary (main) bronchi. The structure of the primary bronchi is similar to that of the trachea. One bronchus enters each lung. Inside the lung, each bronchus branches again and again like the branches of a tree. The branches give rise to smaller and smaller bronchi and finally to very small bronchioles. Each lung has more than a million bronchioles. The network of branching air passageways within the lungs is referred to as the **bronchial tree.**

The Lungs Provide a Large Surface Area for Gas Exchange

The lungs are large, paired organs that occupy the thoracic cavity. They are separated medially by the *mediastinum* (which contains the heart, esophagus, thymus gland, and parts of other organs). The right lung is divided into three lobes; the left lung into two lobes (see Figure 14-1). Each primary bronchus enters its lung at a depression called the **hilus** (hi′-lus). Blood vessels and nerves also enter and leave the lung at the hilus.

Each lung is covered with a **pleural (ploor'-al) membrane,** which forms a sac enclosing the lung and continues as the lining of the thoracic cavity. The part of the pleural membrane that covers the lung is the **visceral pleura;** the portion that lines the thoracic cavity is the **parietal pleura.** The pleural membrane is a **serous membrane.** Recall from Chapter 2 that a serous membrane lines a body cavity that does not open to the outside of the body.

The **pleural cavity** is a potential space between the visceral and parietal pleura. A film of fluid secreted by the pleural membranes fills the pleural cavity. This fluid lubricates and reduces the friction between the two pleural membranes during breathing. Inflammation of the pleural membrane, called *pleurisy,* may be caused by infection or injury. A symptom of pleurisy is pain during breathing, when the swollen membranes contact each other.

The thoracic cavity is completely enclosed. It is bounded on the front and sides by the chest wall, which contains the ribs. Its floor is a strong, dome-shaped muscle, the **diaphragm.**

The lungs contain all the air passageways below the primary bronchi and they are also rich in blood vessels. The lungs also have lymph tissue and nerves. Because there are millions of tiny air passageways, each lung has a very large surface area through which gases can be exchanged. Its surface area is about the size of a tennis court! The lungs are spongy and soft because they consist mainly of air sacs and elastic tissue surrounding them.

Each terminal bronchiole leads into a cluster of microscopic air sacs—the alveoli (Figure 14-2). The wall of an alveolus consists of a single layer of epithelial cells and elastic fibers,

which permit it to stretch and contract during breathing. Each alveolus is surrounded by a network of capillaries, and gases diffuse easily between the alveolus and blood. Alveoli are coated with a thin film of **pulmonary surfactant**—a substance that prevents the alveoli from collapsing.

Quiz Yourself

• What is the sequence of passageways through which air passes on it way from the nasal cavities to the alveoli?

VENTILATION MOVES AIR INTO AND OUT OF THE LUNGS

LEARNING OBJECTIVE

3. Compare and contrast inspiration and expiration.

Pulmonary ventilation, the movement of air into and out of the lungs, is normally accomplished by breathing. **Inspiration** (inhalation) is the process of taking air into the lungs, or breathing in. **Expiration** (exhalation) is the process of breathing out.

The thoracic cavity is closed, so no air can enter except through the trachea. During inspiration, the diaphragm contracts and flattens and **external intercostal muscles** contract (Figure 14-3). As the diaphragm contracts, it moves downward and as the external intercostals muscles contract, they pull each rib up and out. These actions increase the size of the chest

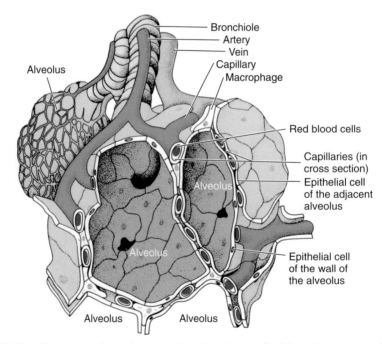

FIGURE 14-2 • Structure of an alveolus. Note that the wall of the alveolus consists of extremely thin epithelium that permits gas exchange. Capillary networks surround each alveolus.

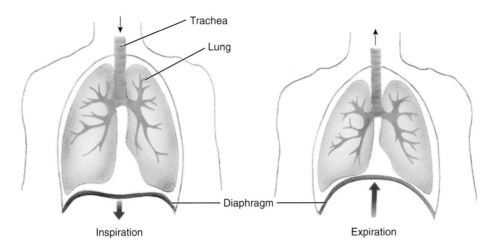

Inspiration

Expiration

(A) During inspiration, the diaphragm contracts, increasing the volume of the thoracic cavity. Air moves into the lungs.

(B) During expiration, the diaphragm relaxes, decreasing the volume of the thoracic cavity. Air moves out of the lungs.

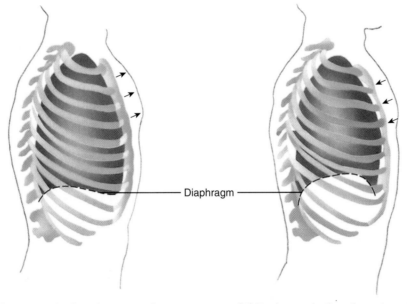

(C) During inspiration, the external intercostal muscles contract, pulling the rib cage upward and outward. The volume of the thoracic cavity increases.

(D) During expiration, the external intercostal muscles relax, decreasing the volume of the thoracic cavity.

FIGURE 14-3 • The mechanics of breathing. Changes in the position of the diaphragm and rib cage during inspiration and expiration result in changes in volume of the chest cavity.

cavity. As the chest cavity expands, the film of fluid on the pleural membranes holds the lung surfaces against the chest wall. This causes the lungs to move outward along with the chest walls. As a result, the space within each lung increases.

The air in the lungs at first tends to spread out to fill the larger space. However, the pressure of the air in the lungs falls below the pressure of the air outside the body (this creates a partial vacuum). As a result, air from the outside rushes in through the respiratory passageways and fills the lungs until

Diaphragm and external intercostal muscles contract → volume of chest cavity increases → lungs expand → volume of lungs increases → air pressure in lungs decreases → air moves into lungs

the two pressures are again equal. During deeper inspiration, additional muscles contract.

Expiration occurs when the diaphragm and external intercostal muscles relax, permitting the elastic tissues of the lung to recoil. The size of the thoracic cavity decreases, increasing the pressure inside the lung. As pressure increases, elastic fibers push against the air, forcing it to rush out of the lung. The millions of alveoli deflate, and the lung is ready for another inspiration. During *forced* expiration (also called active expiration), several sets of muscles contract, including the **internal intercostal muscles**.

> Diaphragm and intercostal muscles relax→ volume of thoracic cavity decreases → lungs recoil → lung volume decreases → pressure in alveoli increases → air rushes out of lungs

Pressure in the space between the visceral and the parietal pleura is lower than atmospheric pressure. This pressure difference prevents the air sacs from completely deflating at the end of each expiration. If the chest wall is punctured, air enters this space and the pressure there becomes equal to atmospheric pressure. When this happens, the air sacs collapse like so many deflated balloons. This condition, referred to as a *collapsed lung,* blocks the movement of air.

Ⓠ Quiz Yourself

- Which muscles contract during inspiration?
- What causes air to rush out of the lungs during expiration?

GAS EXCHANGE OCCURS BY DIFFUSION

LEARNING OBJECTIVE

4. **Compare the process of oxygen and carbon dioxide exchange in the lungs with gas exchange in the tissues.**

Breathing delivers oxygen to the alveoli of the lungs. However, if oxygen merely remained in the lungs, all the other body cells would die. The vital link between the alveoli and the body cells is the circulatory system. Each alveolus serves as a depot from which oxygen is loaded into the blood of the pulmonary capillaries.

Recall from Chapter 2 that **diffusion** is the net movement of molecules from a region of higher concentration to a region of lower concentration. Because the alveoli contain a greater concentration of oxygen than the blood entering the pulmonary capillaries, oxygen molecules diffuse from the alveoli into the blood (Figure 14-4). Carbon dioxide moves from the blood, where it is more concentrated, to the alveoli, where it is less concentrated. Each gas diffuses through the thin lining of the capillary and the thin lining of the alveolus.

Table 14-1 shows the percentages of oxygen and carbon dioxide present in expired air compared with inspired air. Expired air has more than 100 times more carbon dioxide than

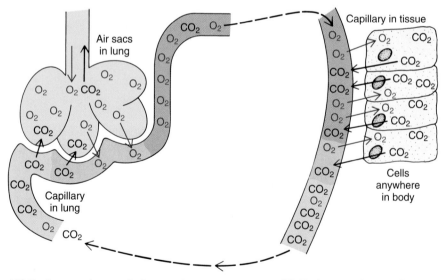

(A) Exchange of gases between air sacs and blood in pulmonary capillaries. The concentration of oxygen (O_2) is greater in the air sacs than in the capillary, so oxygen moves from the air sacs into the blood. Carbon dioxide (CO_2) is more concentrated in the blood, so it moves out of the capillary and into the air sacs.

(B) Exchange of gases between capillary and body cells. Oxygen is more concentrated in the blood, so it moves out of the capillary and into the cells. Carbon dioxide is more concentrated in the cells, so it diffuses out of the cells and into the blood.

FIGURE 14-4 • Gas exchange in the lung and in the tissues.

TABLE 14-1	COMPOSITION OF INHALED AIR COMPARED WITH THAT OF EXHALED AIR		
	% Oxygen	% Carbon Dioxide	% Nitrogen
Inhaled air (atmospheric air)	20.9	0.04	79
Exhaled air (alveolar air)	14.0	5.60	79

As indicated, the body uses up about one third of the inhaled oxygen. The amount of carbon dioxide increases more than 100-fold because it is produced during cellular respiration.

air inspired from the environment. This is because carbon dioxide is produced by the cells of the body during cellular respiration (the process by which cells capture energy from fuel molecules).

As blood circulates through the tissues, oxygen moves from the blood (where it is more concentrated) into the cells (where it is less concentrated). Carbon dioxide is more concentrated in the cells than in the blood. As a result, carbon dioxide diffuses from the cells into the blood and is transported to the lungs.

Quiz Yourself

- Why does oxygen diffuse from the alveoli into the blood?
- As blood circulates through tissues, what is the direction of carbon dioxide diffusion?

GASES ARE TRANSPORTED BY THE CIRCULATORY SYSTEM

LEARNING OBJECTIVE

5. **Compare the transport of oxygen and carbon dioxide in the blood.**

When oxygen diffuses into the blood, it enters the red blood cells and forms a weak chemical bond with hemoglobin, forming **oxyhemoglobin** (ok′-see-**he**′-mow-glow-bin).

$$\text{Hemoglobin} + \text{Oxygen} \rightarrow \text{Oxyhemoglobin}$$

Because the chemical bond linking the oxygen with the hemoglobin is weak, this reaction is readily reversible. In tissues that are low in oxygen, oxyhemoglobin dissociates, releasing oxygen. The oxygen then diffuses out of the capillaries and into the cells.

$$\text{Oxyhemoglobin} \rightarrow \text{Oxygen} + \text{Hemoglobin}$$

Carbon dioxide is transported in the blood in three ways. A small amount (7% to 10%) of carbon dioxide is simply dissolved in plasma. About 20% is transported attached to hemoglobin. Most of the carbon dioxide is transported as **bicarbonate ions (HCO_3^-).**

In the plasma, carbon dioxide slowly combines with water to form carbonic acid. This reaction proceeds much more rapidly inside red blood cells because of the action of an enzyme (carbonic anhydrase). Carbonic acid dissociates, forming hydrogen ions and bicarbonate ions.

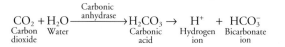

$$\underset{\substack{\text{Carbon} \\ \text{dioxide}}}{CO_2} + \underset{\text{Water}}{H_2O} \xrightarrow{\text{Carbonic anhydrase}} \underset{\substack{\text{Carbonic} \\ \text{acid}}}{H_2CO_3} \rightarrow \underset{\substack{\text{Hydrogen} \\ \text{ion}}}{H^+} + \underset{\substack{\text{Bicarbonate} \\ \text{ion}}}{HCO_3^-}$$

Most of the hydrogen ions released from carbonic acid combine with hemoglobin, which is a very effective *chemical buffer* (a substance that lessens the change in hydrogen ion concentration). Many of the bicarbonate ions diffuse into the plasma.

Quiz Yourself

- How is hemoglobin transported in the blood?
- What is the main way that carbon dioxide is transported?

RESPIRATION IS REGULATED BY THE BRAIN

LEARNING OBJECTIVE

6. **Describe how the body regulates respiration.**

Breathing is a rhythmic, involuntary process regulated by **respiratory centers** in the brainstem (see Figure 14-1). Groups of neurons in the dorsal region of the medulla regulate the basic rhythm of breathing. These neurons send a burst of impulses to the diaphragm by way of the **phrenic nerves** and to the external intercostal muscles by way of the **intercostal nerves,** causing them to contract. After several seconds, these neurons become inactive, the muscles relax, and expiration occurs.

Respiratory centers in the pons help control the transition from inspiration to expiration. These centers can stimulate or inhibit the respiratory centers in the medulla. The cycle of activity and inactivity repeats itself so that at rest we breathe about 14 times per minute. A group of neurons in the ventral region of the medulla becomes active only when we need to breathe forcefully. Overdose of certain medications such as barbiturates depresses the respiratory centers and may lead to respiratory failure.

The basic rhythm of respiration can be altered in response to changing needs of the body. When you are engaged in a strenuous game of tennis, you require more oxygen than when studying anatomy and physiology. During exercise the rate of cellular respiration increases, producing more carbon dioxide. The body must dispose of this carbon dioxide through increased ventilation.

Carbon dioxide concentration is the most important chemical stimulus for regulating the rate of respiration. Specialized **chemoreceptors** (chemical receptors) in the medulla are sensitive to changes in carbon dioxide concentration. These chemoreceptors are also sensitive to the pH (degree of acidity) of the fluid that bathes the brain. Recall that when carbon dioxide level increases, more hydrogen ions are produced. The hydrogen ions lower the pH of the blood and the extracellular fluid, including the fluid surrounding the brain. (Lower pH means increased acidity.) When stimulated, the chemoreceptors signal the respiratory centers, leading to an increase in the breathing rate and in the depth of breathing. As carbon dioxide is removed by the lungs, the hydrogen ion concentration in the extracellular fluid decreases and the body returns to homeostasis. A decrease in carbon dioxide concentration has the opposite effect. It inhibits the chemoreceptors, resulting in slower breathing.

Chemoreceptors in the walls of the aorta (called aortic bodies) and carotid arteries (called carotid bodies) are also sensitive to changes in hydrogen ion concentration and carbon dioxide concentration. Even a slight decrease in the pH of arterial blood stimulates these chemoreceptors to signal the respiratory centers. The breathing rate increases, and the excess carbon dioxide is removed by the lungs. The hydrogen ion concentration in the blood decreases and the pH returns to normal. Surprisingly, oxygen concentration normally does not play an important role in regulating respiration. However, if the oxygen concentration falls to the point of being life threatening, the chemoreceptors in the aorta and carotid arteries become stimulated and signal the respiratory centers to take emergency action.

Although breathing is an involuntary process, we can consciously influence the action of the respiratory centers for a short time by stimulating or inhibiting them. For example, you can inhibit respiration by holding your breath. You cannot hold your breath indefinitely, however, because eventually you feel a strong urge to breathe. Even if you were able to ignore this, you would eventually pass out and resume breathing.

Underwater swimmers and some Asian pearl divers voluntarily hyperventilate before going under water. By taking a series of deep inhalations and exhalations, they "blow off" carbon dioxide, markedly reducing the carbon dioxide content of the alveolar air and of the blood. As a result, it takes longer before the urge to breathe becomes irresistible.

When hyperventilation is continued for a long period, dizziness and sometimes unconsciousness may occur. This is because a certain concentration of carbon dioxide in the blood is needed to maintain normal blood pressure. (This mechanism operates by way of the vasoconstrictor center in the brain,

which maintains the muscle tone of blood vessel walls.) Furthermore, if divers hold their breath too long, the low concentration of oxygen may result in unconsciousness and drowning.

Individuals who have stopped breathing because of drowning, smoke inhalation, electric shock, or cardiac arrest can sometimes be sustained by mouth-to-mouth resuscitation until their own breathing reflexes are initiated again. **Cardiopulmonary resuscitation (CPR)** is a method for aiding victims who have had respiratory and cardiac arrest. CPR must be started immediately because irreversible brain damage may occur within about 4 minutes of respiratory arrest. A number of organizations offer training in CPR.

Quiz Yourself

- Where are the respiratory centers?
- What are the functions of the chemoreceptors that are important in respiration?
- What is the role of carbon dioxide in regulating respiration?

THE RESPIRATORY SYSTEM DEFENDS ITSELF AGAINST POLLUTED AIR

LEARNING OBJECTIVE

7. **Describe defense mechanisms that protect the lungs from pollutants in the air and describe some effects of breathing pollutants.**

We breathe about 20,000 times each day, inhaling about 35 pounds of air—six times more than the food and drink we take in. Most of us breathe dirty urban air containing carbon monoxide, particles of dirt, and many other harmful substances. The respiratory system has a number of defense mechanisms that help protect the delicate lungs from damage.

The hair in the nose and the ciliated, mucous lining of the respiratory passageways help trap foreign particles in inspired air. Recall that the cilia-propelled mucus elevator moves foreign particles away from the lungs. When we breathe dirty air, the bronchial tubes narrow. This **bronchial constriction** increases the chances that inhaled particles land on the sticky mucous lining. Unfortunately, during bronchial constriction, less air can pass through to the lungs, thus decreasing the amount of oxygen available to body cells. Fifteen puffs on a cigarette during a 5-minute period increase airway resistance as much as threefold, and this added resistance to breathing lasts more than 30 minutes. Chain smokers and those who breathe heavily polluted air may remain in a chronic state of bronchial constriction.

The smallest bronchioles and the alveoli are not equipped with cells with cilia or with mucus. Foreign particles that slip through the respiratory defenses and find their way into the alveoli may remain there indefinitely or may be engulfed by macrophages. The macrophages may then accumulate in the lymph tissue of the lungs. Lung tissue of chronic smokers and of those who work in dirty industries contains large, blackened areas where carbon particles have been deposited.

Continued insult to the respiratory system results in disease. *Chronic bronchitis* and *emphysema* are chronic pulmonary dis-eases that have been linked to smoking and breathing polluted air. Cigarette smoking is also the main cause of *lung cancer.* More than 69 of the 4800 chemical compounds in tobacco smoke cause cancer. These carcinogenic substances irritate the cells lining the respiratory passages and interfere with their metabolic activities. Normal cells are transformed into cancer cells, which then multiply rapidly and invade surrounding tissues.

⟳ SUMMARY

LO 1. Trace a breath of air through the respiratory system from nose to alveoli.
- **Respiration** is the exchange of gases between the body and its environment. **Cellular respiration** is the process by which cells capture energy from nutrients. Oxygen is required, and carbon dioxide is released as a waste product.
- Air passes through the **nostrils** into the **nasal cavities** and then through the **pharynx.**
- The pharynx has specific regions. From the nasal cavities, air passes through the **nasopharynx,** through the **laryngopharynx,** and through the **glottis** into the **larynx.** Air that enters through the mouth passes through the **oropharynx.**
- From the larynx, inhaled air passes into the **trachea** (windpipe) and then into the right or left **primary bronchus,** which enters the **lung.** Air then passes into bronchioles and finally, into the **alveoli,** or **air sacs.**

LO 2. Describe the structure and functions of the respiratory organs, including the lungs.
- The **nasal cavities** are separated by a partition—the **nasal septum.** The **nasal conchae,** bony projections from the lateral walls of the nose, increase the surface area over which air flows. The nose filters and moistens inspired air and brings it to body temperature.
- The larynx, which also contains the **vocal cords,** protects the lungs by initiating a cough reflex when it is touched by foreign matter. During swallowing, a flap of tissue, the **epiglottis,** closes the larynx so that food and fluid cannot enter the lower airway.
- Within the lungs, the bronchi branch and rebranch, giving rise to an extensive system of bronchioles. Each terminal bronchiole gives rise to a cluster of alveoli—the air sacs through which gases are exchanged with the blood. **Pulmonary surfactant** coating the alveoli prevents the alveoli from collapsing.
- The **lungs** are large, spongy organs covered with **pleural membranes.** The **visceral pleura** cover the lungs; the **parietal pleura** line the thoracic cavity. The potential space between them is the **pleural cavity.**

LO 3. Compare and contrast inspiration and expiration.
- **Pulmonary ventilation** is the process of moving air into and out of the lungs. We ventilate the lungs by breathing. **Inspiration** is breathing in; **expiration** is breathing out.
- During inspiration, the **diaphragm** and **intercostal muscles** contract, causing the thoracic cavity to expand. The lungs expand, causing a decrease in pressure, and air rushes into the lungs.
- When the diaphragm and intercostal muscles relax, pressure in the lung increases and air rushes out of the lungs.

LO 4. Compare the process of oxygen and carbon dioxide exchange in the lungs with gas exchange in the tissues.
- **Diffusion** is the net movement of molecules from a region of higher concentration to a region of lower concentration. Because oxygen is more concentrated in the lungs than in the pulmonary capillaries, oxygen diffuses from the alveoli into the blood. Oxygen diffuses from the blood into the tissues.
- Carbon dioxide is produced by cells during cellular respiration. It diffuses into the blood. In the lungs, carbon dioxide diffuses from the blood in the pulmonary capillaries into the alveoli and then is expired.

LO = Learning Objective

LO 5. Compare the transport of oxygen and carbon dioxide in the blood.
- Oxygen is transported to the body cells in the form of **oxyhemoglobin.** As oxygen is needed by the cells, oxyhemoglobin dissociates and oxygen diffuses from the blood into the cells.
- Carbon dioxide is transported mainly in the form of **bicarbonate ions.** A small amount (7% to 10%) of carbon dioxide is dissolved in plasma, and about 20% is transported attached to hemoglobin.

LO 6. Describe how the body regulates respiration.
- Breathing is normally regulated by **respiratory centers** in the medulla and pons. Impulses are transmitted from the medulla to the diaphragm by the **phrenic nerves** and from the medulla to the external intercostal muscles by the **intercostal nerves.**
- **Chemoreceptors** in the medulla and in the walls of the aorta and carotid arteries are sensitive to changes in the concentration of carbon dioxide in the blood. When carbon dioxide concentration increases, hydrogen ion concen-

tration increases and pH decreases. An increase in carbon dioxide concentration or hydrogen ion concentration stimulates these receptors to signal the respiratory centers. Breathing rate increases and excess carbon dioxide is removed by the lungs. A life-threatening decrease in oxygen concentration also stimulates the chemoreceptors in the aorta and carotid arteries to signal the respiratory centers.

LO 7. Describe defense mechanisms that protect the lungs from pollutants in the air and describe some effects of breathing pollutants.
- Hairs in the nostrils and the ciliated mucous lining of the upper airway trap foreign particles in inspired air. **Bronchial constriction** is a rapid narrowing of the bronchial tubes which increases the chance that inhaled particles will land on the sticky mucous lining. Macrophages are also important in removing foreign matter.
- Continued insult to the respiratory system may result in chronic bronchitis, emphysema, or lung cancer.

CHAPTER QUIZ

Fill in the Blank

1. From the pharynx, inhaled air passes through an opening, the _____, and into the _____, and then passes through the _____.

2. The process by which cells capture energy from nutrients is _____ _____.

3. The floor of the thoracic cavity is formed by the _____.

4. The _____ seals off the larynx during swallowing.

5. When foreign matter contacts the _____, it may initiate a cough reflex.

6. The part of the pleural membrane that encloses the lung is the _____ pleura.

7. Pulmonary _____ is the process of moving air into and out of the lungs.

8. Breathing in is called _____; breathing out is called _____.

9. Oxygen is transported in the blood chemically bound to _____.

10. Impulses from the medulla reach the diaphragm by way of the _____ nerves.

Multiple Choice

11. Gas exchange takes place through the walls of the: a. bronchi; b. bronchioles; c. alveoli; d. laryngopharynx.

12. You would *not* expect to find the following in the lung: a. trachea; b. bronchioles; c. alveoli; d. elastic tissue.

13. As blood moves through the pulmonary capillaries: a. carbon dioxide moves from the alveoli into the blood; b. oxygen moves from the blood into the alveoli; c. carbon dioxide moves from the blood into the alveoli; d. the carbon dioxide concentration of the blood does not change.

14. Carbon dioxide is transported mainly: a. as bicarbonate ions; b. as oxyhemoglobin; c. dissolved in the plasma; d. attached to macrophages.

15. The rate of respiration is mainly determined by: a. oxygen concentration of the blood; b. voluntary effort; c. hydrogen concentration; d. carbon dioxide concentration.

REVIEW QUESTIONS

1. Trace a breath of inspired air from nose to alveoli. List each structure in sequence through which the air passes.

2. What are the advantages of having millions of alveoli rather than a pair of simple, balloonlike lungs?

3. Compare inspiration with expiration.

4. The larynx is sometimes referred to as the watchdog of the lungs. Why do you think this is appropriate?

5. What are the advantages of breathing through the nose?

6. How is the structure of the respiratory system especially designed to permit gas exchange? (Hint: consider the thickness of alveolar and capillary walls as part of your answer.)

7. How is breathing regulated?

8. Describe several defense mechanisms that the respiratory system uses to protect itself from harmful pollutants in the air we breathe.

9. Label the diagram. (See Figure 14-1 to check your answers.)

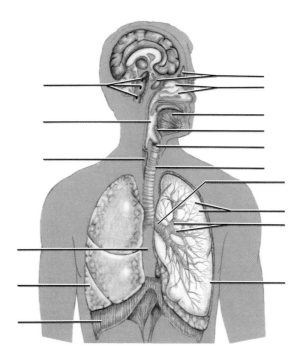

15 The Digestive System

Chapter Outline

I. The digestive system processes food
  A. The wall of the digestive tract has four layers
  B. Folds of the peritoneum support the digestive organs

II. Specific structures of the digestive system have specific functions
  A. The mouth ingests food
    1. The teeth break down food
    2. The salivary glands produce saliva
  B. The pharynx is important in swallowing
  C. The esophagus conducts food to the stomach
  D. The stomach digests proteins
  E. Most digestion takes place in the small intestine
  F. The pancreas secretes enzymes
  G. The liver secretes bile

III. Digestion occurs as food moves through the digestive tract
  A. Glucose is the main product of carbohydrate digestion
  B. Bile emulsifies fat
  C. Proteins are digested to free amino acids

IV. Absorption takes place through the intestinal villi

V. The large intestine eliminates wastes

VI. A balanced diet is necessary to maintain health

VII. Energy metabolism is balanced when energy input equals energy output

Nutrients are the substances in food that are used as building blocks to make new cells and tissues and as ingredients to make the chemical compounds needed for metabolism. Some nutrients serve as an energy source to run the machinery of the body. The process of taking in and using food is **nutrition.**

The food we eat consists of large pieces and large molecules. It is not in a form that can reach the cells of the body or that can be used for nourishment. The **digestive system** processes the food and breaks it down into a form that can be delivered to the cells and then used by the cells. This chapter focuses on the long, eventful journey that food takes through the digestive tract. We discuss the nutrients required for a balanced diet and we describe basic energy metabolism.

THE DIGESTIVE SYSTEM PROCESSES FOOD

LEARNING OBJECTIVES

1. Describe in general terms the following steps in processing food: ingestion, digestion, absorption, and elimination.
2. List in sequence each structure through which a bite of food passes on its way through the digestive tract; label a diagram of the digestive system.
3. Describe the wall of the digestive tract; distinguish between the visceral peritoneum and the parietal peritoneum, and describe their major folds.

The digestive system is responsible for processing food. Four major processes are involved:

1. **Ingestion** involves taking food into the mouth, chewing it, and swallowing it.
2. **Digestion** is the breakdown of food into smaller molecules. The food we ingest undergoes both mechanical digestion and chemical digestion. **Mechanical digestion** is the process of breaking down pieces of food by chewing and by churning and mixing movements in the stomach. **Chemical digestion** is the process of breaking down large molecules, including carbohydrates, proteins, and fats, into smaller molecules that can be absorbed from the digestive tract and used by the cells of the body. Each reaction is regulated by a specific **enzyme**—a chemical catalyst, usually a protein.
3. **Absorption** is the transport of digested food through the wall of the stomach or intestine and into the circulatory system. The circulatory system transports the food molecules, or nutrients, to the liver, where many are removed and stored. Those remaining in the blood are transported to the cells of the body. Each cell requires nutrients for its metabolic activities.
4. **Elimination** removes undigested and unabsorbed food from the body.

The **digestive tract,** also called the **alimentary canal,** is a long tube about 8 meters (m) (23 feet) long. It extends from the mouth, where food is taken in, to the anus, through which unused food is eliminated (Figure 15-1). Below the diaphragm, the digestive tract is often referred to as the **GI (gastrointestinal) tract.** The digestive tube is like a long, coiled hose. Some sections of the tube are narrow; others are wide.

The parts of the digestive tract through which food passes in sequence are the mouth, pharynx (throat), esophagus, stomach, small intestine (subdivided into duodenum, jejunum, and ileum), and large intestine (subdivided into cecum, colon, rectum, and anal canal). Food is eliminated through the anus.

> Mouth → pharynx → esophagus → stomach → small intestine → large intestine → anus

The **accessory digestive glands** are not part of the digestive tract. They secrete digestive juices into it. Three types of accessory glands are the salivary glands, liver, and pancreas.

The Wall of the Digestive Tract Has Four Layers

From esophagus to anus, the wall of the digestive tract consists of four main layers (Figure 15-2):

1. The **mucosa** (mew-**koe'**-sah) is the lining of the digestive tract. It consists of epithelial tissue resting on a layer of loose connective tissue. In the esophagus and anal canal, the epithelium is specialized for protection of underlying tissues. The epithelium in other regions of the digestive tract is specialized for secretion of mucus or digestive juices or for absorption of nutrients. In the stomach and small intestine, the mucosa is thrown into folds, which greatly increase its surface area for digestion and absorption.
2. Beneath the mucosa lies a layer of connective tissue, the **submucosa,** rich in blood vessels and nerves.
3. A muscle layer (*muscularis*) surrounds the submucosa. This layer consists of two sublayers of smooth muscle. This muscle contracts in a wavelike motion called **peristalsis** (per-ih-**stal'**-sis) that pushes food along through the digestive tract.
4. The outer coat of the wall of the digestive tract consists of connective tissue. Above the level of the diaphragm this layer is called the **adventitia.** Below the level of the diaphragm this layer is the **visceral peritoneum** (per'-ih-tow-**nee'**-um). By various folds it connects to the **parietal peritoneum**—the sheet of connective tissue that lines the walls of the abdominal and pelvic cavities. Between the visceral and the parietal peritoneum is a potential space, the **peritoneal cavity.** Inflammation of the peritoneum, called *peritonitis,* can have very serious consequences because infection can easily spread to all the adjoining organs.

Folds of the Peritoneum Support the Digestive Organs

A large double fold of peritoneal tissue, the **mesentery** (**mez'**-en-ter-ee), extends from the parietal peritoneum and attaches to the small intestine (Figure 15-3). The mesentery is shaped somewhat like a fan. The handle part of the fan anchors the intestine to the posterior abdominal wall. Blood and lymph vessels and nerves that supply the intestine are present between the folds of the mesentery.

Other important folds of peritoneum are the greater omentum, the lesser omentum, and the mesocolon (see Figure

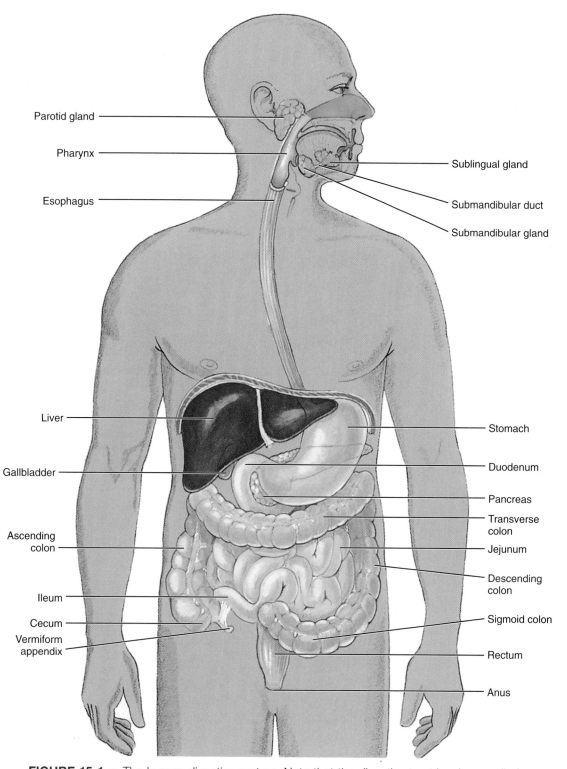

Parotid gland

Pharynx

Esophagus

Sublingual gland

Submandibular duct

Submandibular gland

Liver

Stomach

Gallbladder

Duodenum

Pancreas

Transverse colon

Ascending colon

Jejunum

Descending colon

Ileum

Cecum

Sigmoid colon

Vermiform appendix

Rectum

Anus

FIGURE 15-1 • The human digestive system. Note that the digestive tract is a long, coiled tube extending from mouth to anus. Locate the three types of accessory glands.

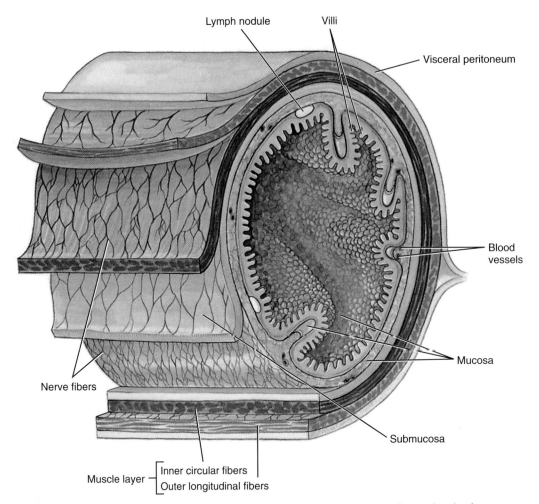

FIGURE 15-2 • Cross section through the wall of the small intestine illustrating its four main layers: mucosa, submucosa, muscle layer, and visceral peritoneum.

15-3). The **greater omentum** (o-**men′**-tum), also known as the *fatty apron,* is a large double fold of peritoneum attached to the stomach and intestine. It hangs down over the intestine like an apron. The greater omentum contains large deposits of fat. It also contains lymph nodes that help prevent spread of infection to the peritoneum. The **lesser omentum** suspends the stomach and duodenum from the liver (see Figure 1-11). The **mesocolon** is a fold of peritoneum that attaches the colon to the posterior abdominal wall.

Quiz Yourself

- What is chemical digestion?
- What is the sequence of structures through which food passes from mouth to anus?
- What are the four main layers that make up the wall of the small intestine?

SPECIFIC STRUCTURES OF THE DIGESTIVE SYSTEM HAVE SPECIFIC FUNCTIONS

LEARNING OBJECTIVES

4. Describe the structures of the mouth, including the teeth, and give their functions.
5. Describe the structure and function of the pharynx and esophagus.
6. Describe the structure of the stomach and its role in processing food.
7. Identify the three main regions of the small intestine and describe the functions of the small intestine.
8. Summarize the functions of the pancreas and liver.

Each region of the digestive tract is specialized to process food in specific ways. The accessory glands are also adapted to perform specific digestive functions.

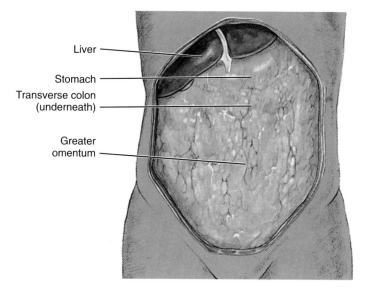

(A) Greater omentum. The greater omentum hangs down over the intestine like an apron. Frontal view of the abdomen.

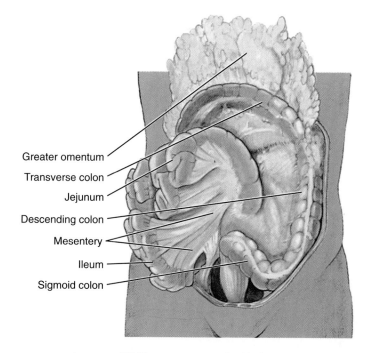

(B) The mesentery. In this frontal view of the abdomen, the greater omentum and transverse colon have been lifted to show the mesentery.

FIGURE 15-3 • Folds of the peritoneum anchor the digestive organs to the abdominal wall and to one another.

The Mouth Ingests Food

The mouth, or **oral cavity,** ingests food and begins the process of digestion. Mechanical digestion begins as you bite, grind, and chew food with your teeth. The flexible, muscular tongue on the floor of the mouth pushes the food about to aid in chewing and swallowing. Taste buds on the tongue enable us to taste foods as sweet, sour, salty, bitter, or savory (meaty; rich in glutamates; see Chapter 8). The tongue is also important in speech.

The Teeth Break Down Food

The teeth are rooted in sockets (alveoli) of the alveolar processes—bony ridges that project from the mandible and maxilla. Each tooth consists of a **crown,** the region above the gum, and one or more **roots,** the portion beneath the gum line (Figure 15-4). A section through a tooth, or an x-ray film of it, shows that it is composed mainly of **dentin**—a calcified connective tissue that imparts shape and rigidity to the tooth. In the crown region the dentin is protected by a tough covering of **enamel.** The bonelike enamel is the hardest substance in

the body, comparable in hardness to quartz. Enamel helps protect the tooth against the wear and tear of chewing and against chemical substances that might dissolve the dentin.

The dentin encloses a **pulp cavity** filled with **pulp**—an extremely sensitive connective tissue containing blood vessels and nerves. Narrow extensions of the pulp cavity, called **root canals,** pass through the roots of the tooth. Each root canal has an opening at its base through which nerves and blood and lymph vessels enter the tooth.

By about 6 months of age, the first of the temporary **deciduous** (dee-**sid′**-you-us) **teeth,** also called *baby teeth,* show their crowns above the gums. After that, new teeth erupt every few weeks so that a full set of 20 deciduous teeth is present by the time a child is about 2 years old (Figure 15-5, *A*). These teeth are fairly small, and between the ages of 6 and 13 years they are slowly shed and replaced by larger **permanent teeth.**

The adult set of teeth consists of 32 teeth (Figure 15-5, *B*). We can describe the number of each type of tooth in one quadrant of the mouth. Closest to the midline are two **incisors** (a total of eight: four on the top and four on the bottom). The incisors are specialized for biting and cutting. Lateral to them

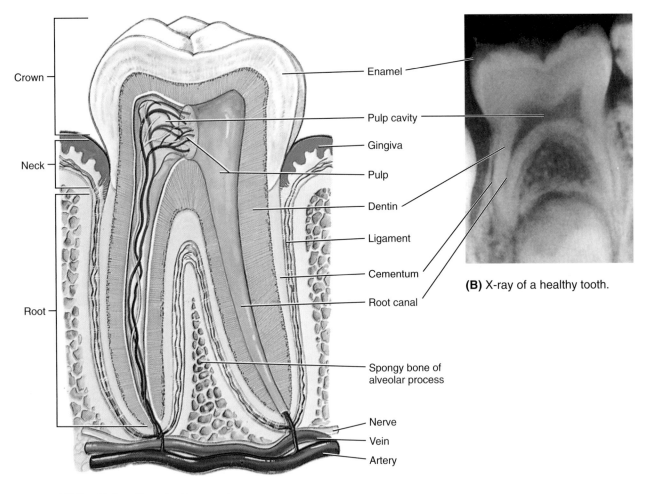

Crown

Neck

Root

Enamel

Pulp cavity

Gingiva

Pulp

Dentin

Ligament

Cementum

Root canal

Spongy bone of alveolar process

Nerve

Vein

Artery

(A) Sagittal section of a lower molar.

(B) X-ray of a healthy tooth.

FIGURE 15-4 • Structure of a tooth.

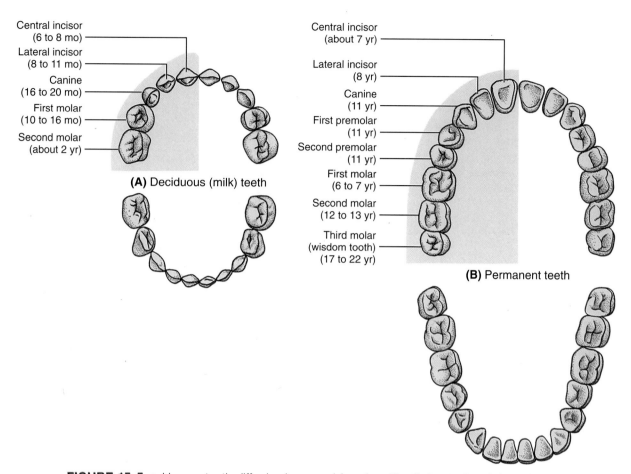

Central incisor
(6 to 8 mo)
Lateral incisor
(8 to 11 mo)
Canine
(16 to 20 mo)
First molar
(10 to 16 mo)
Second molar
(about 2 yr)

(A) Deciduous (milk) teeth

Central incisor
(about 7 yr)
Lateral incisor
(8 yr)
Canine
(11 yr)
First premolar
(11 yr)
Second premolar
(11 yr)
First molar
(6 to 7 yr)
Second molar
(12 to 13 yr)
Third molar
(wisdom tooth)
(17 to 22 yr)

(B) Permanent teeth

FIGURE 15-5 • Human teeth differ in shape and function. The first set of teeth is replaced by permanent teeth during the time from about age 7 years to late adolescence. Approximate time of eruption of each type of tooth is shown in parentheses.

are the **canines**—one in each quadrant. In humans the canines assist the incisors in biting, but in many mammals they are enlarged and are adapted for stabbing and tearing prey.

The more posterior teeth are modified for grinding and crushing. Each quadrant has two **premolars** and three **molars.** The third molars are the wisdom teeth, which often appear after age 18. In many persons, the jaw is too small to accommodate the wisdom teeth. They may remain embedded (impacted) in the jawbone. Sometimes they cause pain and must be surgically removed.

The Salivary Glands Produce Saliva

There are three main pairs of **salivary glands:**

1. The **parotid** (pah-**rot′**-id) **glands** are the largest salivary glands. They are located in the tissue inferior and anterior to the ears. The parotid glands become infected and swollen as a result of some infections, including mumps (a viral infection).
2. The **submandibular** (sub′-man-**dib′**-you-lar) **glands** lie below the jaw.
3. The **sublingual** (sub-**ling′**-gwal) **glands** are located under the tongue.

Saliva consists of two main components: (1) a thin, watery secretion containing **salivary amylase,** a digestive enzyme that begins the chemical digestion of starches (large carbohydrates), and (2) a mucous secretion that lubricates the mouth. Salts, antibodies, and other substances that kill bacteria are present in saliva.

Saliva lubricates the tissues of the mouth and pharynx, making it easier to talk and chew. By moistening food, saliva helps the tongue convert the mouthful of food to a semisolid mass called a **bolus** (**bow′**-lus) that can be swallowed easily.

The Pharynx Is Important in Swallowing

After a bite of food has been tasted, chewed, moistened, and formed into a bolus, it must be swallowed. Swallowing moves the bolus from the mouth through the pharynx and down into the esophagus. The **pharynx,** or throat, is a muscular tube about 12 centimeters (cm) (4.8 inches) long that serves as the hallway of both the respiratory and digestive systems. As noted in Chapter 14, the three regions of the pharynx are the **oropharynx,** posterior to the mouth; the **nasopharynx,** posterior to the nose; and the **laryngopharynx,** which opens into the larynx and esophagus.

The oropharynx and nasopharynx are partitioned by the **soft palate,** which hangs down like a curtain between them. The muscular soft palate is a posterior extension of the bony **hard palate,** which serves as the roof of the mouth. A small mass of tissue, the **uvula,** hangs from the lower border of the soft palate. During swallowing, the bolus is forced into the oropharynx by the tongue. Reflex contractions of muscles in the wall of the pharynx propel the food into the esophagus. During swallowing, the opening to the larynx is closed by the **epiglottis**—a small flap of tissue that prevents food from entering the respiratory passageways.

The Esophagus Conducts Food to the Stomach

The esophagus extends from the pharynx through the thoracic cavity, passes through the diaphragm, and empties into the stomach. The bolus is swept through the pharynx and into the esophagus by peristalsis—waves of muscle contraction. As the bolus enters the esophagus, peristaltic contractions continue pushing the food down toward the stomach. Two layers of muscle in the wall of the esophagus work together in pushing the bolus downward.

At the lower end of the esophagus is a sphincter muscle—the **cardiac sphincter.** This circular muscle constricts the tube so that the entrance to the stomach is generally closed. Normally, the highly acidic gastric juice does not splash up into the esophagus. In gastroesophageal reflux disease (GERD), gastric juice does spurt up into the esophagus, irritating its wall and causing spasms. A common symptom of this condition is "heartburn" (probably so named because the pain seems to occur in the general region of the heart).

The Stomach Digests Proteins

When a peristaltic wave passes down the esophagus, the cardiac sphincter relaxes, permitting the bolus to enter the **stomach.** The stomach is a large, muscular organ that, when empty, is shaped like the letter J (Figure 15-6). When the stomach is empty, its lining has many folds, called **rugae** (**roo'**-jee). As food fills the stomach, the rugae gradually smooth out, increasing the stomach's capacity to more than a quart. As it fills, the stomach begins to look like a football.

Contractions of the stomach mix the food thoroughly. The stomach mashes and churns food and also moves it along by peristalsis. The stomach is lined with simple epithelium that secretes large amounts of mucus. Tiny pits mark the entrance to millions of **gastric glands,** which extend deep into the wall of the stomach.

Parietal cells in the gastric glands secrete **hydrochloric acid** and a substance known as **intrinsic factor,** needed for adequate absorption of vitamin B_{12}. The hydrochloric acid kills bacteria and breaks down the connective tissues in meat. Even after mixing with mucus and food, the stomach is very acidic.

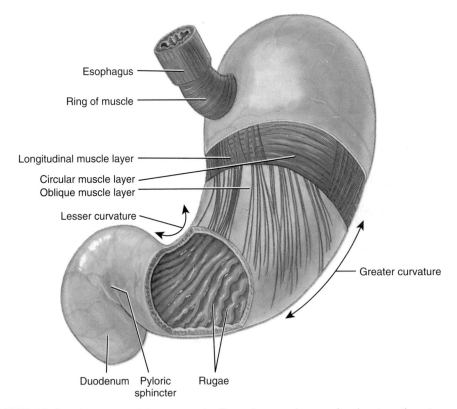

Esophagus
Ring of muscle
Longitudinal muscle layer
Circular muscle layer
Oblique muscle layer
Lesser curvature
Greater curvature
Duodenum   Pyloric sphincter   Rugae

FIGURE 15-6 • Structure of the stomach. From the esophagus, food enters the stomach, where it is broken down mechanically. Protein digestion begins in the stomach.

Chief cells in the gastric glands secrete **pepsinogen,** an inactive form of the enzyme **pepsin,** which begins the digestion of proteins. When pepsinogen comes in contact with the acidic gastric juice in the stomach, it is converted to pepsin.

Small amounts of water, salts, and fat-soluble substances such as alcohol are absorbed through the stomach mucosa. As food is digested over a 3- to 4-hour period, it is converted into a soupy mixture called **chyme** (kime). The exit of the stomach is guarded by the **pyloric** (pie-**lor'**-ik) **sphincter,** a strong ring of muscle. When this sphincter relaxes, chyme passes into the small intestine.

Most Digestion Takes Place in the Small Intestine

The small intestine is a long, coiled tube more than 5 to 6 m (about 17 feet) long by 4 cm (1.5 inches) in diameter. The first 22 cm (about 9 inches) or so of the small intestine make up the **duodenum** (do'-o-dee'-num), which is curved like the letter C (Figure 15-7). As the tube turns downward, it is called the **jejunum** (jeh-**joo'**-num), which extends for about 2 m (6 feet). The jejunum is continuous with the third part of the small intestine, the **ileum** (il'-ee-um), which is about 3.5 m (about 11 feet) long.

The lining of the small intestine has millions of tiny finger-like projections, called **villi** (**vil'**-ee) (Figure 15-8). The villi increase the surface area of the small intestine, providing a greater surface area for digestion and absorption of nutrients. The intestinal surface is further expanded by **microvilli,** tiny projections of the plasma membrane of each of the epithelial cells of the villi. If the lining of the intestine could be completely unfolded and spread out, its surface would approximate the size of a tennis court!

Between adjacent villi, **intestinal glands** extend downward into the mucosa. These glands secrete large amounts of fluid that help keep the chyme in a fluid state so that nutrients can be easily absorbed. **Goblet cells** in the mucosa secrete alkaline mucus that helps protect the intestinal wall from the acidic chyme and from the action of digestive enzymes.

Most digestion takes place in the duodenum rather than in the stomach. The liver and pancreas release digestive juices into the duodenum. Then enzymes produced by the epithelial cells lining the duodenum complete the job of breaking down food molecules so they can be absorbed.

The Pancreas Secretes Enzymes

The **pancreas** is a large, long gland that lies in the abdomen posterior to the stomach (see Figure 15-7). The pancreas is

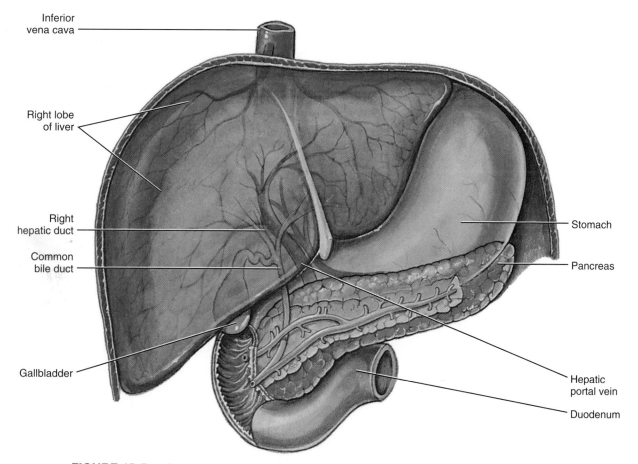

Inferior vena cava

Right lobe of liver

Right hepatic duct

Common bile duct

Gallbladder

Stomach

Pancreas

Hepatic portal vein

Duodenum

FIGURE 15-7 • Structure of the duodenum, liver, and pancreas. Note the gallbladder and ducts.

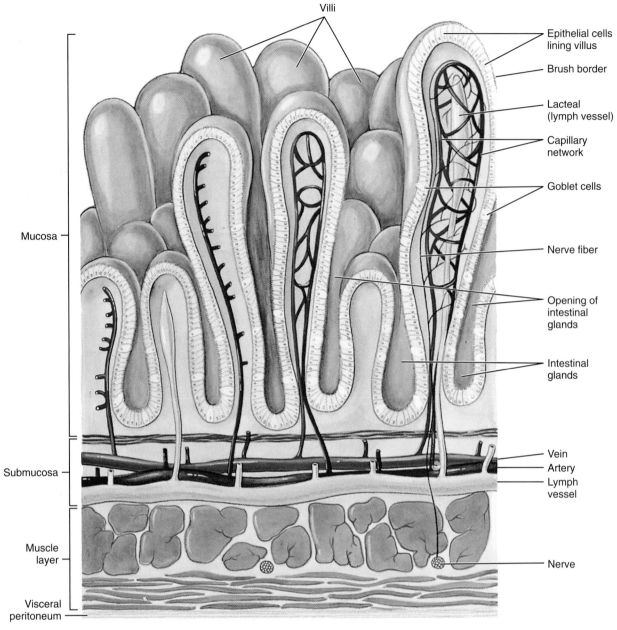

FIGURE 15-8 • The surface of the small intestine is studded with villi and openings into the intestinal glands. Here some of the villi have been opened to show the blood and lymph vessels within.

both an endocrine and an exocrine gland. Recall that its endocrine cells secrete the hormones *insulin* and *glucagon,* which regulate glucose concentration (see Chapter 9). The exocrine portion secretes **pancreatic juice,** which contains a number of digestive enzymes. The pancreatic duct from the pancreas joins the common bile duct coming from the liver, forming a single duct that passes into the duodenum. An accessory pancreatic duct is often present as well.

If the pancreas becomes damaged, its ducts may become blocked. When this happens, the pancreas may be digested by its own enzymes. This condition, called *acute pancreatitis,* is frequently associated with alcoholism.

The Liver Secretes Bile

The **liver** is the largest and one of the most complex organs in the body (see Figure 15-7). The right lobe of the liver is larger than the left lobe and has three main parts. Oxygen-rich blood is brought to the liver by the **hepatic arteries.** However, the liver also receives blood from the **hepatic portal vein.** Recall that the hepatic portal vein delivers nutrients absorbed from the intestine.

Bile is stored and concentrated in the pear-shaped **gallbladder** (see Figure 15-7). The hormone **cholecystokinin (CCK)** is secreted by the intestinal mucosa, mainly when fat is present in the duodenum. This hormone stimulates the gallbladder to contract, releasing bile into the **cystic duct.** The cystic duct from the gallbladder joins the **hepatic duct** from the liver to form the **common bile duct,** which (together with the duct from the pancreas) opens into the duodenum.

A single liver cell can carry on more than 500 separate metabolic activities. The liver performs these important functions:

1. Produces and secretes **bile,** which is important in the mechanical digestion of fats. **Bilirubin** (bil-ee-**roo′**-bin) and other pigments are released from hemoglobin when red blood cells are broken down; these pigments are secreted into the bile.
2. Helps maintain homeostasis by removing nutrients from or adding nutrients to the blood.
3. Converts the simple sugar **glucose** to **glycogen** and stores it; then when glucose is needed, it breaks down the glycogen and releases glucose into the blood.
4. Stores iron and certain vitamins.
5. Converts excess amino acids to fatty acids and urea.
6. Performs many important functions in the metabolism of proteins, fats, and carbohydrates.
7. Manufactures many of the plasma proteins found in the blood.
8. Detoxifies alcohol and many other drugs and toxins that enter the body.
9. Phagocytizes bacteria and worn-out red blood cells.

Quiz Yourself

- What are the functions of teeth? Of saliva?
- What are the functions of the gastric glands?
- What are the functions of the small intestine?
- What are three functions of the liver?

DIGESTION OCCURS AS FOOD MOVES THROUGH THE DIGESTIVE TRACT

LEARNING OBJECTIVE

9. Summarize carbohydrate, lipid, and protein digestion.

Secretion of digestive juices is stimulated by hormones and by chyme. For example, the hormone **gastrin,** which is released by the stomach mucosa, stimulates the gastric glands to secrete pepsinogen. The intestinal glands are stimulated to release their fluid mainly by local reflexes that occur when the small intestine is stretched by chyme.

Glucose Is the Main Product of Carbohydrate Digestion

Large carbohydrates such as **starch** and glycogen consist of long chains of glucose molecules. Starch digestion begins in the mouth. There the enzyme *salivary amylase* begins breaking down some of the long starch molecules to smaller compounds and then to the sugar **maltose.**

$$\text{Starch} \xrightarrow{\text{Salivary amylase}} \text{Smaller carbohydrates} + \text{Maltose}$$

In the duodenum, **pancreatic amylase,** an enzyme in the pancreatic juice, splits the remaining starch molecules to maltose.

$$\text{Carbohydrates} \xrightarrow{\text{Pancreatic amylase}} \text{Maltose}$$

Then the enzyme **maltase** (released by the epithelial cells lining the duodenum) breaks down each maltose molecule to two molecules of glucose. **Sucrose,** the sugar we use in our coffee, and **lactose** (milk sugar) are also broken down to simple sugars in the duodenum. Glucose is the major product of carbohydrate digestion.

$$\text{Maltose} \xrightarrow{\text{Maltase}} \text{Glucose} + \text{Glucose}$$

Many plant foods are rich in starch. However, this starch is not readily available to us because it is encased within the tough **cellulose** cell walls of plant cells. We do not have enzymes that digest cellulose, so much of the starch in plant cells passes through the digestive tract without being digested. Cooking destroys the cellulose walls so that the starch can be more easily reached by amylase and other enzymes. Carbohydrate digestion is summarized in Table 15-1.

Bile Emulsifies Fat

Digestion of **fat** takes place mainly in the duodenum. Bile **emulsifies** (mechanically breaks down) fat by a detergent action that breaks large fat droplets down into smaller droplets.

$$\text{Large fat droplets} \xrightarrow{\text{Bile}} \text{Emulsified fat (small fat droplets containing triglycerides)}$$

These droplets are acted on by an enzyme in the pancreatic juice called **lipase.** Pancreatic lipase breaks down **triglycerides** (fat molecules) to free **fatty acids** and **glycerol.**

$$\text{Triglycerides} \xrightarrow{\text{Lipase}} \text{Fatty acids} + \text{Glycerol}$$

Fat (lipid) digestion is summarized in Table 15-2.

Proteins Are Digested to Free Amino Acids

Proteins consist of smaller molecules called **amino acids.** The amino acid subunits are linked together by chemical bonds called **peptide bonds.** During protein digestion peptide bonds are broken and free amino acids are released.

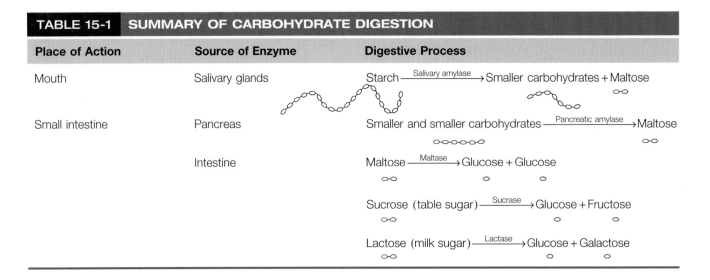

TABLE 15-1	SUMMARY OF CARBOHYDRATE DIGESTION	
Place of Action	**Source of Enzyme**	**Digestive Process**
Mouth	Salivary glands	Starch $\xrightarrow{\text{Salivary amylase}}$ Smaller carbohydrates + Maltose
Small intestine	Pancreas	Smaller and smaller carbohydrates $\xrightarrow{\text{Pancreatic amylase}}$ Maltose
	Intestine	Maltose $\xrightarrow{\text{Maltase}}$ Glucose + Glucose
		Sucrose (table sugar) $\xrightarrow{\text{Sucrase}}$ Glucose + Fructose
		Lactose (milk sugar) $\xrightarrow{\text{Lactase}}$ Glucose + Galactose

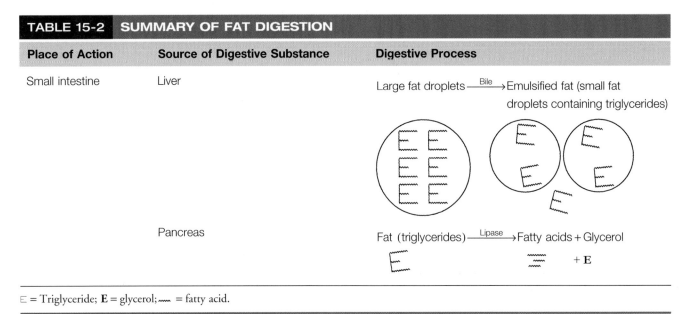

TABLE 15-2	SUMMARY OF FAT DIGESTION	
Place of Action	**Source of Digestive Substance**	**Digestive Process**
Small intestine	Liver	Large fat droplets $\xrightarrow{\text{Bile}}$ Emulsified fat (small fat droplets containing triglycerides)
	Pancreas	Fat (triglycerides) $\xrightarrow{\text{Lipase}}$ Fatty acids + Glycerol + **E**

E = Triglyceride; **E** = glycerol; ⌇⌇ = fatty acid.

Protein digestion begins in the stomach where the enzyme *pepsin* breaks down most proteins to smaller molecules called **polypeptides.** In the duodenum, the enzyme **trypsin** (and other enzymes) in the pancreatic juice break down proteins and polypeptides to smaller protein fragments called peptides.

Proteins and polypeptides $\xrightarrow{\text{Pepsin, Trypsin}}$ Peptides
(small protein fagments)

The peptides are digested by enzymes called **peptidases,** secreted by epithelial cells lining the intestine. Peptidases split peptides into free amino acids, which are the products of protein digestion.

Peptides $\xrightarrow{\text{Peptidases}}$ Free amino acids

Protein digestion is summarized in Table 15-3.

Quiz Yourself

- What is the main product of carbohydrate digestion?
- What is the function of bile?
- What are the products of protein digestion?

ABSORPTION TAKES PLACE THROUGH THE INTESTINAL VILLI

LEARNING OBJECTIVE

10. Describe the structure of an intestinal villus and explain the role of villi in absorption of nutrients.

TABLE 15-3	SUMMARY OF PROTEIN DIGESTION	
Place of Action	**Source of Enzyme**	**Digestive Process**
Stomach	Stomach (gastric glands)	Protein ——Pepsin——→ Polypeptides A-A-A-A-A-A A-A-A-A-A-A A-A-A-A-A-A A-A-A-A-A-A A-A-A-A-A-A A-A-A-A-A-A
Small intestine	Pancreas	Protein, polypeptides ——Trypsin——→ Peptides (smaller protein fragments) A-A-A-A-A-A A-A-A-A-A-A A-A-A-A-A-A A-A-A A-A-A A-A-A-A-A-A A-A A-A A-A
	Small intestine	Peptides ——Peptidases——→ Free amino acids A-A-A-A-A-A A A A A A A A-A-A A A A A-A A-A A A A A

A = Amino acids.

After food has been digested, the nutrients are absorbed by the intestinal villi. The structure of a villus is illustrated in Figure 15-8. Within each villus, there is a network of capillaries that branches from an arteriole and empties into a venule. Each villus also has a central lymph vessel, called a **lacteal** (**lak′**-tee-al).

To reach the blood or lymph, a nutrient must pass through the single layer of epithelial cells lining the villus and through the single layer of cells forming the wall of the capillary or the lacteal. Amino acids and simple sugars are absorbed into the blood. They are transported directly to the liver by the hepatic portal vein. Fatty acids are absorbed into the lacteals. They circulate through the lymph system before entering the blood.

Quiz Yourself

• How are amino acids and simple sugars absorbed?
• How are fatty acids absorbed?

THE LARGE INTESTINE ELIMINATES WASTES

LEARNING OBJECTIVE

11. **Describe the structure and functions of the large intestine.**

After chyme has moved through the stomach and small intestine, it consists mainly of water and indigestible wastes such as cellulose. The small intestine is normally shut off from the large intestine by a sphincter muscle called the **ileocecal** (il′-ee-o-**see′**-kal) **valve.** When a peristaltic contraction brings chyme toward it, the ileocecal valve opens, allowing the chyme to enter the large intestine.

Although only about 1.3 m (about 4 feet) long, the large intestine is called "large" because its diameter is much greater than the diameter of the small intestine. The small intestine joins the large intestine about 7 cm above the end of the large intestine. This creates a pouch called the **cecum** (**see′**-kum) (see Figure 15-1). The **vermiform appendix,** a worm-shaped blind tube, hangs down from the end of the cecum. The function of the appendix is unknown, but it is rich in lymph tissue. Inflammation of the appendix, known as *appendicitis,* can lead to peritonitis and other complications if not diagnosed and treated promptly.

From the cecum to the rectum the large intestine is known as the **colon** (**koe′**-lon). The **ascending colon** extends from the cecum straight up to the lower border of the liver. As it turns horizontally, it becomes the **transverse colon.** The transverse colon extends across the abdomen below the liver and stomach. On the left side of the abdomen the **descending colon** turns downward. It empties into the S-shaped **sigmoid colon,** which empties into the short **rectum.** The rectum is the last 12 cm or so of the digestive tract. It ends in the **anus**—the opening for elimination of **feces.** The last 4 cm of the rectum is called the **anal canal.**

One to 3 days or even longer may be required for the slow journey through the large intestine. The mucosa of the large intestine lacks villi and produces no digestive enzymes. Its surface epithelium consists of cells specialized for absorption and goblet cells that secrete mucus. Because the movements of the large intestine are quite sluggish, bacteria have time to grow and reproduce there. Bacteria that live in the large intestine nourish themselves on the last remnants of the meal. In exchange, these bacteria produce vitamins K and certain B-complex vitamins that we can absorb and use.

As the chyme slowly passes through the large intestine, water and sodium are absorbed from it and what remains becomes feces. Thus undigested and unabsorbed foods are eliminated from the body by the large intestine in the form of feces. Bile pigments, which are excreted by the large intestine, give feces their characteristic brown color.

After meals, contractions of the large intestine increase. This stimulates the desire to **defecate** (expel feces). Two sphincters, an internal anal sphincter and an external anal sphincter in the wall of the anal canal, guard the anal opening. When the rectum fills with feces, the internal sphincter relaxes but the external sphincter remains contracted until relaxed voluntarily. Thus defecation is a reflex action that can be voluntarily inhibited by keeping the external sphincter contracted.

The functions of the large intestine may be summarized as follows:

1. Absorption of sodium and water
2. Incubation of bacteria that produce vitamin K and some of the B-complex vitamins, and absorption of these vitamins
3. Elimination of wastes

In Western countries, *colorectal cancer*, which is cancer of the colon or rectum, is the third most common type of cancer. Risk factors include a diet high in red meat and low in fresh fruit, vegetables, fish, and poultry; smoking; family history; and physical inactivity.

⊚ Quiz Yourself

- What are the main regions of the large intestine?
- What are three functions of the large intestine?

A BALANCED DIET IS NECESSARY TO MAINTAIN HEALTH

LEARNING OBJECTIVE

12. **Describe the components of a balanced diet and summarize the functions of each.**

A balanced diet includes water, minerals, vitamins, carbohydrates, lipids, and proteins. A group of biologically active plant compounds called *phytochemicals* also appear necessary for good health. Carbohydrates, lipids, and proteins are nutrients that can be used as energy sources.

1. **Water** is one of the main components of the body. It is used by the body to transport materials. All the chemical reactions in the body take place in a watery medium. An average adult requires a daily intake of about 2.4 liters (2.5 quarts) of water. About two thirds of this amount is ingested in the form of water or other fluids. The rest comes from solid foods, which actually contain quite a bit of water. For example, a raw apple is actually about 85% water by weight.

2. **Minerals** are inorganic nutrients ingested in the form of salts dissolved in food and water. Some required minerals and their functions are listed in Table 15-4.

3. **Vitamins** are organic compounds required for certain reactions to take place. Many vitamins serve as **coenzymes**—compounds that work with enzymes to regulate chemical reactions. Table 15-5 lists essential vitamins and their functions.

4. **Carbohydrates** are ingested mainly as starch or cellulose, both **polysaccharides** (large carbohydrates). Nutritionists refer to polysaccharides as *complex carbohydrates.* Foods rich in complex carbohydrates are potatoes, rice, corn, and other cereal grains. Sugars (which are simple carbohydrates) account for about 25% of the carbohydrates we ingest. Large carbohydrates are digested to glucose or other simple sugars that can be absorbed into the blood. Glucose is an important energy source for cells. Excess glucose can be stored in the liver and muscles as glycogen.

5. **Lipids** include fats and cholesterol. Most of the lipids we ingest are fats—mainly triglycerides. Lipids provide energy and are needed to make cell membranes, steroid hormones, and bile salts. Diets high in triglycerides and cholesterol have been associated with cardiovascular disease.

6. **Proteins** are digested into their component amino acids. These smaller molecules are then assembled to make the types of proteins the body needs. Of the 20 or so amino acids, nine (10 in children) are considered **essential amino acids** because they must be provided in the diet. (The other amino acids can be synthesized in the body from other nutrients.) Proteins are essential building blocks of cells, and many serve as enzymes. Other vital proteins are hemoglobin and muscle proteins.

7. **Phytochemicals** (**fy′**-tow-kem-ih-kals) are biologically active compounds found in plants that promote health. Diets rich in fruits and vegetables appear to lower the incidence of cancer and heart disease. **Oxidants** are highly reactive molecules produced during cell activities; they can damage DNA and other cell molecules by snatching electrons. Some phytochemicals function as **antioxidants**—substances that destroy oxidants. Phytochemicals that are antioxidants include the lycopenes responsible for the red color of tomatoes and the flavonoids responsible for the blue color of blueberries and the red color of raspberries and red cabbage. A flavonoid antioxidant is also found in dark chocolate.

⊚ Quiz Yourself

- What are the functions of proteins in the body?
- What are the functions of lipids?

TABLE 15-4	SOME IMPORTANT MINERALS AND THEIR FUNCTIONS	
Mineral	**Functions**	**Sources, Comments**
Calcium	Component of bones and teeth; essential for normal blood clotting and for normal muscle and nerve function	Milk and other dairy products, fish, green leafy vegetables; bones serve as calcium reservoir
Phosphorus	Performs more functions than any other mineral; structural component of bone; component of adenosine triphosphate, DNA, RNA, and phospholipids	Meat, dairy products, cereal
Sulfur	Component of many proteins and vitamins	High-protein foods such as meat, fish, legumes, nuts
Potassium	Principal positive ion within cells; influences muscle contraction and nerve function	Fruit, vegetables, grains, fish
Sodium	Principal positive ion in interstitial fluid; important in fluid balance; neural transmission	Many foods, table salt; too much ingested in average American diet; excessive amounts may contribute to high blood pressure
Chloride	Principal negative ion of interstitial fluid; important in fluid balance and in acid-base balance	Many foods; table salt
Magnesium	Needed for normal muscle and nerve function	Nuts; whole grains; green, leafy vegetables, seafood, dairy products, chocolate
Copper	Component of many enzymes; essential for hemoglobin synthesis	Liver, eggs, fish, whole-wheat flour, beans
Iodide	Component of thyroid hormones (hormones that increase metabolic rate); deficiency results in goiter (abnormal enlargement of thyroid gland)	Seafood, iodized salt, vegetables grown in iodine-rich soils
Manganese	Necessary to activate arginase, an enzyme essential for urea formation; activates many other enzymes	Whole-grain cereals, nuts, egg yolks, green vegetables; poorly absorbed from intestine
Iron	Component of hemoglobin, myoglobin, important respiratory enzymes (cytochromes), and other enzymes essential to oxygen transport and cellular respiration	Mineral most likely to be deficient in diet; good sources: meat (especially liver), nuts, fish, egg yolk, legumes, dried fruit; deficiency results in anemia and may impair cognitive function
Fluoride	Component of bones and teeth; makes teeth resistant to decay; excess causes tooth mottling	Fish; in areas where it does not occur naturally, fluoride may be added to municipal water supplies (fluoridation)
Zinc	Cofactor for at least 70 enzymes; helps regulate synthesis of certain proteins; needed for growth and repair of tissues	Meat, milk, yogurt, some seafood, chocolate; deficiency may impair cognitive function
Selenium	Antioxidant (breaks down peroxides)	Seafood, nuts, eggs, liver and other meat, garlic, mushrooms; may protect men against prostate cancer

ENERGY METABOLISM IS BALANCED WHEN ENERGY INPUT EQUALS ENERGY OUTPUT

LEARNING OBJECTIVES

13. **Contrast basal metabolic rate with total metabolic rate and write the basic energy equation for maintaining body weight.**
14. **Define malnutrition and give two examples.**

Metabolic rate is the amount of energy released by the body in a given time as a result of breaking down fuel molecules. Metabolic rate may be expressed either in kilocalories (kcal) of

heat energy used per day or as a percentage above or below a standard normal level. Much of the energy expended by the body is ultimately converted to heat.

The **basal metabolic rate (BMR)** is the rate at which the body releases heat under resting conditions. BMR is the body's basic cost of living—that is, the rate of energy used during resting conditions. This energy is needed to maintain body functions such as heart contraction, breathing, and kidney function. An individual's **total metabolic rate** is the sum of the BMR and the energy used to carry on all daily activities. Someone who performs physical labor has a greater metabolic rate than does an executive whose job requirements do not include a substantial amount of movement and who does not exercise regularly.

TABLE 15-5 THE VITAMINS

Vitamins and U.S. RDA*	Actions	Effect of Deficiency	Sources
FAT-SOLUBLE			
Vitamin A, retinol 5000 IU[†]	Converted to retinal; essential for normal vision; essential for normal growth and differentiation of cells; reproduction; immunity	Growth retardation; night blindness; worldwide 250 million children are at risk of blindness from vitamin A deficiency	Liver, fortified milk, yellow and green vegetables such as carrots and broccoli
Vitamin D, calciferol 400 IU	Promotes calcium and phosphorus absorption from digestive tract; essential for normal growth and maintenance of bone	Weak bones, bone deformities: rickets in children, osteomalacia in adults	Fish oils, egg yolk, fortified milk, butter, margarine
Vitamin E, tocopherols 30 IU	Antioxidant; protects unsaturated fatty acids and cell membranes	Increased catabolism of unsaturated fatty acids, so that not enough are available for maintenance of cell membranes; prevents normal growth; nerve damage	Vegetable oils, nuts, leafy greens
Vitamin K about 80 mcg[‡]	Essential for blood clotting	Prolonged blood clotting time	Normally supplied by intestinal bacteria; leafy greens, legumes
WATER-SOLUBLE			
Vitamin C, ascorbic acid 60 mg[§]	Collagen synthesis; antioxidant; needed for synthesis of some hormones and neurotransmitters; important in immune function	Scurvy (wounds heal very slowly, and scars become weak and split open; capillaries become fragile; bone does not grow or heal properly)	Citrus fruits, strawberries, tomatoes, leafy vegetables, cabbage
B-complex vitamins			
Vitamin B$_1$, thiamine 1.5 mg	Active form is a coenzyme in many enzyme systems; important in carbohydrate and amino acid metabolism	Beriberi (weakened heart muscle, enlarged right side of heart, nervous system and digestive tract disorders); common in alcoholics	Liver, yeast, whole and enriched grains, meat, leafy vegetables
Vitamin B$_2$, riboflavin 1.7 mg	Used to make coenzymes essential in cellular respiration	Dermatitis, inflammation and cracking at corners of mouth; confusion	Liver, milk, eggs, green leafy vegetables, enriched grains
Niacin 20 mg	Component of important coenzymes; essential to cellular respiration	Pellagra (dermatitis, diarrhea, mental symptoms, muscular weakness, fatigue)	Liver, chicken, tuna, milk, green leafy vegetables, enriched grains
Vitamin B$_6$, pyridoxine 2 mg	Derivative is coenzyme needed in amino acid metabolism	Dermatitis, digestive tract disturbances; convulsions	Meat, whole grains, legumes, green leafy vegetables
Pantothenic acid 10 mg	Constituent of coenzyme A (important in cellular metabolism)	Deficiency extremely rare	Meat, whole grains, legumes
Folic acid 400 mcg	Coenzyme needed for nucleic acid synthesis and for maturation of red blood cells	A type of anemia; certain birth defects; increased risk of cardiovascular disease; deficiency in alcoholics, smokers and pregnant women	Liver, legumes, dark-green leafy vegetables, orange juice
Biotin 30 mcg	Coenzyme important in metabolism	—	Produced by intestinal bacteria; liver, chocolate, egg yolk
Vitamin B$_{12}$ 2.4 mcg	Coenzyme important in metabolism; contains cobalt	A type of anemia	Liver, meat, fish, dairy products

*RDA, Recommended dietary allowance, established by the Food and Nutrition Board of the National Research Council to maintain good nutrition for healthy adults; [†]IU, international unit, the amount that produces a specific biological effect and is internationally accepted as a measure of the activity of the substance; [‡]mcg, microgram; [§]mg, milligram.

An average-size person who does not exercise and who sits at a desk all day expends about 2000 kcal daily. If the food the individual eats each day also contains about 2000 kcal, the body will be in a state of energy balance; that is, energy input will equal energy output. This is an extremely important concept because body weight remains constant when:

Energy input = Energy output

When energy output is greater than energy input, stored fat is burned and body weight decreases. On the other hand, people gain weight when they take in more energy (calories) in food than they expend in daily activity, in other words, when:

Energy (calorie) input > Energy output

Malnutrition, or poor nutritional status, can result from dietary intake that is either above or below required needs. Millions of individuals suffer from **undernutrition,** in which their calorie (energy) intake is too low or their diet is deficient in needed nutrients. Essential amino acids, iron, calcium, and vitamin A are the nutrients most often deficient in the diet. **Obesity** is a serious nutritional problem in which energy imbalance results in the deposit of an excess amount of fat in fat tissues. Obesity is the second leading preventable cause of death in the United States. (It is second only to smoking.) Obesity is a major risk factor for many disorders, including heart disease, diabetes mellitus, osteoarthritis, and certain types of cancer.

Quiz Yourself

- What is basal metabolic rate?
- What happens when energy input is greater than energy output?

SUMMARY

LO 1. Describe in general terms the following steps in processing food: ingestion, digestion, absorption, and elimination.

- **Nutrients** are the substances in food that are used to make new cells and tissues and needed chemical compounds. Some nutrients are fuel molecules that provide energy. The process of taking in and using food is referred to as **nutrition.** The first step in processing food is **ingestion,** taking food into the mouth, chewing it, and swallowing it.
- **Digestion,** the process of breaking food down into smaller molecules, includes **mechanical digestion,** the process of breaking down food by chewing and by churning and mixing movements in the digestive tract, and **chemical digestion,** which is regulated by **enzymes.**
- **Absorption** is the process of transferring nutrients through the wall of the stomach or intestine and into the blood. **Elimination,** the function of the large intestine, is the process of removing unabsorbed food from the body.

LO 2. List in sequence each structure through which a bite of food passes on its way through the digestive tract; label a diagram of the digestive system.

- A bite of food passes through the mouth, pharynx, esophagus, stomach, small intestine (duodenum, jejunum, ileum), and large intestine (cecum, colon, rectum, anal canal), and unabsorbed food passes out through the anus.

LO 3. Describe the wall of the digestive tract; distinguish between the visceral peritoneum and the parietal peritoneum, and describe their major folds.

- The lining of the digestive tract is its **mucosa.** A layer of connective tissue, the **submucosa,** lies beneath the mucosa. A **muscle layer** (muscularis) surrounds the submucosa. The outer connective tissue layer is the **adventitia.** Below the diaphragm, the outer layer is called the **visceral peritoneum.** By various folds it connects to the **parietal peritoneum**—the sheet of connective tissue that lines the walls of the abdominal and pelvic cavities. The **peritoneal cavity** is a potential space between the visceral and the parietal peritonea.
- The two peritonea are connected by various folds. The **mesentery** anchors the intestine to the posterior abdominal wall. The **greater omentum,** which hangs over the intestine, contains fat deposits and lymph nodes. The

LO = Learning Objective

lesser omentum suspends the stomach and duodenum from the liver. The **mesocolon** attaches the colon to the posterior abdominal wall.

LO 4. **Describe the structures of the mouth, including the teeth, and give their functions.**

- Digestion begins in the **mouth**, or **oral cavity.** The teeth grind and crush the food. Young children have a set of 20 **deciduous teeth.** Adults have 32 **permanent teeth.** Each quadrant of the mouth has two **incisors,** one **canine,** two **premolars,** and three **molars.**

- The **crown** of a tooth is covered by tough **enamel.** Beneath the enamel is the **dentin** that makes up most of the tooth. The **roots** are embedded in sockets (alveoli) of the alveolar processes. The **pulp cavity** contains blood vessels and nerves.

- Three main pairs of **salivary glands** are the **parotid glands, submandibular glands,** and **sublingual glands. Saliva** contains the enzyme **salivary amylase,** which begins the digestion of carbohydrates. In the mouth the food is converted to a semisolid mass called a **bolus.**

LO 5. **Describe the structure and function of the pharynx and esophagus.**

- In swallowing, reflex movements propel the bolus through the **pharynx** and into the **esophagus. Peristaltic contractions** push the food through the esophagus to the stomach.

LO 6. **Describe the structure of the stomach and its role in processing food.**

- The **stomach** mechanically and chemically digests food. The lining of the large muscular stomach has folds called **rugae.** The stomach mechanically digests food by churning it, reducing it to **chyme.**

- **Parietal cells** in the **gastric glands** secrete **hydrochloric acid** and **intrinsic factor,** which is needed for vitamin B_{12} absorption. **Chief cells** secrete **pepsinogen,** an inactive form of the enzyme **pepsin.** The **pyloric sphincter,** a ring of muscle at the exit of the stomach, relaxes to allow chyme to pass into the small intestine.

LO 7. **Identify the three main regions of the small intestine and describe the functions of the small intestine.**

- The three sections of the **small intestine** are the **duodenum, jejunum,** and **ileum.** Most chemical digestion takes place in the duodenum. **Bile** from the **liver** and **pancreatic juice** from the **pancreas** are released into the duodenum. Cells lining the small intestine produce enzymes needed for the final digestion of proteins and carbohydrates.

LO 8. **Summarize the functions of the pancreas and liver.**

- The pancreas releases pancreatic juice containing enzymes that digest proteins, lipids, and carbohydrates.

- The liver produces bile which mechanically digests fats. Bile is stored in the **gallbladder. Bilirubin** and other pigments from the breakdown of hemoglobin are found in the bile.

- The liver also stores the sugar **glucose** as **glycogen** and stores and metabolizes many other nutrients. It makes plasma proteins and detoxifies drugs.

LO 9. **Summarize carbohydrate, lipid, and protein digestion.**

- Carbohydrate digestion begins in the mouth, where salivary amylase breaks down **starch** to smaller carbohydrates and **maltose.** In the duodenum, pancreatic amylase continues the digestion of carbohydrates to maltose. Then maltase and other specific enzymes in the duodenum break down maltose and other sugars to simple sugars, mainly **glucose.**

- Fat digestion begins in the duodenum when bile **emulsifies** (mechanically breaks down) large fat droplets. Then **lipase** from the pancreas digests the fat to fatty acids and glycerol.

- Protein digestion begins in the stomach with the action of pepsin. In the duodenum, enzymes from the pancreas continue to reduce proteins to smaller molecules called **polypeptides** and then to smaller protein fragments called peptides. Finally, **peptidases** produced by the epithelial cells lining the duodenum break down the peptides to free amino acids.

LO 10. **Describe the structure of an intestinal villus and explain the role of villi in absorption of nutrients.**
- Most absorption takes place through the **villi** of the small intestine. The villi greatly expand the surface area for absorption. Glucose and amino acids are absorbed through the villi, enter the blood, and are transported to the liver by the **hepatic portal vein.** Fatty acids are absorbed through the villi into **lacteals** and are transported by the lymph system; eventually they enter the blood.

LO 11. **Describe the structure and functions of the large intestine.**
- Indigestible material such as cellulose and unabsorbed nutrients pass through the **ileocecal valve** into the large intestine. The large intestine consists of the **cecum, ascending colon, transverse colon, descending colon, sigmoid colon, rectum, anal canal,** and **anus.** The **vermiform appendix** hangs down from the **cecum.**
- Excess water and sodium are absorbed from the chyme as it passes through the large intestine. The large intestine incubates bacteria that produce vitamin K and some of the B-complex vitamins.
- Indigestible material and unabsorbed food are eliminated by the large intestine as feces. Bilirubin and other bile pigments are excreted by the large intestine.

LO 12. **Describe the components of a balanced diet and summarize the functions of each.**
- Water is needed to transport materials and is the medium in which chemical reactions take place. **Minerals** are inorganic nutrients. See Table 15-4. **Vitamins** are organic nutrients required for many reactions (see Table 15-5, p. 256). **Carbohydrates** are energy sources.
- **Lipids** (fats) are an energy source and are used to make cell membranes and certain hormones. Many **proteins** are enzymes. The amino acid subunits of proteins are building blocks of cells. **Essential amino acids** must be included in the diet. **Phytochemicals** are biologically active plant compounds that promote health. Many are **antioxidants,** substances that destroy **oxidants,** which are reactive molecules that damage cells.

LO 13. **Contrast basal metabolic rate with total metabolic rate and write the basic energy equation for maintaining body weight.**
- **Basal metabolic rate** is the body's energy cost of metabolic living. **Total metabolic rate** is the BMR plus the energy used to carry on daily activities.
- When energy input equals energy output, body weight remains constant.

LO 14. **Define malnutrition and give two examples.**
- When energy input and output are not balanced, **malnutrition** can occur. In **undernutrition,** energy input may be less than energy output or essential nutrients may be deficient in the diet. In **obesity,** energy (calorie) input is greater than energy output.

CHAPTER QUIZ

Fill in the Blank

1. The process of taking food into the mouth, chewing it, and swallowing it is called _____.

2. _____ _____ includes chewing and churning to break down food into molecules small enough to be absorbed; _____ _____ involves breakdown of large food molecules by enzymes.

3. The inner lining of the wall of the digestive tract is the _____.

4. Inferior to the diaphragm, the outer layer of the wall of the digestive tract is called the _____ _____.

5. Waves of contraction that push food along through the digestive tract are referred to as _____.

6. The double fold of peritoneum that hangs down over the intestine like an apron is called the _____ _____.

7. The normal maximum number of teeth in the adult mouth is _____.

8. The portion of a tooth above the gum is the _____; the part below the gum is the _____.

9. Each tooth is composed mainly of _____, which in the crown region is covered by _____.

10. The largest salivary glands are the _____ _____.

11. Salivary amylase begins the digestion of _____.

12. The folds in the mucosa of the stomach are called _____.

13. The enzyme produced by the gastric glands is _____.

14. The three divisions of the small intestine are the _____, _____, and _____.

15. The energy cost of metabolic living is referred to as _____ _____ rate.

Multiple Choice

16. The function of the gallbladder is to: a. break down proteins; b. produce bile; c. store bile; d. produce bile pigments.

17. The end products of protein digestion are: a. glucose and glycerol; b. glucose and maltose; c. fatty acids; d. amino acids.

18. Nutrients are absorbed mainly by the: a. intestinal villi; b. rugae in the stomach; c. lacteals; d. hepatic arteries.

19. Chyme passing through the transverse colon would next enter the: a. ascending colon; b. cecum; c. descending colon; d. sigmoid colon.

20. Nutrients that are ingested mainly in the form of salts are: a. proteins; b. minerals; c. vitamins; d. carbohydrates.

REVIEW QUESTIONS

1. Trace the journey of a bite of food containing mainly carbohydrate through the digestive tract, listing each structure through which it must pass and describing what happens to the carbohydrate in each place.

2. Trace the journey of a protein food through the digestive tract, describing how it changes along the way. Do the same for a lipid.

3. Describe (or label on a diagram) the structure of a tooth.

4. The inner wall of the small intestine is not smooth like the inside of a hose. Instead, it has folds and millions of villi. Why is this important?

5. Draw a diagram of a villus and label its parts.

6. List the functions of the three types of accessory glands that release secretions into the digestive tract and identify their secretions.

7. Describe four functions of the liver.

8. What are the functions of the large intestine?

9. What are the components of a balanced diet?

10. What happens when the basic energy equation is shifted in either direction?

11. Label the diagram. (See Figure 15-1 to check your answers.)

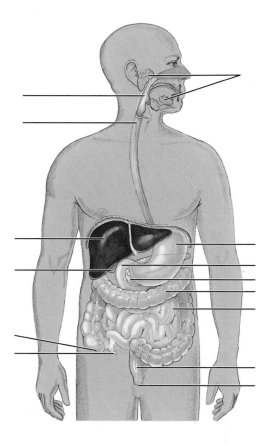

16

The Urinary System and Fluid Balance

Chapter Outline

Whether you drink a pint of water or a gallon and whether you are on a salt-restricted diet or eat a bag of potato chips, the fluid and salt content of your body must be kept within homeostatic limits. The body must replace water and salt losses and excrete excesses. The **urinary system** helps regulate the volume and composition of body fluids.

As cells carry on metabolic activities, they produce waste products such as water and carbon dioxide. The body also produces urea and other nitrogenous waste products as it processes excess nutrients such as amino acids. The body must get rid of these metabolic waste products because, if they are permitted to accumulate, they could reach toxic concentrations.

In this chapter we examine the role of the urinary system in excreting metabolic wastes and in helping maintain the volume and composition of the body fluids. We discuss the important role of hormones in regulating the urinary system and we describe how the body maintains acid-base balance.

METABOLIC WASTE PRODUCTS INCLUDE WATER, CARBON DIOXIDE, AND NITROGENOUS WASTES

LEARNING OBJECTIVE

1. Identify the principal metabolic waste products and the organs that excrete them.

Excretion is defined as the discharge from the body of metabolic wastes products and excess solutes and other substances. Excretion is different from **elimination,** the discharge of undigested or unabsorbed food from the digestive tract.

The principal metabolic waste products are water, carbon dioxide, and **nitrogenous** (ni-**troj′**-uh-nus) **wastes,** those that contain nitrogen. Amino acids and nucleic acids (deoxyribonucleic acid [DNA] and ribonucleic acid [RNA]) contain nitrogen. When excess amino acids are broken down in the liver, the nitrogen-containing amino group is removed. The amino group is chemically converted to **ammonia,** which is then converted to **urea.** Somewhat similarly, **uric acid** is formed from the breakdown of nucleic acids. Urea and uric acid are transported from the liver to the kidneys by the circulatory system.

Although metabolic wastes are excreted mainly by the urinary system, the skin, lungs, and digestive system also function in waste disposal (Figure 16-1). Sweat glands in the skin excrete 5% to 10% of all metabolic wastes. Sweat contains the same substances—water, salts, and nitrogenous wastes—as urine but is much more dilute.

The lungs excrete carbon dioxide and water (in the form of water vapor). **Bile pigments,** which are breakdown products of hemoglobin, pass from the liver into the intestine as part of the bile. These pigments are excreted by the large intestine as part of the feces.

Quiz Yourself

- What are the three main nitrogenous wastes?
- Which organs excrete metabolic wastes?

THE URINARY SYSTEM HAS MANY REGULATORY FUNCTIONS

LEARNING OBJECTIVE

2. Summarize the functions of the urinary system in maintaining homeostasis.

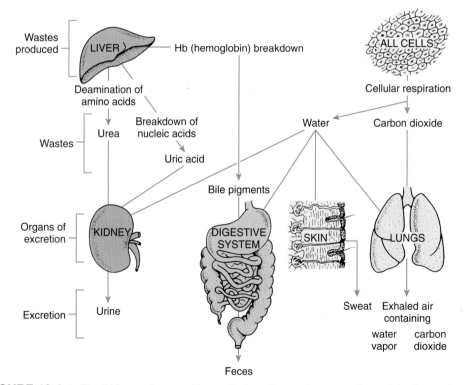

FIGURE 16-1 • The kidneys, lungs, skin, and digestive system excrete metabolic wastes and excess water and salts. Wastes containing nitrogen are produced by the liver and transported to the kidneys. The kidneys excrete these wastes in the urine. All cells produce carbon dioxide and some water during cellular respiration.

The urinary system helps maintain homeostasis by performing the following functions:

1. Maintains fluid homeostasis by adjusting the salt and water content of the urine
2. Excretes metabolic waste products such as urea and uric acid
3. Regulates the concentrations of many electrolytes (inorganic salts, acids, and bases)
4. Regulates the acid-base (pH) level of the blood and body fluids
5. Secretes the enzyme **renin,** which is important in regulating blood pressure
6. Secretes the hormone **erythropoietin** (eh-rith′-row-**poy′**-eh-tin), which regulates production of red blood cells
7. Secretes a hormone that stimulates calcium absorption by the intestine

Quiz Yourself

- What are six functions of the urinary system that help maintain homeostasis?

THE URINARY SYSTEM CONSISTS OF THE KIDNEYS, URINARY BLADDER, AND THEIR DUCTS

LEARNING OBJECTIVES

3. Describe the anatomy of the urinary system and give the function of each of its structures. (Be able to label a diagram of the urinary system.)
4. Describe the structure and function of a nephron. (Be able to label a diagram of a nephron.)
5. Trace a drop of filtrate from glomerulus to urethra, listing in sequence each structure through which it passes.

The principal organs of the urinary system are the paired **kidneys,** which play a vital role in regulating the volume and composition of body fluid. The kidneys remove metabolic wastes and excess water and salts from the blood and produce **urine** (Figure 16-2). From the kidneys, urine passes through the paired **ureters** (yoo-**ree′**-ters) to the **urinary bladder**. The single urinary bladder temporarily stores urine. Eventually,

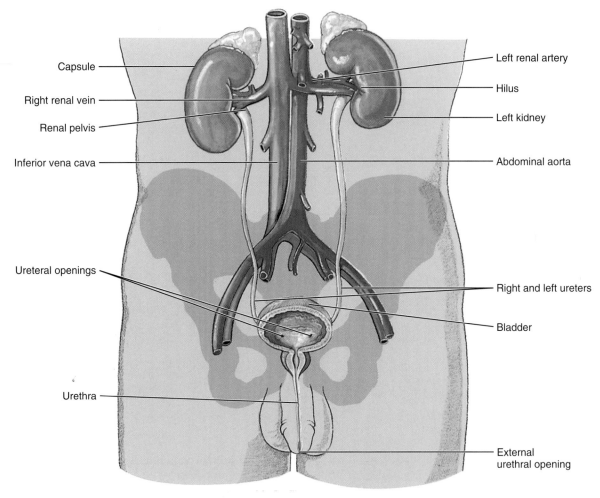

Capsule
Right renal vein
Renal pelvis
Inferior vena cava
Ureteral openings
Urethra

Left renal artery
Hilus
Left kidney
Abdominal aorta
Right and left ureters
Bladder
External urethral opening

FIGURE 16-2 • The urinary system.

urine is discharged from the body through the single **urethra** (yoo-**ree'**-thruh).

> Kidney → ureter → urinary bladder → urethra

The Kidney Has an Outer Cortex and Inner Medulla

The kidneys are located behind the peritoneum lining the abdominal cavity and so are described as **retroperitoneal** (reh'-trow-per'-ih-tow-**nee'**-al). They are located near the posterior body wall just below the diaphragm. The lower ribs protect the kidneys. Each kidney receives blood from a **renal artery** and is drained by a **renal vein.**

Each kidney looks something like a large, dark-red lima bean about the size of a fist. The ureters and blood vessels connect with the kidney at its **hilus** (**hi'**-lus), the notch on its medial border. Covering the kidney is a tough capsule of fibrous connective tissue, the **renal capsule.**

The kidney consists of an outer **renal cortex** and an inner **renal medulla** (Figure 16-3). The renal medulla contains between 5 and 18 triangular structures, the **renal pyramids.** The tip of each pyramid is called a **renal papilla.** Each renal papilla has several pores, the openings of **collecting ducts.** Urine passes from a collecting duct through a renal papilla and into a small tube called a **minor calyx** (**kay'**-liks). Several minor calyces unite to form a **major calyx.** The major calyces join to form a large cavity, the **renal pelvis.** As urine is pro-

duced, it flows into the renal pelvis. From the renal pelvis, urine passes into the ureter. In summary, urine moves through these structures in the following sequence:

> Collecting duct → renal papilla → minor calyx → major calyx → renal pelvis → ureter

The Nephrons Are the Functional Units of the Kidney

Each kidney contains more than a million microscopic units called **nephrons** (**nef'**-rons). The nephrons filter the blood and produce urine. Each nephron consists of two main structures: (1) a **renal corpuscle** and (2) a **renal tubule.** Blood is filtered in the renal corpuscle. Then the filtered fluid, referred to as the **filtrate,** passes through the long, partially coiled renal tubule. As the filtrate moves through the renal tubule, substances needed by the body are returned to the blood. Waste products, excess water and salts, and certain other solutes pass into the collecting ducts and leave the body as urine.

Each renal corpuscle consists of a cluster of capillaries, the **glomerulus** (glow-**mer'**-you-lus), surrounded by a cuplike structure known as **Bowman's capsule** (also referred to as the *glomerular capsule*) (Figure 16-4). Blood from the renal artery flows into the glomerulus through a small **afferent arteriole** and leaves the glomerulus through an **efferent arteriole.** This arteriole conducts blood to a second set of capillaries—the **peritubular capillaries** that surround the renal tubule.

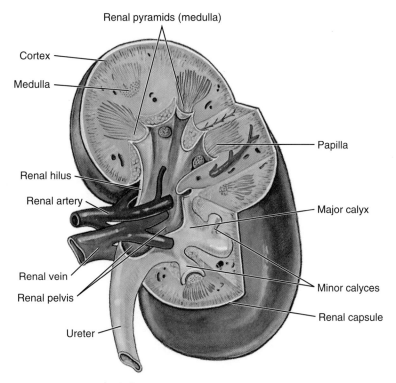

FIGURE 16-3 • Structure of the kidney.

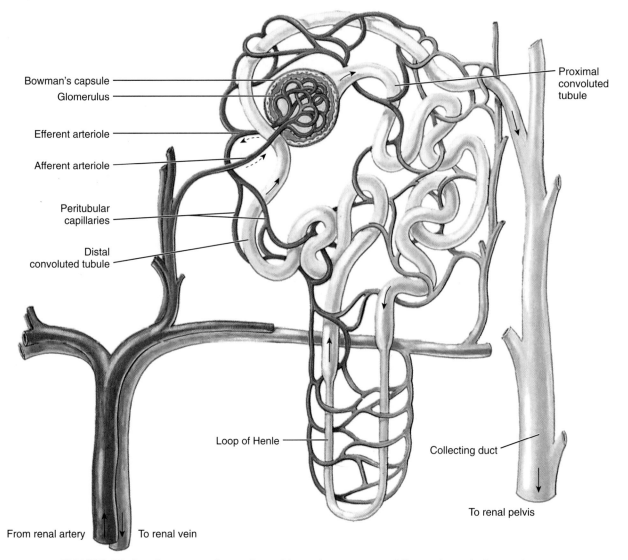

FIGURE 16-4 • Structure of a nephron. Trace the passage of filtrate through the nephron and trace the flow of blood from the renal artery to the renal vein.

Afferent arteriole → capillaries of glomerulus → efferent arteriole → peritubular capillaries

Bowman's capsule has an opening in its bottom through which filtrate passes into the renal tubule. The first part of the renal tubule is the coiled **proximal convoluted tubule.** After passing through the proximal convoluted tubule, filtrate flows into the **loop of Henle** (Hen′-lee) and then into the **distal convoluted tubule.** Urine from the distal convoluted tubules of several nephrons drains into a collecting duct. Thus the filtrate flows through the following structures:

Bowman's capsule → proximal convoluted tubule → loop of Henle → distal convoluted tubule → collecting duct

Part of the distal convoluted tubule curves upward and contacts the afferent arteriole. The cells that make this contact form the **juxtaglomerular** (jux-tah-glow-**mer′**-you-lar) **apparatus** (Figure 16-5). Some of the cells of the juxtaglomerular apparatus secrete the enzyme *renin,* which is important in regulating blood pressure.

The renal corpuscle, the proximal convoluted tubule, and the distal convoluted tubule of most nephrons (cortical nephrons) are located within the renal cortex. Their loops of Henle may dip down into the outer region of the medulla. Other nephrons (juxtamedullary nephrons) have large glomeruli and very long loops of Henle that extend deep into the medulla.

Urine Is Transported by Ducts and Stored in the Bladder

Urine passes from the kidneys through the paired ureters—ducts about 25 centimeters (10 inches) long. Urine is forced

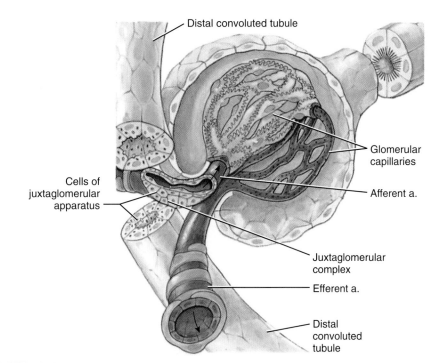

FIGURE 16-5 • Close-up view of the glomerulus and Bowman's capsule. Note the juxtaglomerular apparatus. *a.,* Arteriole.

along through the ureter by peristaltic contractions and is delivered to the urinary bladder.

The urinary bladder is a temporary storage sac for urine. The bladder is lined with a mucous membrane that (like the stomach) has folds called *rugae.* This lining and smooth muscle in its wall permit the bladder to stretch so that it can hold up to 800 milliliters (ml) (about a pint and a half) of urine.

When urine leaves the bladder, it flows through the urethra—a duct leading to the outside of the body. In the male, the urethra is lengthy and passes through the prostate gland and the penis. The male urethra transports semen as well as urine. In the female, the urethra is short and transports only urine. Its opening to the outside is just above the opening into the vagina. Bladder infections are more common in females than in males because the long male urethra is a barrier to bacterial invasion.

Urination Empties the Bladder

Urination, or **micturition** (mik-tyoo-**rish′**-un), is the process of emptying the bladder and expelling urine. When the volume of urine in the bladder reaches about 300 ml, stretch receptors in the bladder wall are stimulated. These receptors send neural messages to the sacral region of the spinal cord, initiating a **urination reflex.** This reflex contracts smooth muscle fibers (detrusor muscle) in the bladder wall and also relaxes the **internal urethral sphincter**—a ring of smooth muscle at the upper end of the urethra. These actions stimulate a conscious desire to urinate.

The **external urethral sphincter** (located inferior to the internal urethral sphincter) is composed of skeletal muscle and can be voluntarily controlled. When the time and place are appropriate, the external urethral sphincter is voluntarily relaxed, allowing urination to occur. However, if the urinary bladder becomes too full, urination may occur despite conscious inhibition.

Voluntary control of urination cannot be exerted by an immature nervous system. That is why most babies under the age of about 2.5 years automatically urinate every time the bladder fills. By age 3 years, most young children learn to control urination.

⊚ Quiz Yourself

- What is the function of the ureter? Of the urethra?
- What are the two main regions of a nephron?
- What is the sequence of structures through which filtrate flows from Bowman's capsule to the collecting duct?

URINE IS PRODUCED BY FILTRATION, REABSORPTION, AND SECRETION

LEARNING OBJECTIVE

6. Describe the process of urine formation and give the composition of urine.

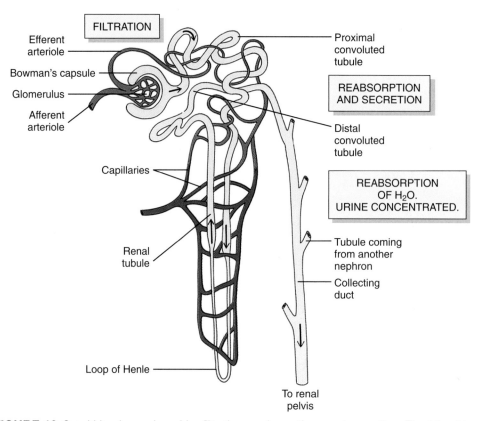

FIGURE 16-6 • Urine is produced by filtration, reabsorption, and secretion. The blood is filtered in the glomeruli. The filtrate is adjusted as it passes through the tubules that drain the glomeruli. Needed materials are reabsorbed into the blood. Certain ions are secreted from the peritubular capillaries into the filtrate in the tubules.

Urine is produced by a combination of three processes: (1) glomerular filtration; (2) tubular reabsorption; and (3) tubular secretion (Figure 16-6).

Glomerular Filtration Is Not Selective With Regard to Small Molecules and Ions

The first step in urine production is **glomerular filtration.** Blood flows through the glomerular capillaries under high pressure, forcing more than 10% of the plasma out of the capillaries and into Bowman's capsule. Glomerular filtration is similar to the mechanism whereby **interstitial fluid** (tissue fluid) is formed as blood flows through other capillary networks in the body. However, blood flow through glomerular capillaries is at much higher pressure than in other capillaries. As a result, more plasma is filtered in the kidney and a large amount of **glomerular filtrate** is produced.

The glomerular capillaries have higher pressure because the afferent arteriole is larger in diameter than the efferent arteriole. As a result, blood enters the glomerulus more rapidly than it can leave. The high pressure forces plasma and substances dissolved in the plasma out of the capillaries and into Bowman's capsule.

Another factor that contributes to the large amount of glomerular filtrate is that the highly coiled glomerular capillaries provide a large surface area for filtration. A third factor is the great permeability of the glomerular capillaries. Numerous small pores are present between the endothelial cells that form their walls, making the glomerular capillaries more leaky than typical capillaries.

The filtrate consists of blood plasma containing ions (charged particles) and small, dissolved molecules. Glomerular filtration is not a selective process. Substances needed by the body, such as glucose, amino acids, and salts, are present in the filtrate. Blood cells and proteins are too large to pass through the walls of the capillary and capsule. When blood cells or proteins do appear in the urine, they signal a problem with glomerular filtration. A number of related chronic kidney diseases in which the glomeruli are damaged are referred to as *glomerulonephritis* (glow′-mer-you-low-neh-**fry**′-tis). Protein in the urine is a common symptom of this disorder.

The total volume of blood passing through the kidneys is about 1200 ml per minute, or about one fourth of the entire cardiac output. Thus, every 4 minutes the kidneys receive a volume of blood equal to the total volume of blood in the body! Every 24 hours about 180 liters (L) (45 gallons) of filtrate are produced. Common sense suggests that we could not excrete urine at the rate of 45 gallons per day. If we were losing fluid that quickly, dehydration would become a life-threatening problem within a few moments.

Tubular Reabsorption Is Highly Selective

The threat to homeostasis caused by the vast amounts of fluid filtered by the kidneys is avoided because **tubular reabsorption** returns about 99% of the filtrate to the blood. This leaves only about 1.5 L to be excreted as urine during a 24-hour period. Tubular reabsorption is the job of the renal tubules and collecting ducts.

Unlike glomerular filtration, tubular reabsorption is highly selective. Wastes, surplus salts, and excess water are kept as part of the filtrate and are excreted as urine. Glucose, amino acids, and other needed substances are returned to the blood. Each day the tubules reabsorb more than 178 L of water, 1200 grams (gm) (2.6 lb) of salt, and about 250 gm (0.5 lb) of glucose. Most of this, of course, is reabsorbed many times over.

Some Substances Are Secreted From the Blood Into the Filtrate

In **tubular secretion,** certain substances are actively transported from the blood in the peritubular capillaries into the filtrate in the renal tubules. Potassium, hydrogen ions, ammonium ions, and some organic ions such as the waste product *creatinine* are secreted into the filtrate. Secretion of hydrogen ions is an important homeostatic mechanism for regulating the pH (a measure of the acidity or alkalinity of a solution) of the blood. Certain drugs, such as penicillin, are also removed from the blood by secretion.

Urine Consists Mainly of Water

By the time the filtrate reaches the renal pelvis, its composition has been carefully adjusted. Materials needed by the body have been returned to the blood, and wastes and excess materials have been cleared from the blood. The adjusted filtrate is called urine. It is composed of about 96% water, 2.5% nitrogen wastes (mainly urea), 1.5% salts, and traces of other substances.

Healthy urine is sterile and has been used to wash battlefield wounds when clean water was not available. However, urine rapidly decomposes when exposed to bacterial action, forming ammonia and other products. It is the ammonia that causes diaper rash in infants.

⦿ Quiz Yourself

- What is the function of tubular reabsorption?
- What happens during tubular secretion?

HORMONES REGULATE KIDNEY FUNCTION

LEARNING OBJECTIVE

7. **Summarize the regulation of urine volume including the actions of antidiuretic hormone (ADH), renin, aldosterone, angiotensin II, and atrial natriuretic peptide (ANP).**

By regulating urine volume and composition, the body maintains a steady volume of blood and body fluids. Several hormones help regulate these processes (Table 16-1).

Antidiuretic Hormone Increases Water Reabsorption

When fluid intake is low, the body begins to dehydrate. When the volume of the blood decreases, the concentration of dissolved salts is greater, causing an increase in the **osmotic pressure** of the blood. Osmotic pressure is a measure of the tendency of a solution to take up water when separated by a semipermeable membrane from a solution with a lower solute concentration. Specialized receptors in the hypothalamus are sensitive to increases in osmotic pressure (Figure 16-7). When stimulated, these receptors signal the posterior lobe of the pituitary gland to release **antidiuretic hormone (ADH).** Recall that ADH is a hormone produced in the hypothalamus and stored in the posterior pituitary gland.

ADH transmits information from the brain to the distal convoluted tubules and collecting ducts of the kidneys. It causes the walls of these ducts to become much more permeable to water, so more water is reabsorbed into the blood. Blood volume increases, and homeostasis of the fluid volume is restored. Only a small amount of concentrated urine is produced.

On the other hand, when a great deal of fluid is consumed, the blood becomes diluted and its osmotic pressure falls. Release of ADH by the pituitary gland decreases. This reduces the amount of water reabsorbed from the distal tubules and collecting ducts. As a result, a large volume of dilute urine is produced.

When the pituitary gland does not produce enough ADH, water is not efficiently reabsorbed from the ducts. This results in the production of a large volume of urine. This condition is called **diabetes insipidus** (not to be confused with the more common disorder, *diabetes mellitus*). An individual with severe, untreated diabetes insipidus may excrete up to 25 quarts of urine each day and must drink almost continually to offset this serious fluid loss. Diabetes insipidus can often be controlled by ADH injections or by use of an ADH nasal spray.

Coffee, tea, and alcoholic beverages contain **diuretics** that increase urine volume. Diuretics inhibit reabsorption of water. Some diuretics inhibit secretion of ADH; others act directly on the tubules in the kidneys.

TABLE 16-1	HORMONAL CONTROL OF FLUID BALANCE			
Hormone	**Source**	**Factors That Stimulate Release**	**Target Tissue**	**Actions**
Antidiuretic hormone (ADH)	Produced in hypothalamus; released by posterior pituitary gland	Low fluid intake decreases blood volume and increases osmotic pressure of blood; receptors in hypothalamus stimulate posterior pituitary	Collecting ducts	Increases permeability of the collecting ducts to water; increases reabsorption, and decreases water excretion
Aldosterone	Adrenal glands (cortex)	Angiotensin II (when blood pressure decreases)	Distal tubules and collecting ducts	Increases sodium reabsorption, which raises blood pressure
Angiotensin II	Produced from angiotensin I	Decrease in blood pressure causes renin secretion; renin catalyzes conversion of a plasma protein to angiotensin I, which is then converted to angiotensin II by angiotensin-converting enzyme (ACE)	Blood vessels and adrenal glands	Constricts blood vessels, which raises blood pressure; stimulates aldosterone secretion
Atrial natriuretic peptide (ANP)	Atrium of heart	Stretching of atria caused by increased blood volume	Afferent arterioles; collecting ducts	Dilates afferent arterioles; inhibits sodium reabsorption by collecting ducts; inhibits aldosterone secretion; lowers blood pressure

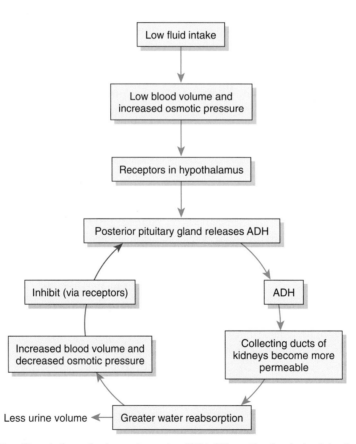

FIGURE 16-7 • Regulation of urine volume by ADH. When the body is dehydrated, the hormone ADH increases the permeability of the collecting ducts to water. More water is reabsorbed, and only a small volume of concentrated urine is produced. Blood volume increases, and homeostasis is restored.

The Renin-Angiotensin-Aldosterone Pathway Increases Sodium Reabsorption

ADH regulates the excretion of water by the kidneys. Salt excretion is regulated mainly by **aldosterone,** secreted by the adrenal glands. Aldosterone secretion can be stimulated by a decrease in blood pressure (which is caused by a decrease in blood volume). Aldosterone acts on the kidney tubules, increasing the reabsorption of sodium. When sodium is reabsorbed, water follows by osmosis; as a result blood volume increases, which raises blood pressure. Aldosterone action results in a lower volume of urine.

When blood pressure falls, cells of the juxtaglomerular apparatus secrete the enzyme renin, activating the **renin-angiotensin-aldosterone pathway.** Renin acts on a plasma protein converting it to a prehormone called angiotensin I. An enzyme known as *ACE* (for *angiotensin-converting enzyme*) converts angiotensin I into its active form, **angiotensin II.** This hormone increases the synthesis and release of aldosterone. It also raises blood pressure directly by constricting blood vessels. These actions help restore extracellular fluid volume and normal blood pressure. In individuals with hypertension, *ACE inhibitors* are sometimes used to block the production of angiotensin II.

> Blood volume decreases → blood pressure decreases → cells of juxtaglomerular apparatus secrete renin → renin catalyzes production of angiotensin I → angiotensin II → stimulates aldosterone secretion and constricts blood vessels → aldosterone increases sodium reabsorption → smaller volume of urine excreted → blood pressure increases

Atrial Natriuretic Peptide Inhibits Sodium Reabsorption

An increase in fluid intake can cause an increase in blood volume, which results in an increase in blood pressure. The atria of the heart are stretched, and in response, they secrete **atrial natriuretic peptide,** or **ANP.** This hormone increases sodium excretion and decreases blood pressure. ANP dilates afferent arterioles, which increases glomerular filtration rate. It inhibits sodium reabsorption by the collecting ducts directly and also indirectly by inhibiting renin and aldosterone. These actions of ANP result in increased urine output by the kidneys and lower blood volume and blood pressure. The renin-angiotensin-aldosterone system and ANP work antagonistically in regulating fluid balance, salt (electrolyte) balance, and blood pressure.

> Increase in blood volume → increase in blood pressure → atria release ANP → inhibits sodium reabsorption → larger volume of urine excreted → decrease in blood volume → decrease in blood pressure

Quiz Yourself

- How does ADH affect urine volume?
- What is the function of aldosterone?
- What is the action of angiotensin II?
- What is the action of ANP?

THE VOLUME AND COMPOSITION OF BODY FLUID MUST BE REGULATED

LEARNING OBJECTIVES

8. Identify the fluid compartments of the body.
9. Summarize the mechanisms that regulate fluid intake and fluid output.
10. Define electrolyte balance and summarize the functions and regulation of five major electrolytes.

We have discussed some aspects of fluid balance earlier in this chapter and also in previous chapters. In this section we integrate some of that information, focusing on electrolyte balance. The human body is about 60% water by weight. All of the chemical reactions in the body take place in a watery medium. Water is used to transport materials throughout the body. It serves as an important **solvent** and is an essential part of many metabolic reactions. A solvent is the dissolving agent of a solution, and the substances dissolved in a solution are called **solutes.**

Body fluid is the water in the body and the substances dissolved in it. Body fluid includes the fluid inside cells, blood plasma, lymph, and interstitial fluid (tissue fluid). These fluids, which consist mainly of water, contain many different substances, including nutrients, gases, wastes, hormones, and inorganic salts, acids, and bases. The concentrations of the many different types of solutes in the body fluid must be continuously adjusted so that they remain within normal limits.

The Body Has Two Main Fluid Compartments

Body fluid is distributed in two principal compartments: the **intracellular compartment** and the **extracellular compartment.** About two thirds of the body fluid is found in the intracellular compartment, that is, within cells (Figure 16-8). This fluid is referred to as **intracellular fluid.** The remaining third is located outside the cells in the extracellular compartment. This **extracellular fluid** includes all fluids in the body that are outside of the cells: interstitial fluid, found in the tissue spaces between cells; blood plasma and lymph; and fluid in special compartments, for example, cerebrospinal fluid.

Fluid constantly moves from one compartment to another. However, in a healthy person the *volume* of fluid in each compartment remains about the same. The movement of fluid

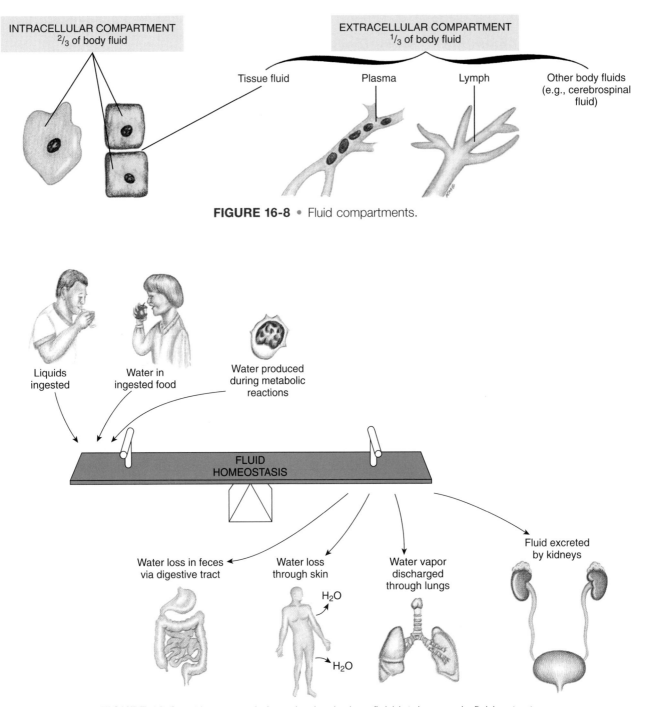

FIGURE 16-8 • Fluid compartments.

FIGURE 16-9 • Homeostasis is maintained when fluid intake equals fluid output.

from one compartment to another depends on blood pressure and osmotic concentration. Blood pressure forces fluid out of the blood at the arterial ends of capillaries. When it leaves the blood, this fluid becomes interstitial fluid. Some of the interstitial fluid returns to the blood at the venous ends of capillaries as a result of osmotic pressure. (Plasma proteins in the plasma exert a pulling force on fluid.) Excess interstitial fluid is also returned to the blood by the lymphatic system. Fluid movement between the intracellular and extracellular compartments

occurs mainly as a result of changes in osmotic pressure. As we will discuss, important differences in composition exist between the intracellular fluid and the extracellular fluid.

Fluid Intake Must Equal Fluid Output

Normally, fluid intake equals fluid output so that the total amount of fluid in the body remains constant (Figure 16-9). The average daily fluid intake is about 2500 ml. Most of this fluid is ingested in the foods we eat and liquids we drink. Water is absorbed from the digestive tract into the blood. Water is also produced during cellular metabolism. Fluid (about 1500 ml per day) is excreted primarily by the kidneys. Fluid is also lost through the skin, lungs, and digestive tract.

When fluid output is greater than fluid intake, **dehydration** occurs. Dehydration can result from too little intake (not drinking enough fluid) or from abnormally high output (profuse sweating, vomiting, diarrhea, abnormally high urine volume).

Fluid intake is regulated by the hypothalamus. Dehydration raises the osmotic pressure of the blood (when there is less fluid, the solute concentration of the blood is greater). The increased osmotic pressure stimulates the **thirst center** in the hypothalamus (Figure 16-10). This results in the sensation of thirst and the desire to drink fluids. Dehydration also leads to a decrease in saliva secretion, which results in dryness in the mouth and throat. This dryness also signals thirst. We feel thirsty when total body fluid is decreased more than 1% to 2%.

The kidneys are primarily responsible for fluid output. Recall that ADH regulates the volume of urine. When the body begins to dehydrate, fluid must be conserved. When the volume of water in the body decreases, the solute concentration of the plasma increases. As a result, ADH secretion increases, and the distal tubules and collecting ducts in the kidneys become more permeable to water. More water is reabsorbed into the blood, and only a small volume of concentrated urine is excreted (see Figure 16-7). As a result, fluid homeostasis is restored. When blood volume increases, less ADH is secreted. Less water is reabsorbed, and a large volume of dilute urine is excreted. Again, fluid homeostasis is restored.

Electrolyte Balance and Fluid Balance Are Interdependent

Among the most important components of body fluids are **electrolytes** (ee-**lek′**-trow-lites)—compounds such as inorganic salts, acids, and bases that form **ions** (electrically charged particles) in solution. Normally, a person obtains adequate amounts of electrolytes in the food and fluid ingested. Most organic compounds dissolved in the body fluid are nonelectrolytes—compounds that do not form ions. Examples of nonelectrolytes in the body fluid are glucose and urea.

Electrolytes produce positively and negatively charged ions. Positively charged ions are referred to as **cations;** negatively charged ions are **anions.** Among the important cations in the body fluid are sodium, potassium, calcium, hydrogen, and magnesium. Important anions include chloride and phosphate.

When the amounts of the various electrolytes taken into the body equal the amounts lost, the body is in **electrolyte balance.** Because electrolytes are dissolved in the body fluid, electrolyte balance and fluid balance are interdependent. When the fluid content decreases, the electrolytes become more concentrated; when fluid content increases, electrolytes are more diluted.

The electrolyte composition varies among body fluids in different compartments, and the concentration of each electrolyte in each compartment must be maintained within narrow limits. Sodium ion concentration is much higher in the extracellular fluid than in the intracellular fluid. In contrast, potassium ion concentration is much higher within cells than in the extracellular fluid. To maintain these differences in ion distribution, cells must pump specific kinds of ions into or out

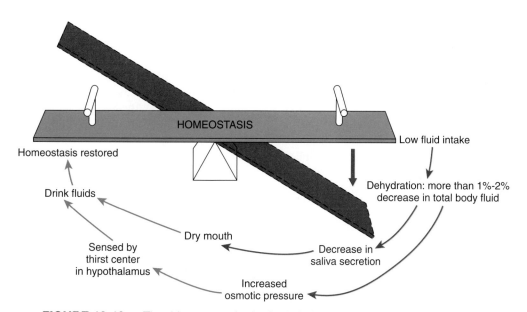

FIGURE 16-10 • The thirst center in the hypothalamus helps regulate fluid intake.

of the cell. This is a form of cellular work known as **active transport.**

Electrolytes Serve Vital Functions

About 90% of the extracellular cations are **sodium** ions. Sodium ions are needed to transmit impulses in neurons and muscle fibers. Low sodium ion concentration can cause headache, mental confusion, rapid heart rate, and low blood pressure. Severe sodium depletion can result in circulatory shock and coma.

Sodium ion concentration is adjusted mainly by regulating the amount of water in the body. When the sodium ion concentration is too high, we feel thirsty and drink water. In addition, sodium ion concentration is regulated by the hormone *aldosterone,* secreted by the adrenal cortex. Aldosterone stimulates the distal convoluted tubules and collecting ducts to increase their reabsorption of sodium ions.

Most of the cations in the intracellular fluid are **potassium** ions. These cations are important in nervous and muscle tissue function. Potassium ions are important also in maintaining the fluid volume within cells, and they help regulate acid-base levels (pH). An abnormally low level of potassium ions may cause mental confusion, fatigue, cramps, and abnormal heart rhythm. When the potassium ion concentration is too high, nerve impulses are not effectively transmitted and the strength of muscle contraction decreases. In fact, a high potassium ion concentration can weaken the heart and lead to death from abnormal heart rhythm or heart failure.

When their concentration is too high, potassium ions are secreted from the blood into the renal tubules and the ions are excreted in the urine. This is because of a direct effect of the potassium ions on the tubules. A high potassium ion concentration also stimulates aldosterone secretion. Aldosterone further stimulates secretion of potassium ions. Loss of potassium ions in the urine brings the potassium concentration in the body back to normal. When the potassium ion concentration becomes too low, aldosterone secretion decreases and potassium secretion decreases almost to zero.

Calcium ions are cations found mainly in the extracellular fluid. **Phosphate** ions are the most abundant intracellular anions. Both calcium and phosphate are important components of bones and teeth. Calcium ions are also essential in blood clotting, transmission of neural impulses, and muscle contraction. Phosphate is needed to make adenosine triphosphate (ATP), DNA, and RNA. The concentration of calcium and phosphate ions is regulated by *parathyroid hormone* and *calcitonin* (see Chapter 9).

Chloride ions are the most abundant extracellular anions. These ions diffuse easily across plasma membranes. Their movement is closely linked to the movement of sodium ions. Chloride ions help regulate differences in osmotic pressure between fluid compartments and are also important in pH balance. The hormone aldosterone indirectly regulates chloride ion concentration.

Magnesium ions are cations found mainly in the intracellular fluid and in bone. They are important in production of bones and teeth and play a role in neural transmission and muscle contraction. Aldosterone increases reabsorption of magnesium ions by the kidneys.

Quiz Yourself

- What are the two main fluid compartments?
- What makes electrolytes important?
- What mechanisms maintain potassium homeostasis?

ACID-BASE HOMEOSTASIS DEPENDS ON HYDROGEN ION CONCENTRATION

LEARNING OBJECTIVE

11. **Describe the mechanisms that maintain acid-base balance and identify causes of acidosis and alkalosis.**

Regulation of acid-base composition in the fluid compartments of the body is critical to health. Acid-base balance depends on the concentration of hydrogen ions. **pH** is a measure of the hydrogen ion concentration of a solution. It is measured on a 0–14 scale. A neutral pH is 7. Lower pH values reflect a higher hydrogen ion concentration and indicate a stronger acidity. Higher pH values indicate a lower hydrogen ion concentration (greater alkalinity). An alkaline solution is also referred to as *basic.*

Blood and most other body fluids are slightly alkaline—pH about 7.4. Even a slight change in hydrogen ion concentration can have a dramatic effect on the distribution of other ions such as sodium, potassium, and calcium. Changes in pH can also affect the rate of chemical reactions and the structure and function of proteins.

The term **acidosis** refers to any condition in which the hydrogen ion concentration of plasma is elevated above the homeostatic range. **Alkalosis** is any condition in which the hydrogen ion concentration is below the homeostatic range. There are two main types of acidosis: metabolic acidosis and respiratory acidosis. There are also two types of alkalosis: metabolic alkalosis and respiratory alkalosis.

Metabolic acidosis refers to any acidosis that is not caused by the respiratory system. Excessive exercise can result in metabolic acidosis caused by a large accumulation of lactic acid. Severe diarrhea can lead to metabolic acidosis resulting from loss of bicarbonate. Acidosis depresses the transmission of neural impulses across synapses. If the pH falls below about 7, coma and death may occur.

Excessive vomiting can lead to **metabolic alkalosis** because hydrochloric acid is lost from the stomach. Alkalosis can cause neurons to fire inappropriately, resulting in muscle twitches, spasms, and convulsions.

About half of all the acid ingested in foods or produced during metabolism is neutralized by the ingestion of alkaline foods. The remaining acid is neutralized by three important mechanisms: chemical buffers, the respiratory system, and the kidneys.

A **chemical buffer** is a substance that minimizes changes in pH when an acid or base is added to a solution. The main buffering systems in the body are the bicarbonate buffer system, the phosphate buffer system, and the protein buffer systems. Hemoglobin is an example of a protein that is a very effective buffer. Recall from Chapter 14 that carbon dioxide in the plasma slowly combines with water to form carbonic acid. Hydrogen ions released from carbonic acid combine with hemoglobin. This mechanism removes hydrogen ions from the blood and so minimizes pH change.

The respiratory system helps regulate acid-base balance by regulating the breathing rate. This changes the carbon dioxide concentration in the blood. **Respiratory acidosis** develops when carbon dioxide is produced more rapidly than it is excreted by the lungs. Decreased ventilation results in a buildup of carbon dioxide. The more carbon dioxide in the blood, the more carbonic acid is formed, resulting in more hydrogen ions. A decrease in breathing rate may occur as a result of respiratory diseases such as emphysema.

Respiratory alkalosis occurs when the respiratory system excretes carbon dioxide more quickly than it is produced. Decreased carbon dioxide in the blood leads to a decrease in hydrogen ions and an increase in pH. Hyperventilation can result in respiratory alkalosis. Hyperventilation may occur as a result of high altitude, stress, or aspirin overdose.

The kidneys help regulate pH by excreting or conserving certain types of ions. For example, when the blood is too acidic, more hydrogen ions are secreted into the filtrate. These ions are buffered and excreted.

Quiz Yourself

- What are three mechanisms that help regulate acid-base balance?
- What is respiratory alkalosis?

SUMMARY

LO 1. Identify the principal metabolic waste products and the organs that excrete them.

- The **urinary system** helps regulate the volume and composition of body fluid. **Excretion** is the discharge of metabolic wastes from the body. The principal metabolic wastes are water, carbon dioxide, and **nitrogenous wastes—urea, uric acid,** and creatinine. The urinary system, skin, lungs, and digestive system excrete metabolic by-products and wastes.

LO 2. Summarize the functions of the urinary system in maintaining homeostasis.

- The **urinary system** helps regulate the volume and composition of body fluid. It adjusts the salt and water content of the **urine;** excretes metabolic waste products; helps regulate electrolyte concentration; helps regulate acid-base (pH) level of blood and body fluids; secretes **renin,** which helps regulate blood pressure; and secretes **erythropoietin,** which regulates red blood cell production.

LO 3. Describe the anatomy of the urinary system and give the function of each of its structures. (Be able to label a diagram of the urinary system.)

- The main organs of the urinary system are the paired **kidneys,** which produce **urine;** the **ureters,** which conduct the urine to the **urinary bladder** where it is temporarily stored; and the **urethra,** which discharges urine from the body.
- The kidney is covered by a **renal capsule.** Each kidney consists of an outer **renal cortex** and an inner **renal medulla.** The renal medulla consists of **renal pyramids.** Urine passes from the **collecting ducts** through the **renal papilla** of a pyramid and flows into a **minor calyx.** Several minor calyces lead into a **major calyx,** which empties into the **renal pelvis.**
- Rugae in its lining and smooth muscle in its wall allow the urinary bladder to stretch as it fills with urine. During **urination,** urine is discharged from the bladder through the urethra to the outside of the body. The **urination reflex** contracts muscle in the bladder wall and relaxes the **internal urethral sphincter.** The **external urethral sphincter** is under voluntary control.

LO = Learning Objective

LO 4. Describe the structure and function of a nephron. (Be able to label a diagram of a nephron.)

- The **nephron** is the functional unit of the kidney. Each nephron consists of a renal corpuscle and a renal tubule. The **renal corpuscle** is composed of a cluster of capillaries, called a **glomerulus,** that fits into a **Bowman's capsule.**
- The **renal tubule** has three main regions: (1) **proximal convoluted tubule,** (2) **loop of Henle,** and (3) **distal convoluted tubule.** The distal convoluted tubules from several nephrons drain into a collecting duct.
- Blood flows into the glomerulus through an **afferent arteriole** and leaves the glomerulus through an **efferent arteriole** that conducts blood to the **peritubular capillaries.**

LO 5. Trace a drop of filtrate from glomerulus to urethra, listing in sequence each structure through which it passes.

- Filtrate passes from Bowman's capsule through the proximal convoluted tubule, through the loop of Henle, and through the distal convoluted tubule, and then passes into the collecting duct. Urine passes from a collecting duct into a renal papilla, then into a minor calyx, the major calyx, and into the renal pelvis. It then passes through the ureter and is stored in the urinary bladder. During urination it leaves the body through the urethra.

LO 6. Describe the process of urine formation and give the composition of urine.

- Urine formation involves **glomerular filtration, tubular reabsorption,** and **tubular secretion.** Blood is delivered to the glomerular capillaries by the afferent arteriole under high pressure; some plasma containing dissolved substances is filtered out of the capillaries and into Bowman's capsule. Glomerular filtration is not a selective process, so needed materials, as well as wastes, become part of the filtrate.
- About 99% of the filtrate is returned to the blood by tubular reabsorption through the renal tubules and collecting ducts. Tubular reabsorption is highly selective. Wastes, excess water, and surplus salts remain in the filtrate, whereas glucose, amino acids, and other needed substances are reabsorbed (returned) into the blood.

- In tubular secretion, some substances including potassium, hydrogen, and ammonium ions are actively transported from the blood into the filtrate.
- The adjusted filtrate is urine; it consists of water, nitrogenous wastes, salts, and traces of other substances.

LO 7. Summarize the regulation of urine volume, including the actions of ADH, renin, aldosterone, angiotensin II, and ANP.

- **ADH,** released by the posterior lobe of the pituitary gland, makes the distal convoluted tubules and collecting ducts more permeable to water so that more water is reabsorbed. When the body begins to dehydrate, the posterior pituitary increases its secretion of ADH and more water is reabsorbed, conserving fluid. When excess fluid is present, ADH secretion decreases and less water is reabsorbed; a large volume of dilute urine is excreted.
- When blood pressure falls, cells of the **juxtaglomerular apparatus** secrete the enzyme *renin,* which activates the **renin-angiotensin-aldosterone pathway. Angiotensin II** raises blood pressure directly by constricting blood vessels. This hormone also raises blood pressure indirectly by increasing **aldosterone** secretion. Aldosterone increases sodium reabsorption. Water follows by osmosis so that blood volume increases, raising blood pressure.
- An increase in blood volume results in a rise in blood pressure. When the atria of the heart are stretched, they secrete **ANP,** which increases sodium excretion, leading to a decrease in blood pressure.

LO 8. Identify the fluid compartments of the body.

- **Body fluid,** the water in the body and the substances dissolved in it, is distributed in the **intracellular compartment,** the fluid inside cells, and **extracellular compartment.** Fluid continuously moves from one compartment to another, but the volume in each compartment remains fairly constant. The extracellular compartment includes the **interstitial fluid** (tissue fluid), the plasma and lymph, and the cerebrospinal fluid.

LO 9. **Summarize the mechanisms that regulate fluid intake and fluid output.**

- Normally, fluid intake equals fluid output. When the body begins to dehydrate, ADH secretion increases and more water is reabsorbed. The renin-angiotensin-aldosterone pathway also increases body fluid. When total body fluid is decreased by 1% to 2%, the **thirst center** in the hypothalamus is stimulated.

LO 10. **Define electrolyte balance and summarize the functions and regulation of five major electrolytes.**

- Body fluid contains **electrolytes**—inorganic salts, acids, and bases that form **ions** (charged particles) in solution. Positively charged ions are **cations;** negatively charged ions are **anions.** When the amounts of the various electrolytes taken into the body equal the amounts lost, the body is in **electrolyte balance.**
- **Sodium** ions, which account for about 90% of the extracellular cations, are essential for nerve and muscle function and for fluid balance. Sodium concentration is regulated by the amount of water in the body and by aldosterone, which stimulates reabsorption of sodium.
- **Potassium ions,** which account for most intracellular cations, are essential for nerve and muscle function, help maintain intracellular fluid volume, and help regulate pH. When the concentration of potassium ions rises above normal, potassium ions are secreted into the renal tubules and excreted in the urine. High potassium ion concentration also stimulates aldosterone secretion, which stimulates potassium excretion.
- **Calcium** and **phosphate** are components of bones and teeth. Calcium ions are essential for blood clotting and for nerve and muscle function. Phosphate ions are essential components of ATP, DNA, and RNA. Calcium and phosphate ion concentration is regulated by parathyroid hormone and calcitonin.

- **Chloride** ions are the most abundant extracellular anions. They are important in osmotic balance and in pH balance. Aldosterone indirectly regulates chloride ion concentration.

LO 11. **Describe the mechanisms that maintain acid-base balance and identify causes of acidosis and alkalosis.**

- Acid-base (**pH**) balance depends on the concentration of hydrogen ions and is regulated by chemical buffers, the respiratory system, and the kidneys.
- A **chemical buffer** is a substance that minimizes changes in pH when an acid or base is added to a solution. Buffering systems in the body include the bicarbonate buffer system, the phosphate buffer system, and protein buffer system.
- The respiratory system helps regulate acid-base balance by changing the breathing rate, and thus excreting more or less carbon dioxide. The kidneys help regulate pH by excreting or conserving certain types of ions, for example, hydrogen ions.
- **Acidosis** is a condition in which the hydrogen ion concentration of plasma is elevated above the homeostatic range. **Respiratory acidosis** develops when carbon dioxide is produced more rapidly than it is excreted by the lungs. **Metabolic acidosis** is caused by metabolic disturbances other than those caused by the respiratory system. Severe diarrhea can cause metabolic acidosis as a result of bicarbonate loss.
- **Alkalosis** is a condition in which the hydrogen ion concentration of plasma is below the homeostatic range. **Respiratory alkalosis** develops when carbon dioxide is expired more rapidly than it is produced. **Metabolic alkalosis** (nonrespiratory alkalosis) is caused by metabolic disturbances other than those caused by the respiratory system. Excessive vomiting can cause metabolic alkalosis as a result of hydrochloric acid loss from the stomach.

CHAPTER QUIZ

Fill in the Blank

1. Two nitrogenous wastes excreted by the kidneys are _____ and _____ _____.

2. Urine is conducted from the renal pelvis to the urinary bladder by the _____.

3. Urine in a major calyx next passes into the renal _____.

4. The outer portion of the kidney is the renal _____, and the inner portion is the renal _____.

5. A nephron consists of two main structures: a renal _____ and a renal _____.

6. The renal corpuscle consists of a cluster of capillaries, the _____ surrounded by _____ _____.

7. Blood flows into capillaries of the glomerulus through an _____ arteriole.

8. From the proximal convoluted tubule, filtrate flows into the _____ _____ _____.

9. Some plasma leaves the glomerular capillaries and passes into _____ _____.

10. The process of returning most of the filtrate to the blood is known as _____ _____.

11. The adjusted filtrate is called _____.

12. The hormone _____ causes the walls of the collecting ducts to be more permeable to water.

Multiple Choice

13. The urinary bladder: a. is a temporary storage sac for urine; b. is the main target of ADH; c. discharges urine into the ureter; d. produces aldosterone.

14. During tubular secretion: a. blood flows through the glomerulus under high pressure; b. urine is discharged into the collecting ducts; c. hydrogen ions and certain other ions are discharged from the peritubular capillaries into the filtrate; d. filtrate is secreted back into the blood.

15. Most body fluid is located in the: a. extracellular compartment; b. extracellular fluid; c. blood; d. intracellular compartment.

16. Compounds such as salts that form ions in solution are called: a. diuretics; b. electrolytes; c. ANPs; d. cations.

17. Aldosterone: a. increases sodium reabsorption by the kidney tubules; b. stimulates water excretion by the proximal tubule; c. results in excretion of a large volume of urine; d. is an enzyme produced by the kidney.

18. The hormone atrial natriuretic peptide (ANP): a. decreases sodium excretion; b. increases blood volume; c. decreases blood pressure; d. activates the renin-angiotensin-aldosterone pathway.

19. Chemical buffers: a. maintain body fluids at a pH below 7; b. dissociate into cations and anions; c. resist changes in pH when an acid or base is added to a fluid; d. maintain respiratory alkalosis.

20. Acidosis: a. can occur when carbon dioxide concentration is too low; b. occurs when the hydrogen ion concentration is too high; c. can result from excessive vomiting; d. causes neurons to fire inappropriately, leading to muscle twitches.

REVIEW QUESTIONS

1. Describe several ways that the kidneys help maintain homeostasis.

2. What are the principal metabolic waste products? Which organs excrete them?

3. Trace a drop of urine from the renal pelvis to its discharge from the body.

4. Describe the structure and functions of each of the following: Bowman's capsule, glomerulus, renal tubule, collecting duct, afferent arteriole, efferent arteriole.

5. Trace a drop of filtrate from the glomerular capillaries to the renal pelvis.

6. What are the main steps in urine production? Where does each occur?

7. How is urine volume and composition regulated? (Include the actions of ADH, aldosterone, renin, angiotensin II, and atrial natriuretic peptide in your answer.)

8. What are the main fluid compartments in the body? Describe each.

9. How are fluid and electrolyte balance related?

10. What are some differences in composition between intracellular and extracellular fluid? How are these differences maintained?

11. How is sodium concentration regulated?

12. How does each of the following help maintain acid-base homeostasis? (a) Chemical buffers? (b) The respiratory system? (c) The kidneys?

13. Identify two causes of acidosis and two causes of alkalosis.

14. Label the diagram. (See Figure 16-4 to check your answers.)

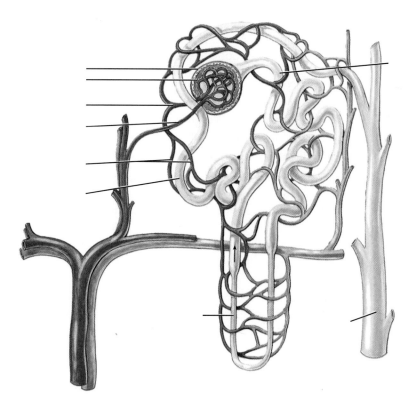

17 Reproduction

Chapter Outline

I. **The male produces sperm**
   A. The testes produce sperm and hormones
   B. The conducting tubes transport sperm
   C. The accessory glands produce semen
   D. The penis delivers sperm into the female reproductive tract
   E. Hormones regulate male reproduction

II. **The female produces ova and incubates the embryo**
   A. The ovaries produce ova and hormones
   B. The uterine tubes transport ova
   C. The uterus incubates the embryo
   D. The vagina functions in sexual intercourse, menstruation, and birth
   E. The external genital structures are the vulva
   F. The breasts contain the mammary glands
   G. Hormones regulate female reproduction
      1. The preovulatory phase consists of the first two weeks of the menstrual cycle
      2. The corpus luteum develops during the postovulatory phase
      3. The menstrual cycle stops at menopause

III. **Fertilization is the fusion of sperm and ovum**

IV. **The zygote gives rise to the new individual**
   A. The embryo develops in the wall of the uterus
   B. Prenatal development requires about 266 days
   C. The birth process includes labor and delivery
   D. Multiple births may be fraternal or identical

V. **The human life cycle extends from fertilization to death**

Reproduction involves several processes including formation of specialized sex cells called **gametes** (gam′-eets) (eggs and sperm), preparation of the female body for pregnancy, sexual intercourse, fertilization (union of sperm and egg), pregnancy, and lactation (producing milk for nourishment of the infant). These events are regulated and coordinated by the interaction of hormones secreted by the anterior lobe of the pituitary gland and by the **gonads** (go′-nads), or sex glands.

In this chapter we discuss the anatomy and physiology of the male and female reproductive systems. We then discuss fertilization and give an overview of development from fertilization to delivery of a baby. Finally, we summarize the developmental stages in the human life cycle.

THE MALE PRODUCES SPERM

LEARNING OBJECTIVES

1. Describe the anatomy of the male reproductive system and describe the functions of each structure.
2. Trace the passage of sperm cells from the tubules in the testes through the conducting tubes and to their ejaculation from the body in semen.
3. Describe the actions of the male gonadotropic hormones and testosterone.

The male's function in reproduction is to produce **sperm cells,** called **spermatozoa** (sper-mah-tow-**zow'**-ah), and to deliver them into the female reproductive tract. The sperm that combines with an egg contributes half the genes of the offspring and determines its sex. Male reproductive structures include the testes and scrotum, the conducting tubes that lead from the testes to the outside of the body, the accessory glands, and the penis (Figure 17-1).

The Testes Produce Sperm and Hormones

In the adult male, millions of sperm cells are manufactured each day within the paired male gonads, the **testes** (**tes'**-teez). Each testis is a small, oval organ about 4 to 5 centimeters (cm) (1.6 to 2 inches) long and 2.5 cm (about 1 inch) wide and thick.

About 1000 threadlike, coiled **seminiferous** (sem'-ih-**nif'**-er-us) tubules fill the testis (Figure 17-2). These tubules are the sperm cell factories, and they also produce male hormones.

The process of sperm production is called **spermatogenesis** (sper-**mat'**-oh-jen'-eh-sis). Undifferentiated sperm cells carry out a special type of nuclear division known as **meiosis** (my-**oh'**-sis). During fertilization, one set of 23 chromosomes is contributed by the mother's ovum and the other set of 23 chromosomes by the father's sperm. Thus the fertilized egg has 23 pairs of chromosomes. The fertilized egg divides hundreds of times by mitosis (see Chapter 2) so that each cell (except the gametes) of the body has an identical set of 23 pairs of chromosomes.

During meiosis, two nuclear and two cell divisions take place. Each undifferentiated sperm cell gives rise to four sperm cells. During the process, the chromosomes are shuffled and the number of chromosomes is reduced to half the normal number. As a result, each sperm cell has one set of 23 chromosomes instead of two sets. Some of these chromosomes were contributed by the mother and others by the father. This reduction division prevents doubling of the chromosome number each time fertilization occurs. The mature sperm is a tiny, elongated cell with a tail (flagellum) that it uses for moving toward an egg.

The testes develop in the abdominal cavity of the male embryo. About 2 months before birth, they *descend* into the **scrotum** (**skrow'**-tum), a skin-covered bag suspended from the groin. As the testes descend, they move through the **inguinal**

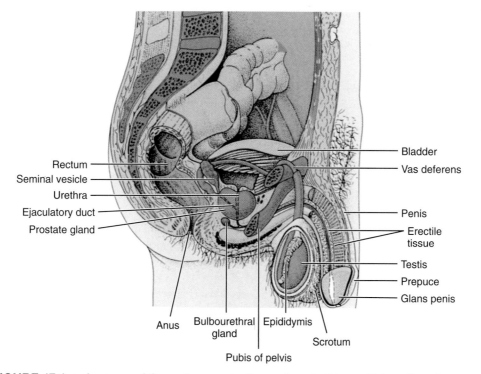

Rectum
Seminal vesicle
Urethra
Ejaculatory duct
Prostate gland
Bladder
Vas deferens
Penis
Erectile tissue
Testis
Prepuce
Glans penis
Anus
Bulbourethral gland
Epididymis
Scrotum
Pubis of pelvis

FIGURE 17-1 • Anatomy of the male reproductive system. In this sagittal section, the scrotum, penis, and pelvic region have been cut to show their internal structure. The penis contains three cylinders of erectile tissue containing blood sinusoids. Identify the accessory glands and trace the conducting tubes from the testis to the urethra.

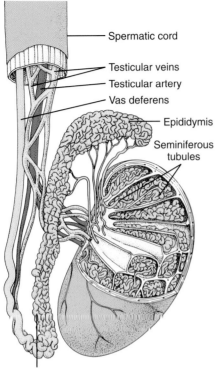

Spermatic cord

Testicular veins

Testicular artery

Vas deferens

Epididymis

Seminiferous tubules

Epididymis

FIGURE 17-2 • Structure of the testis and epididymis. The testis is shown in sagittal section to illustrate the arrangement of the tubules.

canals—the passageways connecting the scrotal and abdominal cavities. The testes pull their arteries, veins, nerves, and conducting tubes after them. These structures, surrounded by muscle and by layers of connective tissue, make up the **spermatic cord.**

The inguinal region remains a weak place in the abdominal wall. Straining the abdominal muscles by lifting a very heavy object may result in a tear in the inguinal tissue. A loop of intestine can then bulge into the scrotum through the tear. This condition is called an *inguinal hernia.*

Sperm cells are not able to develop at body temperature, and the scrotum serves as a cooling unit, maintaining them at about 2° C below body temperature. The wall of the scrotum is rich in sweat glands and blood vessels. These structures promote heat loss and so help maintain the cool temperature.

The Conducting Tubes Transport Sperm

From the tubules inside the testis, sperm pass into a large, coiled tube, the **epididymis** (ep-ih-**did'**-ih-mis) (see Figure 17-2). The epididymis of each testis is located within the scrotum. Sperm mature within the epididymis and are stored there. Each epididymis empties into a straight tube, the **vas deferens** (**def'**-ur-enz), or sperm duct. The vas deferens passes from the scrotum through the inguinal canal as part of the spermatic cord. After entering the pelvic cavity, each vas def-

erens loops over the side and then down the posterior surface of the urinary bladder. The vas deferens is joined by the duct from each of the paired seminal vesicles (discussed in the next section) to form the **ejaculatory duct.** This very short duct passes through the *prostate gland* and then opens into the **urethra.** The single urethra, which conducts both urine and semen, passes through the *penis* to the outside of the body. Thus sperm pass through the following path:

> Seminiferous tubules in the testis → epididymis → vas deferens → ejaculatory duct → urethra

The Accessory Glands Produce Semen

Semen (**see'**-men) is a thick, whitish fluid consisting of sperm cells suspended in secretions of the accessory glands: the seminal vesicles, prostate gland, and bulbourethral glands. The paired **seminal vesicles** are saclike glands. A seminal vesicle empties into each vas deferens. The thick, nutritive fluid secreted by the seminal vesicles contains the sugar *fructose* and other nutrients that provide energy for the sperm cells. Secretions of the seminal vesicles account for about 60% of the semen volume.

The single **prostate** (**pros'**-tate) **gland** surrounds the urethra as the urethra emerges from the urinary bladder. The prostate gland produces a thin, milky secretion that helps keep sperm viable and active. In older men, the prostate gland often enlarges and exerts pressure on the urethra, making urination difficult. Cancer of the prostate is a common disorder in men older than 50 years. **Prostate-specific antigen (PSA)** is a protein produced by the prostate gland. The PSA concentration can be tested in the blood. PSA is a tumor marker because its elevation is associated with prostate cancer. When necessary, the prostate can be removed surgically.

The **bulbourethral** (bul-bow-you-**ree'**-thral) **glands** (also called *Cowper's glands*) are about the size and shape of two peas, one on each side of the urethra. When a male is sexually aroused, these glands release an alkaline mucous secretion that lubricates the penis, facilitating its penetration into the vagina. This secretion also helps neutralize the acidity of the urethra (caused by urine that has passed through it) and the acidity of the vagina.

About 2 milliliters (ml) of semen is discharged from the penis during **ejaculation.** Semen consists of about 40 million sperm cells suspended in the secretions of the accessory glands. Sperm cells are so tiny that they account for very little (less than 1%) of the semen volume. Men with fewer than 20 million sperm/ml of semen may be sterile. Fever or infection of the testes may cause temporary sterility.

The Penis Delivers Sperm Into the Female Reproductive Tract

The **penis,** the male copulatory organ, delivers sperm into the female reproductive tract during sexual intercourse. The penis consists of a long **shaft** that enlarges to form an expanded tip, the **glans** (see Figure 17-1). Part of the loose-fitting skin of the penis folds down and covers the proximal portion of the glans, forming a cuff called the **prepuce** (pre′-pyoos), or foreskin. This cuff of skin is removed during **circumcision,** a procedure commonly performed on male babies for hygienic or religious reasons.

Under the skin, the penis consists of three cylinders of spongy tissue, called **erectile tissue.** Each cylinder, referred to as a **corpus,** contains blood vessels called sinusoids, capillary-like blood vessels that are very leaky. When the male is sexually stimulated, nerve impulses signal the arteries of the penis to dilate. Blood rushes into the sinusoids of the spongy tissue. As this tissue fills with blood, it swells and presses against the veins that conduct blood away from the penis. As a result, more blood enters the penis than can leave and the spongy tissue becomes filled with blood. The penis becomes **erect,** that is, it increases in length, diameter, and firmness. The average penis is about 9 cm long when flaccid (relaxed) and 16 to 19 cm when erect. When the level of sexual excitement reaches a peak, ejaculation occurs. Both erection and ejaculation are reflex actions.

Hormones Regulate Male Reproduction

Male hormones are referred to as **androgens. Interstitial** (in′-ter-**stish′**-al) **cells,** small islands of cells that lie between the tubules in the testes, produce the principal male hormone **testosterone** (tes-**tos′**-teh-rone). Testosterone is responsible for the development of both primary and secondary sex characteristics in the male. **Primary sex characteristics** include the growth and activity of the reproductive structures, including the penis and scrotum. **Secondary sex characteristics** include deepening of the voice, muscle development, and growth of pubic, facial, and underarm hair. Testosterone also stimulates the adolescent growth spurt and stimulates oil glands in the skin (sometimes causing acne).

In boys, **puberty,** the period of sexual maturation, typically begins between ages 10 and 12 years and continues until ages 16 to 18 years. Typically, the first sign of male puberty is enlargement of the testes. At puberty the **hypothalamus** begins to secrete **gonadotropin-releasing hormone (GnRH)** that stimulates the **anterior lobe of the pituitary gland** to secrete gonadotropic hormones. The gonadotropic hormones are **follicle-stimulating hormone (FSH)** and **luteinizing hormone (LH).** FSH stimulates sperm production.

A high concentration of testosterone in the testes is required for spermatogenesis. FSH stimulates **Sertoli cells** to produce **androgen-binding protein (ABP),** which binds to testosterone and concentrates it in the tubules. LH stimulates the testes to secrete testosterone.

Reproductive hormone concentrations are regulated by negative feedback mechanisms (Figure 17-3). Testosterone inhibits mainly LH secretion. It acts on the hypothalamus, decreasing its secretion of GnRH, which results in decreased FSH and LH by the pituitary. Testosterone also directly inhib-

its the anterior lobe of the pituitary by blocking the normal actions of GnRH on LH synthesis and release.

FSH stimulates Sertoli cells in the testes to secrete a peptide hormone called **inhibin.** This hormone is transported by the blood to the pituitary gland, where it inhibits FSH secretion. The endocrine regulation of reproductive function is extremely complex, and other hormones and signaling molecules will almost certainly be identified.

When a male is castrated (i.e., his testes are removed) before puberty, he becomes a eunuch. His sex organs remain childlike, and he does not develop secondary sexual characteristics. If castration occurs after puberty, increased secretion of male hormone by the adrenal cortex helps maintain masculinity.

Quiz Yourself

- What is the sequence of structures through which sperm cells pass from the seminiferous tubules to their ejaculation from the body?
- What are the functions of FSH? Of LH?
- What are the functions of testosterone?

THE FEMALE PRODUCES OVA AND INCUBATES THE EMBRYO

LEARNING OBJECTIVES

4. Describe the anatomy of the female reproductive system and describe the functions of each structure.
5. Trace the development of an ovum and its passage through the female reproductive system.
6. Describe the principal events of the menstrual cycle and summarize the interactions of hormones that regulate the cycle.

The female produces **ova** (eggs), receives the penis and the sperm released from it during sexual intercourse, houses and nourishes the embryo during its prenatal development, and nourishes the infant. Much of the activity of the female reproductive system centers about the **menstrual** (**men′**-stroo-al) **cycle**—the monthly preparation for possible pregnancy.

The organs of the female reproductive system include the ovaries (which produce ova and female hormones), the uterine tubes (where fertilization takes place), the uterus (incubator for the developing baby), the vagina (which receives the penis and serves as a birth canal), the vulva (external genital structures), and the breasts.

The Ovaries Produce Ova and Hormones

The paired **ovaries** are the female gonads. The ovaries produce ova and the female sex hormones *estrogens* and *progesterone.* About the size and shape of large almonds, the ovaries are located close to the lateral walls of the pelvic cavity (Figures

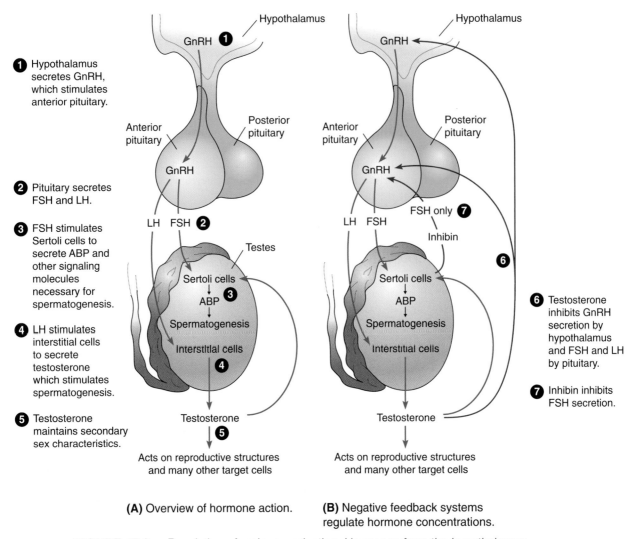

① Hypothalamus secretes GnRH, which stimulates anterior pituitary.

② Pituitary secretes FSH and LH.

③ FSH stimulates Sertoli cells to secrete ABP and other signaling molecules necessary for spermatogenesis.

④ LH stimulates interstitial cells to secrete testosterone which stimulates spermatogenesis.

⑤ Testosterone maintains secondary sex characteristics.

⑥ Testosterone inhibits GnRH secretion by hypothalamus and FSH and LH by pituitary.

⑦ Inhibin inhibits FSH secretion.

(A) Overview of hormone action.

(B) Negative feedback systems regulate hormone concentrations.

FIGURE 17-3 • Regulation of male reproduction. Hormones from the hypothalamus, anterior pituitary gland, and testis interact to regulate sperm production and hormone concentration. Testosterone mainly inhibits LH secretion by the pituitary. Inhibin inhibits FSH secretion. *Red arrows* indicate inhibition. *GnRH,* Gonadotropin-releasing hormone; *FSH,* follicle-stimulating hormone; *LH,* luteinizing hormone; ABP, androgen-binding protein.

17-4 and 17-5). The ovaries are held in position by several connective tissue ligaments. The **ovarian ligament,** for example, anchors the medial end of the ovary to the uterus. Each ovary consists mainly of connective tissue through which developing **ova** (eggs) (singular—*ovum*) are scattered.

The process of ovum development is called **oogenesis** (oh-oh-**jen'**-eh-sis). Like spermatogenesis, it involves meiosis. All undifferentiated ova are produced before birth. By the time of birth, the developing ova are beginning the first division of meiosis. At this stage, they enter a resting period that lasts through childhood and into adult life.

Each developing ovum matures within a little sac of cells and fluid. Together, the developing ovum and its surrounding sac make up a **follicle.** With the onset of puberty, a few follicles develop each month. The developing ovum within each of these follicles completes the first division of meiosis at this

time. Each developing ovum ultimately gives rise to four cells, but the second meiotic division does not take place unless the ovum is fertilized. Three of the four cells produced during oogenesis are **polar bodies,** small cells that eventually disintegrate. Only one of the four cells develops into a mature ovum.

The maturation of ova is controlled by FSH secreted by the anterior lobe of the pituitary gland. Cells of the follicle secrete female hormones, called **estrogens** (**es'**-trow-jens). As a follicle matures, it moves close to the wall of the ovary and can be seen as a fluid-filled bulge on the surface of the ovary. Mature follicles are called *graafian follicles.* Usually, only one follicle matures each month. Several others may develop for about a week and then deteriorate.

In response to FSH and LH from the anterior pituitary gland, the mature follicle ruptures after about 2 weeks of

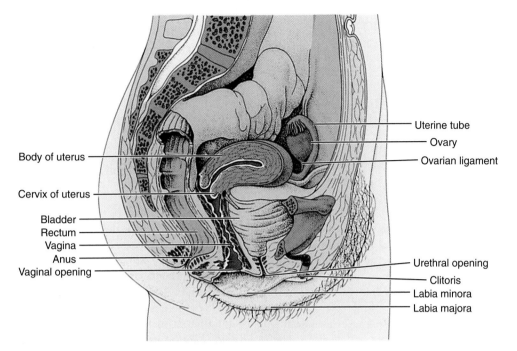

FIGURE 17-4 • Midsagittal section of the female pelvis showing reproductive organs. Note the position of the uterus relative to the vagina.

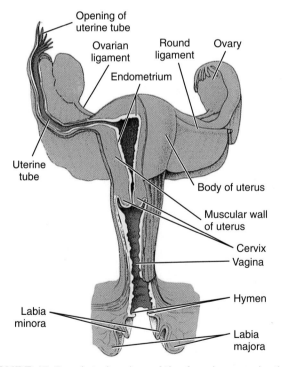

FIGURE 17-5 • Anterior view of the female reproductive system. Some organs have been cut open to expose the internal structure. Connective tissue ligaments help hold the reproductive organs in place.

development. During this process, called **ovulation,** the developing ovum is ejected through the wall of the ovary and into the pelvic cavity. The part of the follicle that remains behind in the ovary develops into an important temporary endocrine structure, the **corpus luteum** ("yellow body").

The Uterine Tubes Transport Ova

Each **uterine tube,** also called the **oviduct** or **fallopian tube,** is about 12 cm long. Its free end is shaped like a funnel and has long, fingerlike projections called **fimbriae (fim′**-bree-ee). At ovulation, the mature ovum is released into the pelvic cavity. Movements of the fimbriae and the current created by the beating of cilia in the lining of the tube draw the ovum into the uterine tube. Action of the cilia helps move the ovum toward the uterus. Unlike sperm, the ovum is not capable of moving by itself. Normally, fertilization takes place in the upper third of the uterine tube. The fertilized egg, or **zygote** (**zye′**-goat), begins its development as it is moved along toward the uterus. If fertilization does not occur, the ovum degenerates in the uterine tube.

Because the uterine tubes open into the peritoneal cavity, bacteria that enter through the vagina can cause serious clinical problems. This route of infection has led to many deaths from abortions performed under nonsterile conditions.

The Uterus Incubates the Embryo

Each month during a woman's reproductive life, the **uterus,** or womb, prepares for possible pregnancy. When pregnancy occurs, the uterus serves as the incubator for the developing embryo. The tiny embryo implants itself in the wall of the uterus and develops there until it is able to live independently. When that time comes, the uterine wall contracts powerfully and rhythmically (the process of labor), expelling the new baby from the mother's body. If pregnancy does not occur, the inner lining of the uterus sloughs off each month and is discarded. This process is called **menstruation** (men-stroo-**ay′**-shun).

The uterus is a single, hollow organ shaped somewhat like a pear. In the nonpregnant condition, it is about the size of a small fist—about 7.5 cm (3 inches) in length and 5 cm (2 inches) in width at its widest region. The uterus lies in the bottom of the pelvic cavity, anterior to the rectum and posterior to the urinary bladder. The main portion of the uterus is its **corpus,** or body. The rounded part of the uterus above the level of the entrance of the uterine tubes is the **fundus** (**fun′**-dus). The lower, narrow portion is the **cervix** (**ser′**-viks). Part of the cervix projects into the vagina (see Figure 17-4).

The uterus is lined by a mucous membrane, the **endometrium** (en′-doe-**me′**-tree-um). Beneath the endometrium, the wall of the uterus consists of a thick layer of muscle. Just as the ovary develops a new ovum each month, the uterus also follows a monthly cycle of activity. Each month, in response to estrogen and progesterone from the ovary, the endometrium prepares for possible pregnancy. The endometrium becomes thick and vascular and develops glands that secrete a nourishing fluid. If pregnancy does not occur, part of the endometrium sloughs off during menstruation.

Cancer of the cervix is one of the most common types of cancer in women. Detection is usually possible by the routine Papanicolaou test (Pap smear), in which a few cells are scraped from the cervix during a routine gynecological examination and studied microscopically. When cervical cancer is detected and treated at very early stages, the prognosis is good. Cervical cancer has been linked to infection with human papillomavirus (HPV). Effective vaccines against HPV are now available. These vaccines also prevent certain other sexually transmitted diseases (certain genital warts) as well as precancers of the vagina and vulva. The vaccines are only effective if administered before a girl or woman is infected with HPV. For this reason the vaccine should be given before the onset of sexual activity.

The Vagina Functions in Sexual Intercourse, Menstruation, and Birth

The vagina receives the penis during sexual intercourse. It serves as an exit through which the discarded endometrium is discharged during menstruation. The vagina is also the lower part of the birth canal.

The vagina is located anterior to the rectum and posterior to the urethra and urinary bladder. An elastic, muscular tube capable of considerable stretching, the vagina extends from the cervix to its orifice (opening) to the outside of the body. The vagina surrounds the end of the cervix. The recesses formed between the vaginal wall and cervix are called **fornices** (**for′**-nee-seez).

Normally, the vagina is collapsed so that its walls touch each other. Two ridges run along anterior and posterior walls, and there are numerous **rugae** (folds). During sexual intercourse (when the penis is inserted into the vagina) and during childbirth (when the baby's head emerges into the vagina), the rugae straighten out, greatly enlarging the vagina.

The External Genital Structures Are the Vulva

The term **vulva** (**vul′**-vah) refers to the external female genital structures. They include the mons pubis, labia, clitoris, hymen, and vestibule of the vagina (Figure 17-6). The **mons pubis** is a mound of fatty tissue that covers the pubic symphysis. At puberty it becomes covered by coarse pubic hair.

The paired **labia** (**lay′**-be-ah) **majora** (meaning large lips) are folds of skin that pass from the mons pubis to the region behind the vaginal opening. Normally, the labia majora meet in the midline, providing protection for the genital structures beneath. After puberty the outer epidermis of the lips is pigmented and covered with coarse hair. Two thin folds of skin, the **labia minora** (small lips), are located just within the labia majora.

The **clitoris** (**klit′**-oh-ris) is a small structure that corresponds to the male glans penis. It projects from the anterior end of the vulva at the anterior junction of the labia minora.

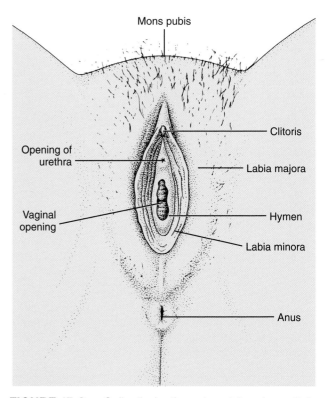

Mons pubis

Clitoris

Opening of urethra

Labia majora

Vaginal opening

Hymen

Labia minora

Anus

FIGURE 17-6 • Collectively, the external female genital structures are referred to as the *vulva*.

However, most of the clitoris is not visible because it is embedded in the tissues of the vulva. The clitoris is a main focus of sexual sensation in the female.

The space enclosed by the labia minora is the **vestibule.** Two openings can be seen in the vestibule—the opening of the urethra anteriorly and the opening of the vagina posteriorly. A thin ring of mucous membrane, the **hymen,** surrounds the entrance to the vagina.

Two small **Bartholin's glands** (greater vestibular glands) open on each side of the vaginal opening. A group of smaller glands (lesser vestibular) open into the vestibule near the opening of the urethra. All of these glands secrete mucus, which helps provide lubrication during sexual intercourse. These glands are vulnerable to infection, especially from the bacterium that causes gonorrhea.

In both male and female the diamond-shaped region between the pubic arch and the anus is the **perineum** (per′-ih-nee′-um). In the female, the region between the vagina and anus is referred to as the *clinical perineum.*

The Breasts Contain the Mammary Glands

The breasts function in **lactation**—production and release of milk for nourishment of the baby. The breasts overlie the pectoral muscles and are attached to them by connective tissue. Fibrous bands of tissue called *ligaments of Cooper* firmly connect the breasts to the skin.

The **mammary glands,** located within the breasts, produce milk. Each breast is composed of 15 to 20 lobes of glandular tissue (Figure 17-7). A duct drains milk from each lobe and opens onto the surface of the nipple. Thus the surface of each nipple has 15 to 20 openings. The amount of adipose tissue around the lobes of the glandular tissue determines the size of the breasts and accounts for their soft consistency. The size of the breasts does not affect their capacity to produce milk.

The nipple consists of smooth muscle that can contract to make the nipple erect in response to sexual stimuli. In the pinkish areola surrounding the nipple, several rudimentary milk glands may be found. In childhood, the breasts contain only rudimentary glands. At puberty, estrogen and progesterone stimulate development of the glands and ducts and the deposit of fatty tissue characteristic of the adult breast.

During pregnancy, high concentrations of estrogen and progesterone stimulate the glands and ducts to develop, resulting in increased breast size. For the first few days after childbirth, the mammary glands produce a fluid called **colostrum** (koe-los′-trum), which contains protein and lactose but little fat. After birth, **prolactin,** secreted by the anterior pituitary, stimulates milk production, and by the third day after delivery, the breasts produce milk. When the infant suckles at the breast, a reflex action results in prolactin and **oxytocin** release from the pituitary gland. Oxytocin stimulates ejection of milk from the glands into the ducts.

Other than skin cancer, **breast cancer** is the most common type of cancer in women and is a leading cause of cancer deaths in women (second only to lung cancer). Breast cancer often spreads to the lymphatic system—to the axillary nodes or the nodes along the internal mammary artery. About two thirds of breast cancers have metastasized (i.e., spread) to the lymph nodes by the time the cancer is first diagnosed.

Because early detection of breast cancer greatly increases the chances of cure and survival, campaigns have been launched to educate women on the importance of self-examination. Mammography, a soft tissue radiological study of the breast, is helpful in detecting small lesions that might not be identified by routine examination. In mammography, lesions show on x-ray film as areas of increased density. Radiologists are increasingly using magnetic resonance imaging (MRI) technology to detect breast cancer in women at high risk.

Hormones Regulate Female Reproduction

The hypothalamus, pituitary gland, and ovaries interact by way of hormones to regulate female reproduction. The hypothalamus produces releasing hormones; the anterior lobe of the pituitary gland secretes FSH and LH; and the ovaries secrete estrogens and **progesterone** (pro-jes′-ter-own).

Like testosterone in the male, estrogens are responsible for the growth of sex organs at puberty (primary sex characteristics) and for the development of secondary sex characteristics. Female secondary sex characteristics include breast development, broadening of the pelvis, and the distribution of fat and muscle that shape the female body.

In girls, puberty typically begins between 10 and 12 years and continues until 14 to 16 years. Breast development is typically the first sign that puberty is imminent. **Menarche** (meh-nar′-kee), the first menstrual period, usually occurs between

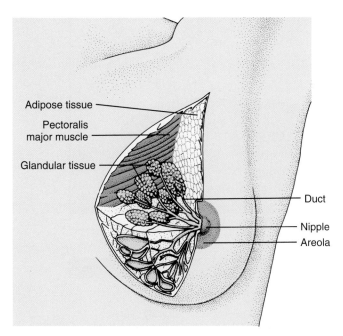

Adipose tissue

Pectoralis major muscle

Glandular tissue

Duct

Nipple

Areola

FIGURE 17-7 • Structure of the mature female breast.

12 and 14 years. As a female approaches puberty, the anterior pituitary gland secretes FSH and LH. These hormones signal the ovaries to begin functioning. Interaction of FSH and LH with estrogens and progesterone from the ovaries regulates the **menstrual cycle.** This cycle occurs every month from puberty until menopause. During the menstrual cycle, estrogens stimulate the growth of follicles and stimulate thickening of the endometrium.

The menstrual cycle stimulates production of an ovum each month and prepares the uterus for pregnancy. Although there is wide variation, a "typical" menstrual cycle is approximately 28 days long. The first day of menstruation marks the first day of the cycle. Menstruation lasts for about 5 days. Ovulation typically occurs about 14 days before the next cycle begins; in a 28-day cycle this would correspond to about the fourteenth day (Figure 17-8). As you read the following description of the menstrual cycle, follow the steps illustrated in Figure 17-9.

The Preovulatory Phase Consists of the First Two Weeks of the Menstrual Cycle

Menstruation occurs during the first 5 or so days of the **preovulatory phase** (pre-**ov′**-u-lah-tor-y). During menstruation, the thickened endometrium of the uterus sloughs off. During the early phase of the menstrual cycle, FSH is the principal hormone released by the pituitary gland. It stimulates a few follicles to develop in the ovary (Figure 17-9). The developing follicles release estrogen, which stimulates the growth of the endometrium once again. Its blood vessels and glands begin to

develop anew. After the first week, typically only one follicle continues to develop.

As the concentration of estrogen in the blood rises, estrogen inhibits secretion of FSH (and LH) from the anterior pituitary gland (and may also inhibit the hypothalamus so that it secretes less GnRH). In addition, cells of the ovary secrete *inhibin,* which inhibits mainly FSH secretion. These negative feedback signals result in a decrease in FSH concentration.

During the late preovulatory phase, estrogen concentration peaks. This increase in estrogen concentration signals the anterior pituitary to secrete LH. This is a positive feedback mechanism. The surge of LH from the anterior pituitary stimulates final maturation of the follicle and ovulation.

The Corpus Luteum Develops During the Postovulatory Phase

The **postovulatory phase** (post-**ov′**-u-lah-tor-y) begins after ovulation. At that time, LH stimulates development of the corpus luteum. This temporary endocrine structure releases progesterone and estrogens. These hormones stimulate continued thickening of the endometrium in preparation for possible pregnancy.

If pregnancy does not occur, the corpus luteum begins to degenerate after about eight days. Progesterone and estrogen levels in the blood fall markedly. Small arteries in the uterine wall constrict, and the part of the endometrium they supply becomes deprived of oxygen. Menstruation begins once again as cells begin to die and damaged arteries rupture and bleed.

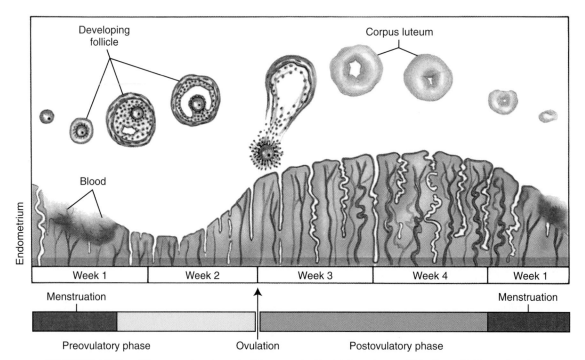

FIGURE 17-8 • The menstrual cycle. The events that take place within the pituitary gland, ovary, and uterus are precisely synchronized by hormonal signals. When fertilization does not occur, the cycle repeats itself about every 28 days.

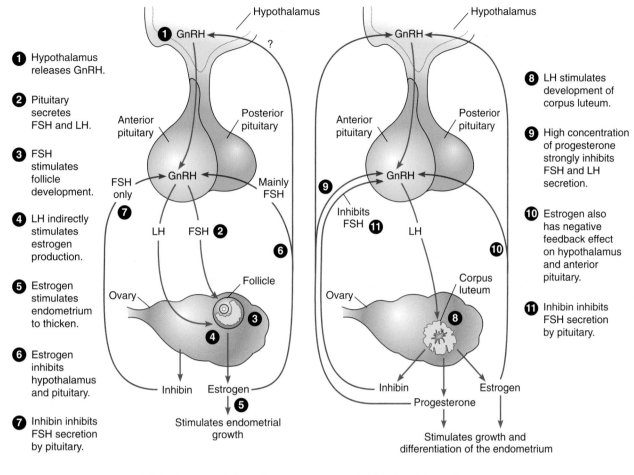

1 Hypothalamus releases GnRH.

2 Pituitary secretes FSH and LH.

3 FSH stimulates follicle development.

4 LH indirectly stimulates estrogen production.

5 Estrogen stimulates endometrium to thicken.

6 Estrogen inhibits hypothalamus and pituitary.

7 Inhibin inhibits FSH secretion by pituitary.

8 LH stimulates development of corpus luteum.

9 High concentration of progesterone strongly inhibits FSH and LH secretion.

10 Estrogen also has negative feedback effect on hypothalamus and anterior pituitary.

11 Inhibin inhibits FSH secretion by pituitary.

(A) Early preovulatory phase.   **(B)** Postovulatory phase.

FIGURE 17-9 • Regulation of female reproduction. Hormones from the hypothalamus, anterior pituitary gland, and ovary interact to regulate the menstrual cycle. **(A)** Early preovulatory phase. During the late preovulatory phase, the high level of estrogen has a positive feedback effect on the pituitary and hypothalamus. A surge of LH stimulates ovulation. **(B)** Postovulatory phase. After ovulation, the corpus luteum secretes progesterone and estrogens. *Red arrows* indicate inhibition. *GnRH*, Gonadotropin-releasing hormone; *FSH*, follicle-stimulating hormone; *LH*, luteinizing hormone.

The Menstrual Cycle Stops at Menopause

At about age 50 years, a woman enters **menopause**—the time when the ovaries become less responsive to gonadotropic hormones and ova are no longer produced. Estrogen and progesterone secretion decreases. The reproductive system gradually stops functioning. The menstrual cycle becomes irregular and eventually halts, and the woman is no longer fertile.

The decrease in hormones can cause a variety of symptoms, including a sensation of heat, referred to as "hot flashes." These sensations may be caused by the effect of decreased estrogen on the temperature-regulating center in the hypothalamus. Menopause does not usually affect a woman's interest in sex or her sexual performance.

Quiz Yourself

- What are the functions of the ovary? Of the uterus?
- Where does fertilization take place?
- What are the functions of estrogen? Of LH?

FERTILIZATION IS THE FUSION OF SPERM AND OVUM

LEARNING OBJECTIVE

7. Describe the process of fertilization.

When sperm are released into the vagina, some find their way into the uterus and uterine tubes. If ovulation has occurred and the ovum is in the uterine tube, **fertilization,** the fusion of sperm and egg, can occur. Fertilization and the establishment of pregnancy together are referred to as **conception.**

Large numbers of sperm are necessary to penetrate the follicle cells surrounding the ovum; however, only one sperm fertilizes the ovum. As soon as one sperm penetrates the ovum, a rapid electrical change takes place, followed by a slower chemical change in the plasma membrane of the ovum. These changes prevent other sperm from entering the ovum. The second meiotic division takes place and the sperm and ovum nuclei fuse to form a fertilized egg, or **zygote.**

After ejaculation, sperm remain viable for about 48 to 72 hours. The ovum remains fertile for about 12 to 24 hours after ovulation. Thus fertilization is most probable when intercourse takes place on the day of ovulation or during the 2 days preceding ovulation. In a very regular 28-day menstrual cycle, sexual intercourse is most likely to result in fertilization and conception on days 12 to 16. However, many women do not have regular cycles and many factors can cause irregular cycles, even in women who are generally regular.

⊚ Quiz Yourself

- What is fertilization?
- How many sperm are needed to fertilize an ovum?

THE ZYGOTE GIVES RISE TO THE NEW INDIVIDUAL

LEARNING OBJECTIVES

8. **Summarize the course of development from fertilization to birth.**

9. **Describe the functions of the amnion and placenta.**
10. **Identify the three stages of the birth process.**

The deoxyribonucleic acid (DNA) of the zygote contains all the genetic information needed to produce a complete individual. The zygote divides to form an **embryo** composed of two cells. Each of these cells then divides, producing four cells. As these first cell divisions take place, the embryo is slowly moved along the uterine tube toward the uterus by the action of cilia (Figure 17-10). By the time the embryo reaches the uterus on the fifth day of development, it is a tiny cluster of about 32 cells.

The Embryo Develops in the Wall of the Uterus

On about the seventh day of development, the embryo begins to *implant* itself in the wall of the uterus. All further *prenatal* (before birth) development takes place within the uterine wall.

Several **fetal membranes** develop around the embryo. These membranes help protect, nourish, and support the developing embryo. They are discarded at birth. One fetal membrane, the **amnion** (**am′**-nee-on), forms a sac around the embryo. The fluid that fills the amnion keeps the embryo moist and cushions it (Figure 17-11).

The **placenta** (plah-**sen′**-tah) is the organ of exchange between the mother and the embryo (see Figure 17-11). Nutrients and oxygen in the mother's blood move through the placenta and into the embryo. Wastes from the embryo move through the placenta and into the mother's blood. During pregnancy, the corpus luteum and the placenta secrete progesterone.

The placenta produces a hormone called **human chorionic gonadotropin (hCG),** which signals the corpus luteum to increase in size and to release large amounts of estrogens and

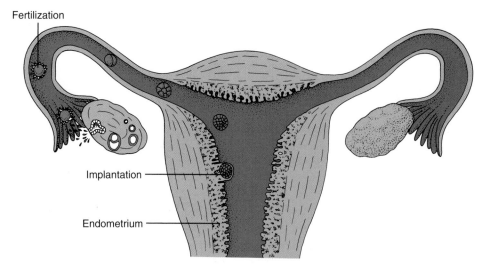

FIGURE 17-10 • The first cell divisions take place as the embryo is moved through the uterine tube to the uterus.

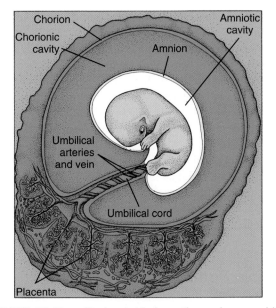

FIGURE 17-11 • At about 45 days, the embryo and its membranes together are about the size of a ping-pong ball and the mother still may be unaware of her pregnancy. The amnion, filled with amniotic fluid, surrounds and cushions the embryo. The umbilical arteries and vein deliver blood to and from the placenta where materials are exchanged between the embryo and the mother. (The chorion and amnion are fetal membranes.)

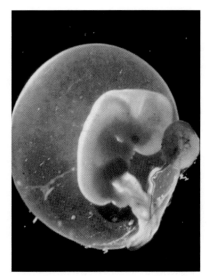

FIGURE 17-12 • Human embryo at 5½ weeks. At this stage, the embryo is about 1 cm (0.4 inch) long. Note the developing limb buds. (From Guigoz, Petit Format, Photo Researchers, Inc.)

progesterone. These hormones stimulate the endometrium and the placenta to continue their development. Without hCG, the corpus luteum degenerates and the embryo is aborted. After about the eleventh week of pregnancy, the placenta itself produces enough estrogens and progesterone to maintain pregnancy. At that time, the corpus luteum begins to deteriorate.

The stalk of tissue that connects the embryo with the placenta is the **umbilical cord** (see Figure 17-11). Two umbilical arteries deliver blood from the embryo to the placenta, and an umbilical vein returns blood to the embryo.

Prenatal Development Requires About 266 Days

From fertilization, about 266 days (38 weeks) is required for the developing baby to complete its prenatal development (Figures 17-11 through 17-14). Obstetricians typically count from the onset of the mother's last menstrual period and consider an average pregnancy 280 days (40 weeks).

By 4 weeks, the rudiments of many organs are present. The brain and spinal cord are among the first organs to develop and by 4 weeks the eyes and ears are visible. A simple circulatory system is working by this time. Small mounds of tissue called *limb buds,* which can be seen by the end of the first month, slowly lengthen, forming the limbs.

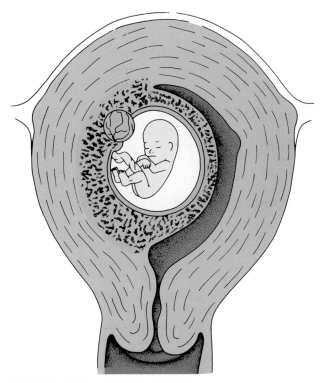

FIGURE 17-13 • At 10 weeks, the human fetus is about 6 cm (2.4 inches) long.

After the second month, the embryo is referred to as a **fetus** (**fee′**-tus) (see Figure 17-13). By the end of the third month, the fetus is more than 6 cm (2.4 inches) long and weighs about 14 grams (gm) (0.5 ounce). By 5 months of development, the fetus moves about in the amniotic fluid. At this time the mother usually becomes aware of fetal movements.

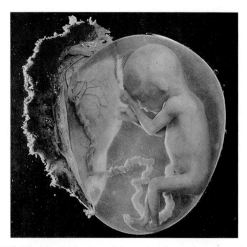

FIGURE 17-14 • Human fetus at 16 weeks, about 16 cm (6.4 inches). (From Nilsson L: *A child is born,* New York, 1977, Dell Publishing.)

The last 3 months (last trimester) of development are a time of rapid growth and specialization of tissues and organs. During the seventh month, the cerebrum grows rapidly and develops convolutions (folds). The grasping and sucking reflexes are present, and the fetus may suck its thumb. Most of the body is covered by downy hair (lanugo), which is usually shed before birth.

A baby born after 30 weeks has a good chance of surviving, but if it is born before 37 weeks, it is considered premature. At birth, the average full-term baby weighs about 3000 gm (7 pounds) and measures about 52 cm (20 inches) in total length.

The Birth Process Includes Labor and Delivery

Several days before birth, the fetus usually assumes an upside-down position, which prepares it to enter the birth canal head first. At the end of pregnancy, the stretching of the uterine muscle by the growing fetus combines with the effects of increased estrogen concentration to produce strong contractions of the uterus. Childbirth, or **parturition,** includes **labor** and **delivery.**

Labor, which begins with a long series of involuntary contractions of the uterus, may be divided into three stages. During the **first stage,** regular uterine contractions occur. At first they may occur at about 30-minute intervals, but then they become more intense, rhythmical, and frequent, occurring as often as every minute (or even less) later in labor. As this stage progresses, the cervix becomes *dilated* to about 10 cm (4 inches) and *effaced* (i.e., continuous with the uterine wall, so it cannot be distinguished from the adjoining portion of the uterus), allowing passage of the fetal head. Rupture of the amnion with release of the amniotic fluid through the vagina may occur during this stage. The first stage

of labor is the longest, often lasting 8 to 24 hours in a first pregnancy.

The **second stage** begins when the cervix is fully dilated and ends with the delivery of the baby. By contracting her abdominal muscles, the mother can help push the baby along through the vagina. When the **neonate** (newborn) emerges, it is still connected to the placenta by the umbilical cord. Most physicians clamp and cut the cord immediately after the infant has been delivered.

During the **third stage** of labor, the placenta separates from the uterus and is expelled. Generally, this occurs within 10 to 20 minutes after the birth of the baby. Now referred to as the *afterbirth,* the placenta is inspected for abnormalities and then discarded.

Multiple Births May Be Fraternal or Identical

Before fertility drugs became available in the United States, twins were born once in about 88 births, triplets once in 88 squared (7744) births, and quadruplets once in 88 cubed (1 in 512,000) births. With the use of fertility drugs, multiple births have become much more common.

Twins (or other multiple births) can be either fraternal or identical. **Fraternal twins** (also called *dizygotic twins*) develop when a woman ovulates two eggs and each is fertilized by a different sperm. Each fertilized egg has its own unique genetic endowment, and the twins who develop are no more genetically alike than any two siblings are.

Identical twins (also called *monozygotic twins*) develop when the tiny mass of cells that makes up the early embryo divides to form two independent groups of cells, and each develops into a baby. Because the cells of each twin have developed from one fertilized egg, they have identical genes and are indeed identical twins. Rarely, the two masses of cells do not separate completely and give rise to **conjoined twins.**

Quiz Yourself

- Where does prenatal development take place?
- What is the function of the placenta?
- What happens during the second stage of labor?

THE HUMAN LIFE CYCLE EXTENDS FROM FERTILIZATION TO DEATH

LEARNING OBJECTIVE

11. **List the stages of human development from fertilization to death.**

Development begins at fertilization and continues through the stages of the human life cycle until death. In this chapter we have briefly examined the development of the **embryo** and **fetus.** The **neonatal period** extends from birth to the end of the first month of postnatal life. **Infancy** follows the neonatal period and lasts until age 2 years. Some consider infancy to end when the infant can assume an erect posture and walk, usually between the ages of 10 and 14 months. **Childhood,** also a period of rapid growth and development, continues from infancy until adolescence.

Adolescence is the time of development between puberty and adulthood. In the United States, adolescence is considered to begin about age 11 and end at age 19 or 20. During adolescence, a young person experiences the physical and physiological changes that result in physical and reproductive maturity.

This is also a time when young people make the psychological adjustments that prepare them to assume the responsibilities of adulthood. **Young adulthood** extends from adolescence until about age 40. **Middle age** is usually considered to be the period between ages 40 and 65. **Old age** begins after age 65.

Quiz Yourself

- What is the neonatal period?
- A 14-year-old girl would be in what stage of the life cycle?

SUMMARY

LO 1. Describe the anatomy of the male reproductive system and describe the functions of each structure.

- The reproductive function of the male is to produce male **gametes,** the **sperm** cells, and to deliver them into the female reproductive tract. **Spermatogenesis,** or sperm cell production, takes place in the **seminiferous tubules** within the **testes.** During spermatogenesis, sperm undergo **meiosis,** a type of cell division (reduction division) in which the chromosome number is reduced to one set of chromosomes, rather than two. Each undifferentiated sperm cell gives rise to four sperm cells, and each sperm cell has only one complete set of chromosomes.
- The testes are located in the **scrotum**—a skin-covered bag suspended from the groin.
- From the tubules in the testes, sperm pass into an **epididymis,** where they complete maturation and may be stored. From the epididymis, they enter the **vas deferens,** or sperm duct. During ejaculation, sperm pass into the **ejaculatory duct** and then into the **urethra,** which extends through the **penis.**
- Most of the volume of the **semen** is produced by the **seminal vesicles** and the **prostate gland.** The **bulbourethral glands** produce a few drops of alkaline fluid before **ejaculation.**
- The penis consists of a long **shaft** that enlarges to form the **glans.** The three columns of spongy tissue (**erectile tissue**) within the penis have large **sinusoids.** When these blood vessels become engorged with blood, the penis becomes erect.

LO 2. Trace the passage of sperm cells from the tubules in the testes through the conducting tubes and to their ejaculation from the body in semen.

- Sperm pass from the seminiferous tubules in the testis to the epididymis and then enter the vas deferens. Sperm then pass through the ejaculatory duct and through the urethra.

LO 3. Describe the actions of the male gonadotropic hormones and testosterone.

- During **puberty,** the period of sexual maturation, the hypothalamus begins to secrete **gonadotropin-releasing hormone** (GnRH), which stimulates the anterior lobe of the pituitary gland to produce the gonadotropic hormones **follicle-stimulating hormone** (**FSH**) and **luteinizing hormone (LH).**
- FSH stimulates sperm production. LH stimulates the testes to secrete testosterone.
- **Testosterone** is responsible for the **primary sex characteristics**—that is, the development and activity of the reproductive structures. This hormone also stimulates development and maintenance of **secondary sex characteristics.**
- The concentrations of reproductive hormones are regulated by negative feedback mechanisms. Testosterone inhibits FSH and LH secretion. **Inhibin,** a hormone secreted by the Sertoli cells in the testis, inhibits FSH secretion.

LO 4. Describe the anatomy of the female reproductive system and describe the functions of each structure.

- The reproductive role of the female includes production of ova, receiving sperm, incubation and nourishment of the developing embryo, and lactation. **Ova** (female gametes) develop in

LO = Learning Objective

the **ovary** as part of **follicles.** The ovary also produces the female hormones estrogens and progesterone.

- Fertilization takes place in the **uterine tube.** The ovum begins to develop as it passes through the uterine tube into the **uterus,** which serves as its incubator.
- The **vagina** is the lower part of the birth canal. It also receives the penis during sexual intercourse and serves as an outlet for menstrual discharge.
- The external female genital structures are collectively referred to as the **vulva.** They include the **mons pubis, labia majora, labia minora, clitoris, vestibule, hymen,** and **Bartholin's glands.**
- The **mammary glands** within the breasts function in **lactation.** After birth, **prolactin** stimulates milk production. **Oxytocin** stimulates ejection of milk from the glands into the ducts.

LO 5. Trace the development of an ovum and its passage through the female reproductive system.

- Beginning at puberty, a few **follicles** begin to develop each month when stimulated by FSH. The ova within these follicles undergo the first meiotic division at this time. At **ovulation,** the ovum is ejected into the pelvic cavity. It then passes into the uterine tube, where it is either fertilized or deteriorates. If fertilized, the ovum begins to develop as it passes through the uterine tube into the uterus.

LO 6. Describe the principal events of the menstrual cycle and summarize the interactions of hormones that regulate the cycle.

- The first day of menstrual bleeding marks the first day of the **menstrual cycle.** In a "typical" 28-day cycle, ovulation occurs on about the 14th day.
- Events of the menstrual cycle are coordinated by the interaction of gonadotropic and ovarian hormones. FSH stimulates follicle growth during the first 2 weeks of the cycle.
- **Estrogens** released from the developing follicles stimulate the **endometrium** of the uterus to thicken. LH released from the anterior pituitary stimulates ovulation and the development of the **corpus luteum,** a temporary endocrine structure.
- The corpus luteum secretes **progesterone** and estrogens. If fertilization does not occur, the corpus luteum begins to degenerate; estrogen

and progesterone levels fall, and the endometrium begins to slough off again (**menstruation**).

- Estrogens are responsible for the growth of sex organs at puberty and for the development and maintenance of secondary sex characteristics. Estrogens and progesterone prepare the endometrium each month for possible pregnancy.

LO 7. Describe the process of fertilization.

- The ovum undergoes the second meiotic division after a sperm enters it. **Fertilization** is the fusion of egg and sperm. Only one sperm actually fertilizes the ovum.

LO 8. Summarize the course of development from fertilization to birth.

- The fertilized ovum is called a **zygote.** The zygote divides to form a two-celled **embryo.** Then each new cell divides again and again, forming the building blocks of the new individual.
- On about the seventh day of development, the embryo implants in the wall of the uterus. Many organs begin to develop by the fourth week. After the second month of development, the embryo is called a **fetus.** The developing baby typically completes its prenatal development in about 266 days (38 weeks) from the time of fertilization.

LO 9. Describe the functions of the amnion and placenta.

- Several **fetal membranes** develop around the embryo. The **amnion** forms a protective sac of fluid around the embryo. The **placenta** is the organ of exchange between the mother and developing embryo. The placenta produces the hormone **human chorionic gonadotropin (hCG),** which signals the corpus luteum to secrete estrogens and progesterone.

LO 10. Identify the three stages of the birth process.

- Childbirth, called **parturition,** includes **labor** and **delivery.** During the **first stage** of labor, the **cervix** dilates; during the **second stage,** the baby is delivered; during the **third stage,** the placenta is expelled.

LO 11. List the stages of human development from fertilization to death.

- The stages of the human life cycle include embryo, fetus, **neonatal period, infancy, childhood, adolescence, young adulthood, middle age,** and **old age.**

CHAPTER QUIZ

Fill in the Blank

1. Sperm cells are produced in tubules within the _____.

2. From the epididymis, sperm pass into the _____ _____.

3. The _____ _____, which surrounds the urethra, contributes a thin, alkaline secretion to the semen.

4. Testosterone is produced by interstitial cells in the _____.

5. The period of sexual maturation is called _____.

6. Hormones produced by the ovary are _____ and _____.

7. The endometrium is the lining of the _____.

8. Ejection of the ovum from the follicle is called _____.

9. During the preovulatory phase, FSH stimulates development of _____.

10. The number of sperm that fertilize an ovum is _____.

11. Lactation is the process of producing _____.

12. A fertilized ovum is called a _____.

13. The _____ is a fluid-filled sac around the embryo.

14. The _____ is the organ of exchange between mother and embryo.

Multiple Choice

15. Fertilization normally takes place in the: a. ovary; b. pelvic cavity; c. uterine tube; d. uterus.

16. The embryo normally implants in the: a. ovary; b. cervix; c. uterine tube; d. uterus.

17. Prolactin signals: a. the ovary to produce follicles; b. the corpus luteum that pregnancy has begun; c. sperm production by the testes; d. the mammary glands to produce milk.

18. The amnion: a. protects the embryo; b. provides the embryo with oxygen; c. is an important source of estrogen; d. secretes progesterone.

19. In the female, secondary sex characteristics are maintained by: a. progesterone; b. estrogens; c. FSH; d. LH.

20. The hormone inhibin: a. inhibits FSH in the male; b. inhibits FSH in the female; c. inhibits FSH in the male *and* female; d. is produced by the anterior pituitary.

REVIEW QUESTIONS

1. The testes are located in the scrotum outside the pelvic cavity. Why?

2. Trace the path traveled by a sperm cell from the seminiferous tubules of the testes until it is discharged from the body.

3. During sexual excitement, the penis becomes erect. Relate this process to the internal structure of the penis.

4. What are the actions of testosterone? Draw a diagram illustrating the regulation of male reproductive function.

5. Trace the fate of the ovum from the time its follicle matures in the ovary until it becomes an embryo.

6. Draw a diagram illustrating the regulation of female reproductive events during the preovulatory phase of the menstrual cycle.

7. What is the function of the corpus luteum? Which hormone is necessary for its development?

8. In a typical 28-day menstrual cycle, when does ovulation occur? When does menstruation occur? When is a woman most likely to become pregnant?

9. What is puberty? What is menopause?

10. Trace the early development of the embryo.

11. Label the diagrams. (See Figures 17-1 and 17-5 to check your answers.)

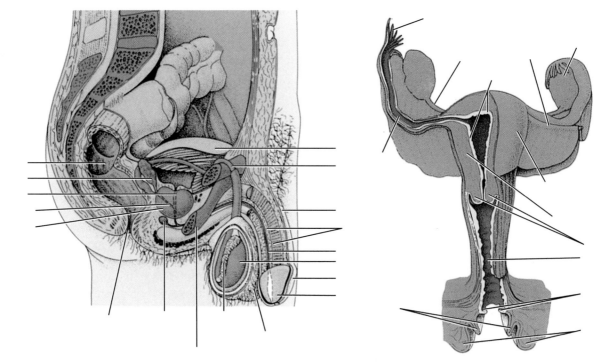

APPENDIX

A

Chapter Quiz Answers

CHAPTER 1

1. anatomy; physiology
2. metabolism
3. catabolism
4. homeostasis
5. molecules
6. cells
7. organs
8. hormones
9. d
10. c
11. a
12. c
13. c
14. a
15. b
16. f
17. e
18. a
19. g
20. b
21. c
22. d
23. e
24. a
25. f

CHAPTER 2

1. d
2. b
3. c
4. f
5. e
6. h
7. g

8. a
9. inside the cell; the solution outside the cell
10. phagocytosis
11. energy
12. anaphase
13. cilia
14. ducts
15. connective tissue
16. b
17. d
18. c
19. b
20. a

CHAPTER 3

1. integumentary
2. epidermis; dermis
3. keratin
4. subcutaneous
5. sebaceous; sebum
6. water; salts
7. hair follicle
8. keratin
9. melanin
10. ultraviolet

CHAPTER 4

1. red marrow
2. periosteum
3. diaphysis
4. osteons (haversian systems)
5. lacunae
6. break down bone
7. axial

8. cranial; facial
9. sagittal suture
10. spinal cord
11. pectoral girdle
12. thoracic
13. centrum
14. suture
15. synovial
16. flexion; abduction
17. hinge
18. b
19. b
20. a
21. a
22. c
23. d
24. c

CHAPTER 5

1. fibers
2. epimysium
3. tendons
4. myosin; actin
5. motor nerve (or motor neuron)
6. calcium
7. ATP
8. energy
9. muscle tone
10. antagonist
11. joints
12. c
13. c
14. b
15. d
16. a
17. b

18. a
19. c
20. d

CHAPTER 6

1. brain; spinal cord
2. peripheral nervous system (PNS)
3. glial
4. neurons
5. cell body
6. axon
7. ganglion; nucleus
8. reception
9. synapse
10. ventricles
11. brainstem
12. gray
13. ascending
14. interneurons; efferent (motor)
15. dura mater
16. cerebrospinal fluid (CSF)
17. c
18. a
19. b
20. c
21. d
22. a

CHAPTER 7

1. somatic
2. optic; vagus
3. hearing
4. 8; 12
5. sensory (afferent)
6. plexus
7. autonomic
8. sympathetic
9. parasympathetic
10. parasympathetic
11. c
12. b
13. a
14. b

CHAPTER 8

1. electrical
2. receptor
3. adaptation
4. rhodopsin
5. accommodation
6. malleus, incus, stapes
7. cochlea
8. saccule, utricle

9. semicircular canals
10. olfactory
11. pain
12. referred
13. muscle spindles
14. b
15. a
16. a
17. b
18. d
19. b
20. d
21. a

CHAPTER 9

1. ducts; hormones
2. chemical messenger (signal) that stimulates a change in some metabolic activity
3. target
4. hypothalamus
5. oxytocin
6. prolactin
7. anterior pituitary
8. hypothalamus
9. posterior pituitary
10. abnormally tall individuals
11. the rate of metabolism
12. calcitonin; lower calcium level in the blood
13. aldosterone
14. insulin
15. glucagon
16. epinephrine; norepinephrine
17. c
18. d
19. a
20. d
21. b
22. b
23. d

CHAPTER 10

1. oxygen
2. plasma
3. antibodies
4. clotting
5. red bone marrow
6. anemia
7. defend the body against disease (destroy bacteria by phagocytosis)
8. platelets
9. fibrin; thrombin
10. B; anti-A

11. Rh; Rh-negative; Rh-positive
12. d
13. b
14. a
15. a

CHAPTER 11

1. pericardium
2. myocardium (cardiac muscle)
3. interventricular septum
4. mitral
5. semilunar
6. coronary
7. sinoatrial node (SA node)
8. bundle
9. systole; diastole
10. diastole
11. cardiac output
12. stroke volume
13. parasympathetic, sympathetic
14. c
15. a
16. b
17. d
18. a

CHAPTER 12

1. arteries
2. capillaries
3. pressure
4. systemic
5. pulmonary
6. oxygen-rich
7. thoracic
8. superior vena cava
9. circle; Willis
10. carotid; vertebral
11. hepatic portal; liver
12. pulse
13. blood pressure
14. lymphatic
15. lymph
16. lymphatics
17. a
18. b
19. c
20. d
21. b
22. c

CHAPTER 13

1. pathogens
2. skin (and other barriers)

3. phagocytic
4. interferons
5. antigens
6. antibodies
7. antibody
8. cell
9. memory
10. antigen
11. a
12. d
13. c
14. b
15. b

CHAPTER 14

1. glottis; larynx; trachea
2. cellular respiration
3. diaphragm
4. epiglottis
5. larynx
6. visceral
7. ventilation
8. inspiration; expiration
9. hemoglobin
10. phrenic
11. c
12. a
13. c
14. a
15. d

CHAPTER 15

1. ingestion
2. mechanical digestion; chemical digestion

3. mucosa
4. visceral peritoneum
5. peristalsis
6. greater omentum
7. 32
8. crown; root
9. dentin; enamel
10. parotid glands
11. carbohydrates (starch)
12. rugae
13. pepsin
14. duodenum; jejunum; ileum
15. basal metabolic
16. c
17. d
18. a
19. c
20. b

CHAPTER 16

1. urea; uric acid
2. ureter
3. pelvis
4. cortex; medulla
5. corpuscle; tubule
6. glomerulus; Bowman's capsule
7. afferent
8. loop of Henle
9. Bowman's capsule
10. tubular reabsorption
11. urine
12. ADH
13. a
14. c
15. d
16. b

17. a
18. c
19. c
20. b

CHAPTER 17

1. testes
2. vas deferens
3. prostate gland
4. testes
5. puberty
6. estrogens, progesterone
7. uterus
8. ovulation
9. follicles
10. one
11. milk
12. zygote
13. amnion
14. placenta
15. c
16. d
17. d
18. a
19. b
20. c

APPENDIX
B

Dissecting Terms

COMMON PREFIXES, SUFFIXES, AND WORD ROOTS

Your task of mastering new terms will be greatly simplified if you learn to dissect each new word. Many terms can be divided into a prefix (the part of the word that precedes the main root), the word root itself, and often a suffix (a word ending that may add to or modify the meaning of the root). As you progress in your study of anatomy and physiology, you will learn to recognize the more common prefixes, word roots, and suffixes. Such recognition will help you analyze new terms so that you can determine their meaning and that will help you remember them.

Here we provide a list of common prefixes, suffixes, and word roots. After each word part, we give you an example in parentheses.

PREFIXES

a-, ab- from, away, apart (*ab*duct, lead away, move away from the midline of the body)

a-, an-, un- less, lack, not (*a*symmetrical, not symmetrical)

ad-, af-, ag-, an-, ap- to, toward (*ad*duct, move toward the midline of the body)

ambi- both sides (*ambi*dextrous, able to use either hand)

ante- forward, before (*ante*flexion, bending forward)

anti- against (*anti*coagulant, a substance that prevents coagulation of blood)

aut-, auto- self (*auto*immune disease, a condition in which the immune system attacks the body's own tissues)

bi- two (*bi*ceps, a muscle with two heads of origin)

bio- life (*bio*logy, the study of life)

brady- slow (*brady*cardia, abnormally slow heart beat)

circum-, circ- around (*circum*cision, a cutting around)

co-, con- with, together (*con*genital, existing with or before birth)

contra- against (*contra*ception, against conception)

crypt- hidden (*crypt*orchidism, undescended or hidden testes)

cyt- cell (*cyt*ology, the study of cells)

di- two (*di*saccharide, a compound made of two sugar molecules chemically combined)

dis-, di-, dif- apart, un-, not (*dis*sect, cut apart)

dys- painful, difficult (*dys*pnea, difficult breathing)

end-, endo- within, inner (*endo*plasmic reticulum, a network of membranes found within the cytoplasm)

epi- on, upon (*epi*dermis, on the dermis)

eu- good, well (*eu*phoria, a sense of well-being)

ex-, e-, ef- out from, out of (*ex*tension, a straightening out)

extra- outside, beyond (*extra*embryonic membrane, a membrane such as the amnion that protects the embryo)

hemi- half (cerebral *hemi*sphere, lateral half of the cerebrum)

hetero- other, different (*hetero*geneous, made of different substances)

homo-, hom- same (*homo*logous, corresponding in structure)

hyper- excessive, above normal (*hyper*secretion, excessive secretion)

hypo- under, below, deficient (*hypo*dermic, below the skin; *hypo*thyroidism, insufficiency of thyroid hormones)

in-, im- not (*im*balance, condition in which there is no balance)

inter- between, among (*inter*stitial, situated between parts)

intra- within (*intra*cellular, within the cell)

iso- equal, like (*iso*tonic, equal osmotic pressure)

mal- bad, abnormal (*mal*nutrition, poor nutrition)

mega- large, great (*mega*karyocyte, giant cell of bone marrow)

meta- after, beyond (*meta*phase, the stage of mitosis after prophase)

micro- small (*micro*scope, instrument for viewing very small objects)

neo- new (*neo*natal, newborn during the first 4 weeks after birth)

oligo- small, deficient (*oli*guria, abnormally small volume of urine)

oo- egg (*oo*cyte, developing egg cell)

para- near, beside, beyond (*para*central, near the center)

peri- around (*peri*cardial membrane, membrane that surrounds the heart)

poly- multiple, complex (*poly*saccharide, a carbohydrate composed of many simple sugars)

post- after, behind (*post*natal, after birth)

pre- before (*pre*natal, before birth)

retro- backward (*retro*peritoneal, located behind the peritoneum)

semi- half (*semi*lunar, half moon)

sub- under (*sub*cutaneous tissue, tissue immediately under the skin)

super-, supra- above (*supra*renal, above the kidney)

syn- with, together (*syn*drome, a group of symptoms that occur together and characterize a disease)

trans- across, beyond (*trans*port, carry across)

SUFFIXES

-able, -ible able (vi*able*, able to live)

-ac pertaining to (cardi*ac*, pertaining to the heart)

-ad used in anatomy to form adverbs of direction (cephal*ad*, toward the head)

-ase indicates an enzyme (lip*ase*, an enzyme that stimulates fat digestion)

-asis, -asia, -esis condition or state of (hemost*asis*, stopping of bleeding)

-cide kill, destroy (bio*cide*, substance that kills living things)

-ectomy surgical removal (append*ectomy*, surgical removal of the appendix)

-emia condition of blood (an*emia*, without enough blood)

-gen something produced or generated or something that produces or generates (patho*gen*, an organism that causes disease)

-gram record, write (electrocardio*gram*, a record of the electrical activity of the heart)

-graph record, write (electrocardio*graph*, an instrument for recording the electrical activity of the heart)

-itis inflammation of (appendic*itis*, inflammation of the appendix)

-logy study or science of (physio*logy*, study of the function of the body)

-oid like, in the form of (thyr*oid*, in the form of a shield)

-oma tumor (carcin*oma*, a malignant tumor)

-osis indicates disease (psych*osis*, a mental disease)

-ous, -ose full of (poison*ous*, full of poison)

-scope instrument for viewing or observing (micro*scope*, instrument for viewing small objects)

-stomy a surgical procedure in which an artificial opening is made (colo*stomy*, surgical formation of an artificial anus)

-tomy cutting or section (appendec*tomy*, cutting out the appendix)

-uria refers to urine (poly*uria*, excessive production of urine)

SOME COMMON ROOTS

aden gland, glandular (*aden*osis, a glandular disease)

alg pain (neur*alg*ia, nerve pain)

angio vessel (*angio*tensin, a hormone that helps regulate blood pressure)

arthr joint (*arthr*itis, inflammation of the joints)

bi, bio life (*bio*logy, study of life)

blast a formative cell, germ layer (osteo*blast*, cell that gives rise to bone cells)

brachi arm (*brachi*al artery, blood vessel that supplies the arm)

bronch branch of the trachea (*bronch*itis, inflammation of the bronchi)

bry grow, swell (em*bry*o, an organism in the early stages of development)

carcin cancer (*carcin*ogenic, cancer producing)

cardi heart (*cardi*ac, pertaining to the heart)

cephal head (*cephal*ad, toward the head)

cerebr brain (*cerebr*al, pertaining to the brain)

cervic, cervix neck (*cervic*al, pertaining to the neck)

chol bile (*chol*ecystogram, an x-ray of the gallbladder)

chondr cartilage (*chondr*ocyte, a cartilage cell)

chrom color (*chrom*osome, deeply staining body in nucleus)

cran skull (*cran*ial, pertaining to the skull)

cyt cell (*cyt*ology, study of the cells)

derm skin (*derm*atology, study of the skin)

duct, duc lead (*duct*, passageway)

ecol dwelling, house (*ecol*ogy, the study of organisms in relation to their environment)

enter intestine (*enter*itis, inflammation of the intestine)

evol to unroll (*evol*ution, descent of complex organisms from simpler ancestors)

gastr stomach (*gastr*itis, inflammation of the stomach)

gen generate, produce (*gen*e, a hereditary factor)

glyc, glyco sweet, sugar (*glyco*gen, storage form of glucose)

gon semen, seed (*gon*ad, an organ producing gametes)

hem, em blood (*hem*atology, the study of blood)

hepat, hepar liver (*hepat*itis, inflammation of the liver)

hist tissue (*hist*ology, study of tissues)

hom, homeo same, unchanging, steady (*homeo*stasis, reaching a steady state)

hydr water (*hydr*olysis, a breakdown reaction involving water)

leuk white (*leuk*ocyte, white blood cell)

macro large (*macro*phage, large janitor cell)

mamm breast (*mamm*ary glands, the glands that produce milk to nourish the young)

micro small (*micro*scope, instrument for viewing small objects)

morph form (*morph*ogenesis, development of body form)

my, mys muscle (*my*ocardium, muscle layer of the heart)

nephr kidney (*nephr*on, microscopic unit of the kidney)

neur, nerv nerve (*neur*algia, pain associated with nerve)

neutr neither one nor the other (*neutr*on, a subatomic particle that is neither positively nor negatively charged)

occip back part of the head (*occip*ital, back region of the head)

ost, oss bone (*ost*eology, study of bones)

path disease (*path*ologist, one who studies disease processes)

ped child (*ped*iatrics, branch of medicine specializing in children)

ped, pod foot (bi*ped*, organism with two feet)

phag eat (*phag*ocytosis, process by which certain cells ingest particles and foreign matter)

phil love (hydro*phil*ic, a substance that attracts water)

phyt plant (*phyt*ochemicals, compounds found in plants that promote health)

proct anus (*proct*oscope, instrument for examining rectum and anal canal)

psych mind (*psych*ology, study of the mind)

scler hard (athero*scler*osis, hardening of the arterial wall)

som body (chromo*som*e, deeply staining body in the nucleus)

stas, stat stand (*stas*is, condition in which blood stands, as opposed to flowing)

thromb clot (*thromb*us, a clot within the body)

ur urea, urine (*ur*ologist, a physician specializing in the urinary tract)

visc pertaining to an internal organ or body cavity (*visc*era, internal organs)

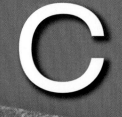

APPENDIX C

Abbreviations

Many technical terms in anatomy and physiology and in the health sciences are both long and difficult to pronounce. For this reason, we use a great many abbreviations. Some common abbreviations are listed here.

A Adenine

ACTH Adrenocorticotropic hormone

AD Alzheimer's disease

ADH Antidiuretic hormone

ADP Adenosine diphosphate

AIDS Acquired immunodeficiency syndrome

AMP Adenosine monophosphate

amu Atomic mass unit (dalton)

ANS Autonomic nervous system

APC Antigen-presenting cell

ATP Adenosine triphosphate

AV node or valve Atrioventricular node or valve (of heart)

BAL Blood alcohol level

B lymphocyte or B cell Lymphocyte responsible for antibody-mediated immunity

BMR Basal metabolic rate

BP Blood pressure

BUN Blood urea nitrogen

C Cytosine

Ca Cancer

CAD Coronary artery disease

cAMP Cyclic adenosine monophosphate; cyclic AMP

CAPD Continuous ambulatory peritoneal dialysis

CBC Complete blood cell count

CD4 T cells Helper T cells (T_h); have a surface marker designated CD4

CD8 T cells T cells with a surface marker designated CD8; include cytotoxic T cells

CF Cystic fibrosis

CHD Coronary heart disease

CNS Central nervous system

CO Cardiac output

COPD Chronic obstructive pulmonary disease

CP Creatine phosphate

CPR Cardiopulmonary resuscitation

C-section Cesarean section

CSF Cerebrospinal fluid

CT scan Scan generated by computed tomography

CVA Cerebrovascular accident

CVS Cardiovascular system; also, chorionic villus sampling

DNA Deoxyribonucleic acid

DNR Do not resuscitate

DX Diagnosis

EBV Epstein-Barr virus

ECF Extracellular fluid

EEG Electroencephalogram

EKG (ECG) Electrocardiogram

EM Electron microscope or micrograph

EPSP Excitatory postsynaptic potential (of a neuron)

ER Endoplasmic reticulum

Factor VIII Blood-clotting factor (absent in hemophiliacs)

FAD/FADH$_2$ Flavin adenine dinucleotide (oxidized and reduced forms, respectively)

FSH Follicle-stimulating hormone

G Guanine

GABA Gamma-aminobutyric acid

GH Growth hormone (somatotropin)

GI Gastrointestinal

GnRH Gonadotropin-releasing hormone

G protein Cell signaling molecule that requires GTP

GTP Guanosine triphosphate

Hb Hemoglobin

hCG Human chorionic gonadotropin

Hct Hematocrit

HD Huntington disease

HDL High-density lipoprotein
hGH Human growth hormone
HIV Human immunodeficiency virus
HLA Human leukocyte antigen
HPV Human papilloma virus
IBD Inflammatory bowel disease
Ig Immunoglobulin, as in IgA, IgG, etc.
IGF Insulin-like growth factor
IM Intramuscular
IPSP Inhibitory postsynaptic potential
IUD Intrauterine device
IV Intravenous
LA Left atrium
LDH Lactic dehydrogenase enzyme
LDL Low-density lipoprotein
LH Luteinizing hormone
LM Light microscope or micrograph
LV Left ventricle
MAO Monoamine oxidase
MG Myasthenia gravis
MHC Major histocompatibility complex
MI Myocardial infarction
mm Hg Millimeters of mercury
MRI Magnetic resonance imaging
mRNA Messenger RNA
mtDNA Mitochondrial DNA
n, 2n The chromosome number of a gamete and of a zygote, respectively
NAD$^+$/NADH Nicotinamide adenine dinucleotide (oxidized and reduced forms, respectively)
NADP$^+$/NADPH Nicotinamide adenine dinucleotide phosphate (oxidized and reduced forms, respectively)
NK cell Natural killer cell
NO Nitric oxide
P53 A tumor suppressor gene
PET Positron emission tomography
PG Prostaglandin
PID Pelvic inflammatory disease
PKU Phenylketonuria
PMS Premenstrual syndrome

PNS Peripheral nervous system
PSA Prostate-specific antigen
PT Prothrombin time
PTH Parathyroid hormone
RA Right atrium
RAS Reticular activating system
RBC Red blood cell (erythrocyte)
RDA Recommended daily allowance
REM sleep Rapid eye movement sleep
Rh factors Red blood cell antigens first identified in Rhesus monkeys
RNA Ribonucleic acid
rRNA Ribosomal RNA
RV Right ventricle
RX Prescription
SA node Sinoatrial node (of heart)
SCID Severe combined immune deficiency
SEM Scanning electron microscope or micrograph
SIDS Sudden infant death syndrome
STD Sexually transmitted disease
SV Stroke volume
T Thymine
T$_3$ Triiodothyronine (a thyroid hormone)
T$_4$ Thyroxine (a thyroid hormone)
TCR T cell antigen receptor
TEM Transmission electron microscope or micrograph
TIA Transitory ischemic attack
T lymphocyte or T cell Lymphocyte responsible for cell-mediated immunity
T$_c$ lymphocyte Cytotoxic T cell
T$_h$ lymphocyte Helper T cell
Tm Tubular transport maximum
TMJ Temporomandibular joint
TNF Tumor necrosis factor
tRNA Transfer RNA
TSH Thyroid-stimulating hormone
U Uracil
UA Urinalysis
UV light Ultraviolet light
WBC White blood cell (leukocyte)

Glossary

abdomen (**ab′**-doe-men) The region of the body between the diaphragm and the pelvis.

abdominal (ab-**dom′**-ih-nal) **cavity** The superior part of the abdominopelvic cavity containing the liver, gallbladder, spleen, stomach, pancreas, small intestine, and part of the large intestine.

abdominopelvic (ab-dom′-ih-no-**pel′**-vic) **cavity** The lower part of the ventral body cavity below the thoracic cavity.

abduction (ab-**duk′**-shun) A movement whereby a body part is drawn away from the main body axis or the axis of a limb.

ABO blood types A system of categorizing blood, based on the presence or absence of specific antigens on the plasma membranes of red blood cells.

abortion (ah-**bor′**-shun) Expulsion of an embryo or fetus before it is capable of surviving outside the uterus.

absorption (ab-**sorp′**-shun) The passage of material into or through a cell or tissue, as in the movement of digested nutrients from the gastrointestinal tract into the blood or lymph.

accommodation The ability to change the curvature of the lens to clearly focus on objects at various distances.

acetylcholine (as′-eh-til-**koe′**-leen) A neurotransmitter released by cholinergic nerves, such as those stimulating skeletal muscle contraction.

Achilles′ (ah-**kil′**-eez) **tendon** The tendon of the gastrocnemius and soleus muscle that inserts on the calcaneus (heel bone).

acid (**as′**-id) A substance that is a hydrogen ion (proton) donor; dissociates in solution to produce hydrogen ions and some type of anion.

acquired immunodeficiency syndrome (AIDS) A serious disease caused by the human immunodeficiency virus (HIV) in which a deficiency develops in helper T cells.

acromegaly (ak′-roe-**meg′**-ah-lee) A condition resulting from hypersecretion of growth hormone in the adult; characterized by enlarged bones in the extremities and face along with the enlargement of other tissues.

actin (**ak′**-tin) A contractile protein found in the thin filaments within a muscle cell.

actin filaments Thin filaments composed mainly of the protein *actin;* actin and myosin filaments make up the myofibrils of muscle fibers.

action potential An electrical signal that results from depolarization of the plasma membrane in a neuron or muscle cell; also called a *nerve* or *muscle impulse.*

active immunity An acquired immunity resulting from the production of antibodies in response to exposure to antigens.

active transport The movement of substances through cell membranes against concentration gradients. Active transport requires energy expenditure.

acute (a-**kyoot′**) Having a short and relatively severe course; not chronic.

Adam′s apple The thyroid cartilage of the larynx. In males, it is pronounced because of enlargement caused by testosterone.

adduction (ad-**duk′**-shun) A movement whereby a body part is drawn toward the main body axis or the axis of a limb.

adenosine triphosphate (a-**den′**-oh-seen try-**fos′**-fate) **(ATP)** See *ATP.*

adipose tissue A type of connective tissue in which fat is stored.

adrenal cortex (ah-**dree′**-nal **kore′**-tekz) The outer part of the adrenal gland; it has three zones, each producing different hormones.

adrenal (ah-**dree**′-nal) **glands** Paired endocrine glands, one located just superior to each kidney. They are also known as the *suprarenal glands.*

adrenal medulla (ah-**dree**′-nal meh-**dul**′-ah) The inner part of the adrenal gland that secretes catecholamines (epinephrine and norepinephrine) in response to sympathetic stimulation.

adrenergic (ad-ren-**er**′-jik) **neuron** A neuron that releases norepinephrine.

adrenocorticotropic (ad-ree′-no-kore-ti-kow-**trope**′-ik) **hormone (ACTH)** A hormone produced by the anterior lobe of the pituitary gland; stimulates the adrenal cortex to release hormones.

adventitia (ad′-ven-**tish**′-eah) The outermost layer or covering of an organ or structure.

aerobic (air-**oh**′-bik) Requiring molecular oxygen.

afferent (**af**′-er-ent) Indicates movement *toward* a structure. Compare with *efferent.*

afferent arteriole (ar-**teer**′-ee-ole) Blood vessel within the kidney that carries blood to the glomerulus.

afferent neuron A nerve cell that carries information toward the central nervous system; also called a *sensory neuron.*

afterbirth The separated placenta and membranes expelled from the uterus after childbirth.

agglutination (a-glue′-tin-**nay**′-shun) The aggregation of particles into masses or clumps, especially in reference to microbes and blood cells.

albumin (al-**byou**′-min) The smallest and most abundant of the plasma proteins.

aldosterone (al-**dos**′-ter-own) The principal mineralocorticoid hormone of the adrenal cortex. It increases sodium reabsorption in the kidneys and also enhances water reabsorption and potassium excretion.

alimentary (al′-ih-**men**′-tah-ree) **canal** The digestive tract.

alkaline (**al**′-kuh-line) Refers to a solution containing more hydroxyl ions than hydrogen ions, resulting in a pH greater than 7.

allergen (**al**′-er-jen) An antigen that produces an allergic reaction.

allergy (**al**′-er-jee) A hypersensitivity of the immune system to some substance in the environment; manifested, for example, as hay fever, skin rash, asthma, or food allergies.

all-or-none response The phenomenon by which a stimulus produces maximal response or no response at all. If the stimulus is subthreshold, no response occurs. If the stimulus is threshold or greater, a maximal response occurs.

alpha (**al**′-fah) **cell** Endocrine cells of the islets of Langerhans of the pancreas; produce the hormone *glucagon.*

alveolar (al-**vee**′-oh-lar) **gland** A type of gland characterized by a small, hollow sac.

alveolus (al-**vee**′-oh-lus) A small, hollow sac. (1) An air sac of the lung through which gas exchange with the blood takes place. (2) A milk-secreting sac of a mammary gland. (Plural—*alveoli.*)

amino (ah-**mee**′-no) **acid** An organic acid possessing both an amine ($-NH_2$) and a carboxyl ($-COOH$) group. Amino acids are the basic units of proteins.

amnion (**am**′-nee-on) An extraembryonic membrane that forms a fluid-filled sac for the protection of the developing embryo.

amphiarthrosis (am′-fee-ar-**throw**′-sis) Joint showing slight movement; the joints between vertebrae.

amygdala (ah-**mig**′-duh-lah) Part of the limbic system; filters incoming sensory information and evaluates its importance in terms of emotional needs and survival.

anabolism (a-**nab**′-o-lizm) The synthesizing or building-up part of metabolism in which small molecules combine to form larger ones.

anaerobic (an-air-**oh**′-bik) Metabolizing in the absence of oxygen.

anal canal The terminal end of the rectum.

anaphase (**an**′-ah-faze) Third stage of mitosis in which the chromatids of each chromosome separate at their centromeres and the two sets of chromosomes move to opposite poles.

anaphylaxis (an′-ah-fih-**lak**′-sis) An acute, serious allergic reaction.

anastomosis (ah-nas′-tow-**mow**′-sis) The union or communication of blood vessels, nerves, or lymphatics.

anatomical (an′-ah-**tom**′-ih-kal) **position** The positioning of the body for descriptive purposes in which the body stands erect, facing the viewer, with upper limbs at sides and palms facing anteriorly.

anatomy (ah-**nat**′-ah-me) The study of the structures of the body and their relationships.

androgen (**an**′-drow-jen) A male hormone, such as testosterone; stimulates or produces male characteristics.

anemia (ah-**nee**′-me-ah) A deficiency of hemoglobin or number of red blood cells.

angiotensin (an-jee-o-**ten**′-sin) **II** A hormone that acts as a powerful vasoconstrictor; important in regulating blood pressure.

anion (**an**′-eye-on) A negatively charged ion such as Cl⁻.

antagonist (an-**tag**′-o-nist) A muscle opposing the action of another muscle, its agonist.

anterior (an-**tee**′-ree-or) Located in front of, or nearer to the front of, the body. Anterior is also ventral or at the belly side.

anterior root The ventral root of a spinal nerve; consists of motor fibers.

antibiotic (an′-ti-bye-**ot**′-ik) A chemical substance produced by a microbe that inhibits growth or kills other microorganisms.

antibody (**an**′-ti-bod′-ee) A specific protein produced by plasma cells (B cells) in response to a specific antigen; recognizes and binds to a specific antigen. Also called an *immunoglobulin.*

antibody-mediated immunity A specific immune response in which specific B cells are activated when they come into contact with specific antigens. Activated B cells multiply and give rise to plasma cells that secrete specific antibodies.

antidiuretic (an′-tie-die-you-**ret**′-ik) A substance that decreases or inhibits the formation of urine.

antidiuretic hormone (ADH) A hormone produced in the hypothalamus and stored in the posterior pituitary. ADH increases water reabsorption in the kidneys.

antigen (**an**′-tih-jen) A molecule (usually a protein) that can be specifically recognized as foreign by cells of the immune system.

antihistamine (an′-ti-**his**′-tah-min) A drug that blocks the effects of histamine.

anus (**ay**′-nus) The distal end and outlet of the digestive tract.

aorta (ay-**or**′-tah) The largest and main systemic artery of the body. It arises from the left ventricle and branches to distribute blood to all parts of the body.

apoptosis (ap′-uh-**toe**′-sis) Programmed cell death; a normal part of development and maintenance.

aqueous humor (**ak**′-wee-us **hyou**′-mor) A serous fluid within the anterior cavity of the eye.

arachnoid (ah-**rak**′-noyd) **membrane** The middle meninx of the central nervous system located between the dura mater and the pia mater.

areola (ah-**ree**′-o-lah) The dark, pigmented area surrounding the nipple of the mammary gland.

arm The region of the upper limb between the shoulder and the elbow.

arrector pili (a-**rek**′-tor **pi**′-lee) The smooth muscle associated with hairs whose contraction causes the hair to assume a more vertical position. The contraction of the arrector pili results in "goose bumps."

arteriole (ar-**teer**′-ee-ole) A small artery that carries blood to capillaries. Vasoconstriction and vasodilation of arterioles help regulate blood pressure and blood distribution to the tissues.

artery (**ar**′-ter-ee) A thick-walled blood vessel that carries blood away from the heart.

arthritis (ar-**thrye**′-tis) The inflammation of a joint.

ascending colon (**koe**′-lon) The part of the large intestine that extends from the cecum upward to the lower border of the liver. The ascending colon is on the right side of the abdomen.

association areas Cortical areas of the cerebrum that link sensory and motor areas; association areas are responsible for thought, learning, memory, and judgment.

association neuron A nerve cell located within the central nervous system that transmits information between sensory and motor neurons. It is also called an *interneuron.*

asthma (**az**′-muh) A disease characterized by airway constriction, often leading to difficult breathing or dyspnea.

astigmatism (ah-**stig**′-mah-tizm) A defect of vision resulting from irregularity in the curvature of the cornea or lens.

atherosclerosis (ath′-er-o-skleh-**roe**′-sis) A progressive disease in which smooth muscle cells and lipid deposits accumulate in the inner lining of arteries, leading to decreased arterial diameters and impairment of circulation.

atom The smallest particle of an element with the chemical properties of that element.

ATP Abbreviation for adenosine triphosphate. The energy currency of the cell. A chemical compound used to transfer energy from those biochemical reactions that yield energy to those that require it.

atrioventricular (a′-tree-oh-ven-**trik**′-u-lar) **node** The part of the cardiac conduction system within the right atrium near the opening of the coronary sinus.

atrioventricular valve A valve between each atrium and its ventricle that prevents backflow of blood.

atrium (**ay**′-tree-um) (of heart) One of two superior chambers of the heart that receives blood from veins.

auditory ossicle (**aw**′-di-toe′-ree **os**′-sih-kul) One of the three bones of the middle ear.

auditory tube The tube connecting the middle ear cavity with the nasopharynx; also called the *eustachian tube.*

auricle (**aw**′-reh-kle) (1) A small, muscular pouch of the atria of the heart. (2) The pinna, or flap, of the outer ear.

autoimmune (aw′-tow-ih-**mune**′) **disease** A disease in which the body produces antibodies against its own cells or tissues.

autonomic division (of the nervous system) The portion of the peripheral nervous system that controls the visceral functions of the body by innervating smooth muscle, cardiac muscle, or glands.

autonomic ganglion (aw′-toe-**nom**′-ik **gang**′-lee-on) A collection of cell bodies of either the sympathetic or parasympathetic nervous systems located outside of the central nervous system.

axilla (ak-**sil**′-ah) The armpit area of the shoulder region of the body.

axon (**ak**′-son) The long, tubular extension of a neuron that transmits nerve impulses away from the cell body.

ball-and-socket joint The type of synovial joint in which the rounded head of one bone moves within a fossa or cup-shaped depression of another.

baroreceptor (bar′-o-re-**sep**′-tor) Receptor found within certain blood vessels that is stimulated by changes in blood pressure.

basal ganglia (**bay**′-sal **gang**′-lee-ah) The cerebral nuclei located deep within the white matter of the cerebrum that play an important role in movement.

basal metabolic rate (BMR) The rate of metabolism measured under standard or basal conditions.

base A substance which when dissolved in water produces a pH greater than 7. Most bases yield hydroxyl ions (OH⁻) when dissolved in water. A base is also referred to as an *alkali.*

basophil (**bay′**-so-fil) A type of white blood cell (leukocyte), stained by basic dyes, that is involved in allergic and inflammatory reactions.

B cell B lymphocyte. A type of white blood cell responsible for antibody-mediated immunity. When stimulated, B cells differentiate to become plasma cells that produce antibodies.

belly (1) The bulge in the middle of a spindle-shaped muscle. (2) The abdomen.

benign (be-**nine′**) Refers to a tumor that is not malignant.

beta (**bay′**-tah) **cell** A cell in the islets of Langerhans of the pancreas that produces insulin.

beta receptor A receptor on visceral effectors innervated by postganglionic fibers of the sympathetic nervous system.

bicuspid (bi-**kus′**-pid) **valve** The left atrioventricular valve separating the left atrium from the left ventricle. It is also known as the *mitral valve.*

bilateral (bye-**lat′**-er-al) Referring to the two sides of the body.

bile (byl) The greenish fluid secreted by the liver containing bile salts and bile pigments. Bile salts emulsify fats in the small intestine.

bilirubin (bil′-ee-**roo′**-bin) A red bile pigment that gives feces their characteristic brown color. Bilirubin is produced by the breakdown of hemoglobin in the liver.

blind spot The area of the retina in which the optic nerve ends and which lacks photoreceptors.

blood The fluid circulating within the heart and blood vessels that provides the main transport of substances throughout the body.

blood-brain barrier The barrier separating the blood from the brain; prevents many substances from entering the cerebrospinal fluid from the blood.

blood pressure The force exerted by the blood against the inner walls of the blood vessels.

blood vessel A tube transporting blood in a circulatory system. The major blood vessels are the arteries, capillaries, and veins.

body cavity A space of the body containing organs.

bolus (**bow′**-lus) A rounded mass of food that has been moistened for swallowing.

bone A hard type of connective tissue containing calcium salts that makes up most of the skeletal system.

bony labyrinth Cavities within the temporal bone forming the chambers of the inner ear.

Bowman's capsule The double-walled, cuplike sac of cells that surrounds the glomerulus of each nephron.

bradycardia (brad′-ee-**kar′**-dee-ah) A slow heart rate of less than 60 beats per minute.

brain A concentration of nervous tissue in the cranial cavity that with the spinal cord makes up the central nervous system.

brainstem The elongated part of the brain located superior to the spinal cord; contains the medulla, pons, and midbrain.

Broca's (**broe′**-kaz) **area** A part of the premotor area of the cerebrum involved with directing the formation of words.

bronchiole (**brong′**-kee-ole) A small branch of a tertiary bronchus whose terminal branches (respiratory bronchioles) divide into alveolar ducts.

bronchitis (brong-**kye′**-tis) An inflammation of the bronchi.

buccal (**buk′**-al) Pertaining to the mouth or the cheek area.

buffer See *chemical buffer.*

bulbourethral (bul-bow-you-**ree′**-thral) **gland** One of two glands located inferior to the prostate gland of the male; secretes an alkaline solution into the urethra during sexual excitation. Also called *Cowper's gland.*

bursa (**bur′**-sah) A small sac lined with synovial membrane and filled with fluid interposed between nearby body parts that move in relation to each other.

bursitis (bur-**sye′**-tis) An inflammation of the bursa.

buttocks (**but′**-okz) A pair of prominences of the lower back formed by the gluteal muscles.

calcaneus (kal-**kay′**-nee-us) The heel bone.

calcitonin (kal′-sih-**tow′**-nin) A thyroid hormone that lowers calcium and phosphate levels in the blood by stimulating calcium absorption by bone and inhibiting the breakdown of bone.

calorie (**kal′**-o-ree) A unit of heat that is used in the study of metabolism and is defined as the amount of heat required to raise the temperature of 1 gram of water 1 degree Celsius.

calyx (**kay′**-liks) A cuplike extension of the renal pelvis of the kidney. (Plural—*calyces.*)

cancer (**kan′**-ser) A group of diseases in which cells become abnormal and multiply in an unregulated way, forming malignant tumors; cancer cells are able to invade other tissues and may spread (metastasize) to distant parts of the body.

canine (**kay′**-nine) The tooth between the incisors and the premolars in each quadrant of teeth.

capillary (**kap′**-ih-lar-ee) Small blood vessel that permits exchanges to take place between the blood and body tissues.

carbohydrate (kar-bow-**hi′**-drate) An organic compound (e.g., sugar, starch) composed of carbon, hydrogen, and oxygen in which the numbers of hydrogen and oxygen atoms are in approximately 2:1 proportion.

cardiac (**kar′**-dee-ak) Pertaining to the heart.

cardiac cycle The sequence of events occurring during one complete heartbeat.

cardiac muscle One of three types of muscle. Cardiac muscle is located within the heart.

cardiac output The volume of blood pumped by one ventricle in one minute. Cardiac output averages about 5 L/min at rest.

cartilage (**kar′**-tih-lij) A specialized fibrous connective tissue that forms most of the temporary skeleton of the embryo. It also serves as the skeletal tissue for certain regions of the body such as the external ear and the tip of the nose.

castration (cas-**tray′**-shun) Surgical removal of the gonads, especially the testes.

catabolism (kah-**tab′**-o-lizm) The breaking-down phase of metabolism in which complex substances are broken down into simpler compounds with the release of energy.

catecholamine (kat′-eh-**kole′**-ah-mean) A class of chemical compounds that includes the neurotransmitters *norepinephrine, serotonin,* and *dopamine.*

cation (**kat′**-eye-on) A positively charged ion.

cecum (**see′**-kum) The blind sac that marks the first part of the large intestine.

cell The basic structural and functional unit of the body, consisting of organelles bounded by a plasma membrane; cells are typically microscopic in size.

cell body The part of a neuron containing the nucleus; most of the materials needed by the neuron are produced there.

cell-mediated immunity A specific immune response in which specific T cells are activated when they come into contact with specific antigens. Activated T cells give rise to a clone of cells; some differentiate to become killer T cells that migrate to the site of infection and kill pathogens. Also called *cellular immunity.*

cellular respiration The process by which cells capture energy from nutrients; one aspect of respiration.

cementum (se-**men′**-tum) A bonelike connective tissue forming the outer layer of the root of a tooth; attaches the root to the jaw bones.

central canal The circular canal running the length of the spinal cord.

central nervous system (CNS) The subdivision of the nervous system containing the brain and the spinal cord.

cephalic (seh-**fal′**-ik) Pertaining to, or directionally close to, the head.

cerebellum (ser-eh-**bel′**-um) The deeply convoluted subdivision of the brain lying beneath the cerebrum that is concerned with the coordination of muscular movements. It is part of the metencephalon.

cerebral aqueduct (seh-**ree′**-bral **ah′**-kweh-duct) The channel running through the midbrain that connects the third and fourth ventricles. It is also called the *aqueduct of Sylvius.*

cerebral cortex The outer part of the cerebrum, composed of gray matter and consisting mainly of nerve cell bodies.

cerebrospinal (seh-ree′-broe-**spy′**-nal) **fluid (CSF)** A clear fluid that circulates within the cavities of the central nervous system and within the subarachnoid space.

cerebrovascular (se-ree′-broe-**vas′**-kyou-lar) **accident (CVA)** Disorders of the blood vessels supplying the brain that result in damage to neural tissues of the brain. Also called a *stroke.*

cerebrum (seh-**ree′**-brum) The largest subdivision of the brain; has centers for learning, voluntary movement, and the interpretation of sensation.

cervical (**ser′**-vih-kul) Pertaining to the neck or cervix.

cervical plexus (**plek′**-sus) A network of the branches of anterior rami of cervical nerves C1-C4 that mainly supplies neck structures.

cervix (**ser′**-viks) Neck or a constricted area of an organ, as in the cervix of the uterus.

chemical buffer (**buf′**-er) A substance that minimizes changes in pH.

chemoreceptors (kee′-mow-ree-**sep′**-tors) Receptors that are sensitive to specific chemicals; for example, chemoreceptors in the medulla and in the walls of the aorta and carotid arteries are sensitive to changes in arterial carbon dioxide concentration.

chiasma (kye-**az′**-mah) An X-shaped crossing, as in the optic chiasma formed by the crossing of the optic nerves.

cholesterol (koe-**les′**-te-rol) The steroid that is a component of cell membranes and is used in the production of steroid hormones and bile salts.

cholinergic (koe′-lin-**er′**-jik) **neuron** A neuron that releases acetylcholine as its neurotransmitter.

cholinesterase (koe′-lin-**es′**-ter-ayz) An enzyme that breaks down acetylcholine.

chondrocyte (**kon′**-droe-site) A mature cartilage cell.

chordae tendineae (**kor′**-dee **ten′**-di-nee) Cords connecting the cardiac papillary muscles with the atrioventricular valves.

choroid (**koe′**-royd) The black, vascular coat of the eye between the sclera and the retina.

choroid plexus Specialized capillary network projecting from the pia mater into the ventricles of the brain; produces cerebrospinal fluid.

chromosomes (**krow′**-ma-sowms) The 46 discrete, rod-shaped bodies in the nucleus of a cell; contain the genes.

chronic (**kron′**-ik) Of a long duration or recurring frequently, as in a chronic disease.

chyme (kime) The semifluid mixture of partially digested food and gastric juices.

cilia (**sil′**-ee-a) Threadlike cellular organelles that project from the surface of some cells and by their movement can propel a stream of fluid.

ciliary muscle Smooth muscle of the ciliary body of the eye; functions in visual accommodation.

circadian (sir-**kay′**-dee-un) **rhythm** An internal rhythm that approximates the 24-hour day (sleep-wake) cycle.

circle of Willis A circular anastomosis at the base of the brain.

circumcision (ser′-kum-**sizh′**-un) Removal of the prepuce (foreskin) of the penis.

circumduction (ser′-kum-**duk**′-shun) The movement of a limb in such a manner that its distal part describes a circle.

climax The time of greatest intensity, as in sexual response or the course of a disease.

clitoris (**klit**′-oh-ris) A small erectile organ located at the top of the vulva that serves as the center of sexual sensation in the female.

clot A semisolid mass. A blood clot results from a cascade of biochemical reactions ending in the conversion of fibrinogen into fibrin.

coccyx (**kok**′-six) The bone formed by the fusion of the four coccygeal vertebrae at the inferior end of the vertebral column.

cochlea (**kok**′-lee-ah) The spiral-shaped portion of the inner ear that contains the auditory receptors (organs of Corti).

coenzyme A small, nonprotein molecule essential for an enzyme to operate.

coitus (**koe**′-i-tus) The act of copulation or sexual intercourse in which the penis is inserted into the vagina.

collagen (**kol**′-a-jen) A fibrous protein found in collagen fibers that is the principal support of many connective tissues.

colon (**koe**′-lon) The part of the large intestine consisting of the ascending, transverse, descending, and sigmoid regions.

color blindness An abnormal perception of one or more colors caused by the absence of one or more of the photopigments in the cones.

commissure (**kom**′-i-shyour) A joining site between corresponding parts, as in the eyelids or lips.

common bile duct The duct formed by the union of the common hepatic duct with the cystic duct; conducts bile to the duodenum.

compact bone Dense skeletal tissue that has tightly joined layers.

complement A group of proteins in plasma and other body fluids activated by an antigen-antibody complex; these proteins destroy pathogens both directly and indirectly.

compound In chemistry, a substance composed of two or more elements combined in a fixed ratio.

concentration gradient A difference in the concentration of a substance from one point to another, for example, across a cell membrane.

conception The process of fertilization and the subsequent establishment of pregnancy.

conchae (**kong**′-kee) Skull bones with a shell-like shape.

condyle (**kon**′-dil) A rounded projection on a bone.

cones The photoreceptors of the retina of the eye involved in color vision.

congenital (kon-**jen**′-i-tal) Refers to a condition existing before or at birth.

conjunctiva (kon′-junk-**tie**′-vah) The membrane covering the eyeball and eyelids.

connective tissue A diverse group of tissues that support and protect the organs of the body and hold body parts together; characterized by a large proportion of intercellular substance through which its cells are scattered.

contralateral (kon′-trah-**lat**′-er-al) Referring to the opposite side of the body or opposite side of a body part.

cornea (**kor**′-nee-ah) The transparent anterior portion of the outer covering of the eyeball.

coronal (koe-**roe**′-nal) **plane** A plane running vertical to the ground and dividing the body into anterior and posterior parts. Also called a *frontal plane*.

coronary (**kor**′-o-na-ree) Pertaining to the heart.

coronary artery disease A disorder in which the cardiac muscle receives an inadequate amount of blood because its blood supply is disrupted.

coronary sinus A large vein on the posterior side of the heart that drains smaller coronary veins and empties into the right atrium.

corpus callosum (kal-**loe**′-sum) A large bundle of nerve fibers that connects the two cerebral hemispheres.

corpus luteum (**loo**′-tee-um) The yellow endocrine body in the ovary that develops from the ruptured follicle after ovulation; secretes progesterone and estrogens.

cortex (**kor**′-teks) The outer portion of an organ, as in the adrenal cortex or outer part of the cerebrum.

cortisol (**kor**′-ti-sol) Principal glucocorticoid secreted by the adrenal cortex.

costal cartilage (**kos**′-tal **kar**′-tih-lij) The hyaline cartilage forming the articulation of the first 10 ribs to the sternum or each other.

cranial nerves The 12 pairs of nerves emerging from the brain that transmit information directly between certain sensory receptors and the brain and between the brain and certain effectors.

cranium (**kray**′-nee-um) The bones of the skull case, including the frontal, parietal, temporal, occipital, ethmoid, and sphenoid bones.

creatine phosphate An intermediate energy-transfer compound found mainly in muscles.

cretinism (**kree**′-tin-izm) A condition in which a person is dwarfed and mentally retarded by severe deficiency of thyroid hormones during childhood.

Cushing's syndrome A condition caused by abnormally large amounts of glucocorticoids; characterized by edema, an abnormal deposition of fat to the face and trunk, and an increased susceptibility to infection.

cutaneous (kyou-**tay**′-nee-us) Referring to the skin.

cytokines (**sigh**′-tow-kines) Signaling proteins that regulate interactions between cells in the immune system. Important groups include interferons and interleukins.

cytoskeleton Network of protein fibers in the cell; provides structural support and plays a role in cell movement.

deamination (dee-am-ih-**na**′-shun) The removal of an amino group from an amino acid.

decibel (**des′**-i-bel) A unit of measurement of sound intensity.

deciduous (dee-**sid′**-you-us) **teeth** The primary teeth or the first set of human dentition. Also called the *milk teeth* or *baby teeth.*

dehydration (dee-hi-**dray′**-shun) A condition caused by excessive water loss from the body or its parts.

dendrite (**den′**-drite) A short branch of a neuron that receives nerve impulses and conducts them to the cell body.

dentin (**den′**-tin) The layer forming the body of the tooth; lies under the enamel and cementum and encloses the pulp.

depolarization (dee-poe′-lar-i-**zay′**-shun) A decrease in the charge difference across a plasma membrane; may result in an action potential in a neuron or muscle cell.

dermis (**der′**-mis) The thick layer of skin composed of irregular, dense connective tissue that is located beneath the epidermis.

descending colon The section of the large intestine located between the transverse colon and sigmoid colon.

diabetes insipidus (die-ah-**be′**-teez in-**sip′**-i-dus) A disease resulting from insufficiency of antidiuretic hormone (ADH); characterized by the production of large volumes of urine.

diabetes mellitus (**mel′**-ih-tus) A disease resulting from insulin deficiency or insulin resistance; results in excessive amount of glucose in the blood and decreased use of glucose by cells.

dialysis (die-**al′**-ih-sis) The diffusion of solutes through a selectively permeable membrane, resulting in separation of solutes.

diaphragm (**die′**-ah-fram) The muscle separating the thoracic cavity from the abdominal cavity; contracts during inspiration, expanding the chest cavity.

diaphysis (dye-**af′**-ih-sis) The shaft of a long bone.

diarthroses (dye-ar-**throw′**-seez) Joint articulations in which the bones are freely movable. Also called *synovial joints.*

diastole (dye-**as′**-tow′-lee) The time during the cardiac cycle in which the ventricles are relaxing.

diencephalon (dye′-en-**sef′**-ah-lon) The part of the prosencephalon (forebrain) of the brain that consists primarily of the thalamus and the hypothalamus.

diffusion (dif-**you′**-zhun) The net movement of particles (atoms, molecules, or ions) from a region of higher concentration to a region of lower concentration, resulting from random motion; results in the tendency of a molecular mixture to attain a uniform composition throughout.

digestion (di-**jes′**-chun) The process of mechanical or chemical breakdown of food into molecules small enough to be absorbed.

digestive system The digestive tract and the accessory digestive structures.

distal (**dis′**-tal) Farther from the midline or point of attachment to the trunk.

diuretic (dye-you-**ret′**-ik) A substance that inhibits the reabsorption of water and thus increases urine output.

DNA Abbreviation for *deoxyribonucleic acid.* The basic storage molecule for genetic information that is coded in specific sequences of its component nucleotides. DNA is a nucleic acid whose pentose sugar is deoxyribose and whose bases are adenine, thymine, guanine, and cytosine.

dopamine (**doe′**-pah-meen) A neurotransmitter.

duodenum (do′-o-**dee′**-num) The first portion of the small intestine.

dura mater (**doo′**-rah **may′**-ter) The outermost of the meninges of the central nervous system.

edema (e-**dee′**-mah) An abnormal accumulation of fluid in the tissues.

effectors (ee-**fek′**-tors) Muscles and glands.

efferent (**ef′**-er-ent) Indicates movement away from a structure.

efferent arteriole The blood vessel taking blood away from the glomerulus.

ejaculation (e-jak-yoo-**lay′**-shun) The reflex expulsion of semen from the penis.

ejaculatory (e-**jak′**-yoo-lah-toe′-ree) **duct** The tube transporting sperm from the vas deferens to the urethra.

electrocardiogram (e-lek′-trow-**kar′**-dee-o-gram) **(ECG or EKG)** A graphic recording of the electrical changes occurring during the cardiac cycle.

electroencephalogram (e-lek′-trow-en-**sef′**-ah-loe-gram) **(EEG)** A graphic recording of the electrical changes associated with the activity of the cerebral cortex.

electrolyte (ee-**lek′**-trow-lite) A compound, such as a salt, that dissociates into ions when dissolved in water.

element Any one of the more than 100 pure chemical substances that in combination make up chemical compounds. An element cannot be changed to a simpler substance by a normal chemical reaction.

elimination The ejection of waste products, especially undigested food remnants from the digestive tract.

emphysema (em-fih-**see′**-mah) A disease in which air accumulates in the respiratory passageways because of decreased alveolar elasticity.

emulsification (ee-**mul′**-si-fi-**kay′**-shun) The process of mechanically breaking down large fat droplets into smaller ones.

enamel (e-**nam′**-el) The bony outer covering of the crown of the tooth.

endocardium (en-doe-**kar′**-dee-um) The inner layer of the heart wall, consisting of an endothelial lining resting on connective tissue.

endocrine (**en′**-doe-krin) **gland** A ductless gland that secretes hormones.

endocrinology (en′-doe-kri-**nol′**-o-jee) The study of the endocrine glands and tissues and their hormones.

endogenous (en-**doj′**-e-nus) Produced within the body or the result of internal causes.

endolymph (**en′**-doe-lymf′) The fluid of the membranous labyrinth of the ear.

endometrium (en′-doe-**me′**-tree-um) The mucous membrane lining the uterus.

endomysium (en′-doe-**mis′**-ee-um) The connective tissue covering each muscle cell.

endoneurium (en′-doe-**nyoo′**-ree-um) The connective tissue covering a neuron.

endoplasmic reticulum (en′-doe-**plaz′**-mik reh-**tik′**-yoo-lum) An intracellular system of membranes continuous with the plasma membrane; functions in transporting material through the cell, and in storage, synthesis, and packaging of materials.

endorphins (en-**dor′**-finz) Peptide neurotransmitters released by some neurons in the central nervous system; block pain signals.

endosteum (en-**dos′**-tee-um) The thin layer of connective tissue that lines the marrow cavity of a bone.

endothelium (en′-doe-**thee′**-lee-um) The simple epithelial tissue that lines the cavities of the heart and of the blood and lymphatic vessels.

enkephalin (en-**kef′**-ah-lin) A peptide of the nervous system that affects pain perception.

enzyme (**en′**-zime) An organic catalyst, usually a protein, that promotes or regulates a biochemical reaction.

eosinophil (ee′-o-**sin′**-o-fil) A type of white blood cell with a granular cytoplasm.

epididymis (ep-i-**did′**-ih-mis) A coiled tube that receives sperm from the testes and conveys it to the vas deferens.

epidural (ep′-ih-**doo′**-ral) **space** Space between the dura mater and the surrounding bone.

epiglottis (ep-ih-**glot′**-is) Cartilage guarding the superior opening into the larynx.

epimysium (ep′-ih-**mis′**-ee-um) The fibrous connective tissue that envelops muscles.

epinephrine (ep′-ih-**nef′**-rin) A hormone secreted by the adrenal medulla; its actions are similar to those produced by stimulation of the sympathetic nervous system. Also known as *adrenaline.*

epineurium (ep′-ih-**nyoo′**-ree-um) Outermost connective tissue covering that surrounds a peripheral nerve.

epiphyseal (ep′-ih-**fiz′**-eal) **plate** Cartilage plate separating the epiphysis from the diaphysis in growing long bones.

epiphysis (eh-**pif′**-ih-sis) The end of a long bone. The two epiphyses are connected by the shaft or diaphysis.

epithelial (ep′-ih-**thee′**-lee-uhl) **tissue** The type of tissue that covers body surfaces, lines the hollow organs, and forms glands. Also called *epithelium.*

erection (ee-**rek′**-shun) Engorgement of the spongy erectile tissue of the penis or clitoris, resulting in enlargement and stiffening of the organ.

erythrocyte (eh-**rith′**-row-site) A red blood cell (RBC).

erythropoiesis (eh-rith′-roe-poy-**ee′**-sis) The formation of red blood cells or erythrocytes.

erythropoietin (eh-rith′-row-**poy′**-eh-tin) A hormone that stimulates red blood cell formation.

esophagus (ee-**sof′**-ah-gus) The portion of the digestive tract that connects the pharynx and stomach.

essential amino acids Amino acids that cannot be synthesized by the body in appropriate amounts and therefore need to be included in the diet.

estradiol (es-trah-**die′**-ol) Most potent of the naturally occurring estrogens in humans.

estrogens (**es′**-trow-jens) Female sex hormones produced by the ovaries. Function in the development and maintenance of the female reproductive organs and of secondary sex characteristics.

eustachian (u-**stay′**-kee-an) **tube** The tube connecting the middle ear with the nasopharynx. Also called the *auditory tube.*

eversion (ee-**ver′**-zhun) Movement of the sole of the foot outward or laterally; opposite of inversion.

excretion (eks-**kree′**-shun) Ejection of metabolic waste products from individual cells, tissues, or the body as a whole.

exocrine (**ek′**-so-krin) **gland** A type of gland that secretes its products into ducts that open onto a free surface such as the skin or lining of the digestive tract. Compare with endocrine gland.

expiration (eks-pih-**ray′**-shun) The process of moving air from the lungs into the atmosphere. Also called *exhalation.*

extension A movement that increases the angle between adjoining bones; opposite of flexion.

exteroceptor (eks′-ter-oh-**sep′**-tor) Receptor specialized for receiving stimuli from the external environment, for example, the eyes.

extracellular (eks-trah-**sell′**-you-lar) Outside a cell.

extracellular fluid (ECF) Fluid, such as plasma and interstitial fluid, that is located outside the body's cells.

eyeball The ball-shaped part or globe of the eye.

face Anterior region of the head.

facet (**fas′**-et) Small planar surface on a bone serving as an articular surface for another bone.

fallopian (fal-**low′**-pee-an) **tube** Also called *uterine tube* or *oviduct.* Passageway through which the fertilized ovum reaches the uterine cavity.

fascia (**fash′**-ee-ah) A band or sheet of fibrous tissue that lies beneath the skin or invests muscles and various organs of the body.

fascicle (**fas′**-ih-kul) A small grouping of nerve or muscle fibers surrounded by a connective tissue envelope.

fat A chemical compound composed of fatty acids combined with glycerol. Fat is stored in adipose tissue.

feces (**fee′**-seez) Bodily waste eliminated from the anus.

feedback Mechanism by which a form of output is used as input to exert some degree of control over a specific process. Classified as *positive* and *negative feedback.* Such mechanisms are used by most of the body's systems to maintain homeostasis.

fertilization Union of an ovum and sperm to form a zygote.

fetus (**fee'**-tus) During intrauterine life, the term applied to the new individual starting at the end of the embryonic period; that is, at the beginning of the ninth week after fertilization.

fever (**fee'**-vur) Condition in which the body temperature is elevated above normal. Normal body temperature is 37° C, or 98.6° F.

fibrillation (fih-brih-**lay'**-shun) Contraction of cardiac muscle at an extremely high rate and in an uncoordinated fashion so that little or no blood is actually pumped by the heart.

fibrin (**fye'**-brin) The protein formed by the action of thrombin on fibrinogen during normal clotting of blood.

fibrinogen (fye-**brin'**-o-jen) Plasma protein converted to fibrin when acted on by thrombin.

fibroblast (**fye'**-bro-blast) A connective tissue cell that produces the fibers of the connective tissue.

fibrocartilage A specific type of cartilage containing numerous collagen fibers in its amorphous matrix. Its characteristics are intermediate between those of hyaline cartilage and dense ordinary connective tissue.

fissure (**fish'**-er) A groove or slit between two bones or between other adjacent structures. For example, the longitudinal fissure partially separates the two cerebral hemispheres.

fixator (**fick'**-say-tor) A muscle that by its action tends to fix a body part in position or to limit its range of motion.

flagellum (flah-**jel'**-um) A whiplike cellular organelle used in movement (e.g., by sperm cells).

flexion (**flek'**-shun) A movement that reduces the angle between two adjoining bones; opposite of extension.

follicle-stimulating hormone (FSH) Hormone secreted by the anterior lobe of the pituitary gland; stimulates development of ovarian follicles in the female and spermatogenesis in the male. Also stimulates ovarian follicles to secrete estrogens.

fontanelle (fon-tah-**nell'**) A gap or interval between adjacent bones that is typically covered by membranous tissue until the bones have completed their growth. Examples include the anterior and posterior fontanelles of the fetal skull.

foramen (foe-**ray'**-men) A hole or opening, especially within a bone.

forearm (**four'**-arm) The region of the upper limb located between the elbow proximally and the wrist distally.

fossa (**faw'**-sah) A depression or hollow located below the surface level of a structure or part of a structure; for example, the fossa ovalis of the heart and the subscapular fossa. (Plural—*fossae*.)

fovea (**foe'**-vee-ah) The location of the sharpest vision within the retina.

free radicals Toxic, highly reactive compounds that interfere with normal cell function.

frontal plane Plane or section directed perpendicular to the midsagittal plane of the body and dividing the body into anterior and posterior parts. Also called a *coronal plane* or *section.*

fundus (**fun'**-dus) In a hollow organ, that part located farthest from its opening or exit. Examples include the fundus of the stomach and the fundus of the uterus.

G protein One of a group of proteins involved in transferring signals across the plasma membrane.

gallbladder Small, pouchlike organ located on the visceral aspect of the liver; stores bile.

gamete (**gam'**-eet) A sperm or ovum.

gamma globulins A group of plasma proteins that serve as antibodies.

ganglion (**gang'**-lee-on) A group of nerve cell bodies usually located outside the central nervous system. (Plural—*ganglia.*)

gastric (**gas'**-trik) **glands** Tiny glands located within the wall of the stomach that secrete gastric juice.

gastrin Hormone released by the stomach mucosa in response to stretching or the presence of substances such as caffeine and partially digested proteins. It stimulates the gastric glands to release gastric juice.

gastrointestinal tract (GI tract) That portion of the digestive tract located inferior to the diaphragm.

gene A segment of deoxyribonucleic acid (DNA) that serves as a unit of hereditary information; a segment of a chromosome.

genetics (jeh-**net'**-iks) The branch of biology that is concerned with the study of heredity.

genitalia (jen'-ih-**tal'**-ee-ah) The external reproductive organs of the male and female.

genome (**gee'**-nome) All of the genetic material in a cell or in an individual organism.

gigantism Clinical condition occurring when the anterior pituitary secretes excessive amounts of growth hormone during childhood.

gland A cell, tissue, or organ that discharges a substance used by or eliminated from the body.

glial (**glee'**-ul) **cells** In nervous tissue, cells that support and nourish neurons.

gliding joint Type of synovial joint in which the participating bones possess flat articulating surfaces, allowing only side-to-side and back-and-forth movement. Examples include joints between the carpal bones.

globulin (**glob'**-u-lin) One type of protein in the blood plasma; some are gamma globulins (antibodies).

glomerular (glow-**mer'**-you-lar) **filtration** Process by which plasma containing dissolved substances is filtered out of renal capillaries and into Bowman's capsule.

glomerulus (glow-**mer'**-you-lus) The cluster of capillaries located at the proximal end of each nephron; the glomerulus is surrounded by Bowman's capsule. Also applies to any spherical mass of blood vessels or nerves.

glottis (**glot'**-iss) The space between the vocal cords; the opening into the larynx.

glucagon (**gloo'**-kuh-gon) Hormone released by the islets of the pancreas; increases the concentration of glucose in the blood.

glucocorticoid (gloo'-koe-**kor'**-tih-koyd) **hormones** Class of hormones secreted by the adrenal cortex that help regulate carbohydrate and fat metabolism; the principal glucocorticoid is cortisol.

glucose (**gloo'**-kose) A simple sugar (monosaccharide) important in many metabolic processes; the principal cellular fuel of the body.

glucosuria (gloo'-koe-**soo'**-ree-uh) Condition characterized by the presence of glucose in the urine.

glycogen (**gly'**-ko-jen) A complex polysaccharide that is the main storage carbohydrate; produced from glucose and stored mainly in the liver and in skeletal muscles.

goiter (**goy'**-ter) An abnormal enlargement of the thyroid gland; may be associated with either hyposecretion or hypersecretion of thyroid hormone.

Golgi (**goal'**-jee) **complex** Organelle composed of stacks of cytoplasmic membranes; processes and packages proteins and produces lysosomes. Also called *Golgi apparatus.*

gonad (**go'**-nad) Generalized term for ovary or testis; an organ that produces gametes.

gonadotropic (gon'-ad-oh-**trow'**-pik) **hormone** Hormone involved in the regulation of the ovaries or testes.

graafian follicle A mature ovarian follicle. Normally only one follicle matures each month in the human female.

graft rejection An immune response launched against a transplanted tissue or organ when the host's immune system regards the graft as foreign.

gray matter Nervous tissue in the central nervous system that consists mainly of cell bodies, dendrites, and unmyelinated axons.

greater omentum (oh-**men'**-tum) Large double fold of peritoneum attached to the duodenum, the greater curvature of the stomach, and a portion of the large intestine. It contains large deposits of adipose and lymphatic tissue.

greater vestibular (ves-**tib'**-yoo-lar) **glands** Mucus-secreting glands that open onto each side of the vaginal orifice; help provide lubrication during sexual intercourse. Also called *Bartholin's glands.*

groin (groyn) Depression located at the junction of the anterior aspect of the thigh with the trunk.

growth hormone An anterior pituitary hormone that stimulates body growth. Also called *somatotropin.*

guanine One of the four nitrogen-containing bases of DNA.

gustatory (**gus'**-tah-toe-ree) Refers to the sense of taste.

gyrus (**jye'**-rus) A convolution of the cerebral cortex. (Plural—*gyri.*)

hair follicle (**fol'**-ih-kul) An epithelial ingrowth of the epidermis that moves down into the dermis and surrounds the root of the hair.

hamstrings Group of posterior thigh muscles consisting of the biceps femoris, semitendinosus, and semimembranosus.

hard palate (**pal'**-at) The anterior hard portion of the roof of the mouth; formed by the fusion of portions of the maxillae and palatine bones.

haversian (hah-**ver'**-shun) **system** Structural unit of bone; consists of concentric rings of bone around a central canal that contains blood vessels and nerves. The system has a general spindle-shaped configuration. Also called an *osteon.*

heart murmur Abnormal heart sound resulting from turbulent blood flow of sufficient magnitude to cause vibrations.

heart rate The number of times the heart beats in 1 minute; normally this is about 72 beats per minute in the adult.

heart sounds Characteristic sounds of the heartbeat typically heard with the assistance of a stethoscope. Specific sounds result from closure of specific valves.

helper T cells Differentiated T lymphocytes that play a role in the activation of B lymphocytes.

hematocrit (hee-**mat'**-o-krit) Percentage of red blood cells present in the total blood volume. The determination of this value is a routine clinical blood test.

hemoglobin (hee'-moh-**glo'**-bin) The respiratory pigment of red blood cells that has the property of taking up oxygen or releasing it.

hemorrhage (**hem'**-or-ij) Loss of blood from the blood vessels; typically refers to excessive bleeding.

hepatic (he-**pat'**-ik) Of or pertaining to the liver.

hepatic portal vein Conducts blood to the liver, where it gives rise to an extensive network of hepatic sinusoids from which the liver cells remove excess nutrients; the sinusoids empty into the hepatic vein.

heredity (heh-**red'**-ih-tee) The transfer of biological information from parent to offspring.

hilus (**hi'**-lus) **of kidney** Region on the concave border of the kidney where the ureter and blood vessels are attached.

hippocampus (hip-eh-**kam'**-pus) A part of the limbic system; important in formation and retrieval of memories.

histamine (**his'**-tah-meen) A substance released from a variety of cells in response to injury; produces vasodilation, bronchiolar constriction, and increased permeability of the blood vessels.

histology (his-**tol'**-oh-jee) The study of tissues.

holocrine (**hole'**-oh-krin) **gland** Specific type of gland, such as a sebaceous gland, in which the secretory product consists not only of the excretory product but also of the cell itself.

homeostasis (ho-me-oh-**stay'**-sis) The relatively constant, balanced internal environment of the body; the automatic tendency to maintain this balance, or steady state.

homeostatic mechanisms The self-regulating control systems that maintain homeostasis; many are negative feedback systems.

horizontal plane Anatomical plane that parallels the ground. It divides the body into inferior and superior portions. Also called a *transverse plane.*

hormone (**hoar′**-moan) Chemical messenger that helps regulate the activity of other tissues and organs. Secreted by endocrine tissues and glands.

human chorionic gonadotropin (ko′-ree-**on′**-ik gon′-ah-do-**trow′**-pin) **(hCG)** Hormone secreted by cells of the trophoblast (a membrane surrounding the embryo); signals the corpus luteum that pregnancy has begun.

human immunodeficiency virus (HIV) The retrovirus that causes acquired immunodeficiency syndrome (AIDS).

hyaline (**high′**-ah-line) **cartilage** A clear, glassy cartilage that is present in synovial joints.

hydrogen (**high′**-droe-jen) **bond** A very weak chemical bond formed between an already bonded hydrogen atom and a negatively charged atom such as oxygen or nitrogen.

hydrolysis (high-**drol′**-ih-sis) A chemical reaction involving water in which a large molecule is broken down into smaller products with the addition of water.

hydrophilic (high′-droe-**fil′**-ik) Attracted to water.

hydrophobic (high′-droe-**fo′**-bik) Repelled by water.

hymen (**high′**-men) A fold of membrane that surrounds the external opening of the vagina.

hypertension (high′-pur-**ten′**-shun) Elevated blood pressure.

hypertonic (high′-pur-**ton′**-ik) Having an osmotic pressure or solute concentration greater than that of some other solution with which it is compared.

hyperventilation (high′-pur-ven′-tih-**lay′**-shun) Abnormally rapid, deep breathing.

hypoglycemia (high′-poe-gly-**see′**-me-ah) Reduction in the blood glucose level to below normal.

hypothalamus (high′-poe-**thal′**-ah-mus) A portion of the brain inferior to the thalamus that functions in the regulation of the pituitary gland, the autonomic nervous system, emotional responses, body temperature, water balance, and appetite.

hypothyroidism (high′-poe-**thigh′**-royd-izm) A condition of deficient thyroid gland activity; results in decreased basal metabolic rate, fatigue, and increased sensitivity to cold temperatures.

hypotonic (high′-poe-**ton′**-ik) Referring to a solution whose osmotic pressure or solute content is less than that of a solution to which it is compared.

hypoxia (high-**pock′**-see-ah) Oxygen deficiency.

ileum (**il′**-ee-um) The terminal portion of the small intestine extending from the jejunum to the cecum.

immune (ih-**mune′**) **response** Any reaction designed to defend the body against pathogens or other foreign substances. Nonspecific immune responses are directed against foreign agents in general, whereas specific immune responses are mobilized against particular pathogens.

immunity (ih-**mu′**-nih-tee) The ability to resist and overcome infection or disease; nonsusceptibility to the pathogenic effects of foreign microorganisms or to the toxic effect of antigenic substances.

immunization (im′-yoo-nih-**zay′**-shun) The process of inducing active immunity by the injection of a vaccine.

immunoglobulins (im′-yoo-no-**glob′**-yoo-lins) Antibodies produced by plasma cells in response to antigenic stimulation. The five classes of immunoglobulin are IgG, IgA, IgM, IgD, and IgE.

immunology (im′-yoo-**nol′**-oh-jee) The study of the body's defense mechanisms.

immunosuppression Inhibition of the body's ability to mount an effective immune response; may be caused by certain drugs or exposure to ionizing radiation.

implantation (im-plan-**tay′**-shun) Attachment, penetration, and embedding of the embryo (blastocyst) within the uterine wall, occurring 7 or 8 days after fertilization.

impotence (**im′**-poe-tence) Chronic inability to sustain an erection; often caused by psychological factors.

infancy (**in′**-fan-see) The first 2 years of life; sometimes defined as the period extending from the end of the neonatal period to the time when the individual is able to assume an erect posture and walk.

infarct (**in′**-farkt) A localized area of dead tissue caused by an inadequate blood supply and the resulting oxygen deprivation.

inferior (in-**fee′**-ree-or) Anatomical directional term describing a structure located below or directed downward compared with another structure or part.

inferior vena cava Large vein returning blood to the right atrium from the abdominopelvic structures and the lower limbs.

inflammation (in-flah-**may′**-shun) The response of the body tissues to injury or infection, characterized clinically by heat, swelling, redness, and pain and physiologically by increased blood vessel dilation, capillary permeability, and phagocytosis.

ingestion (in-**jes′**-chun) The process of eating; taking substances into the mouth and swallowing them.

inguinal (**ing′**-gwih-nal) **canal** One of the two passageways that connect the scrotal and abdominal cavities. The testes descend into the scrotum by way of the inguinal canals.

inhalation See *inspiration.*

inner ear Portion of the ear within the temporal bone consisting of the bony labyrinth, the membranous labyrinth, and the cochlea.

insertion (in-**sir′**-shun) The more movable point of attachment of muscle to bone; contrasts with the origin or less movable point of attachment.

inspiration (in′-spur-**ray′**-shun) The process of drawing air into the lungs. Also called *inhalation.*

insulin (**in'**-suh-lin) A hormone released by the beta cells of the islets of Langerhans of the pancreas that facilitates diffusion of glucose into cells.

integration (in-teh-**gray'**-shun) The process of sorting and interpreting neural impulses to determine an appropriate response.

integumentary system A body system consisting of the skin and its glands, nails, and hair.

interatrial (in'-ter-**a'**-tree-uhl) **septum** Wall located between the right and left atria of the heart.

intercellular Between the cells of a tissue.

interferons (in'-ter-**feer'**-ons) Cytokines (signaling molecules) secreted by certain cells when invaded by viruses and certain intracellular pathogens; stimulate other cells to produce antiviral proteins.

interleukins (in ter **loo'** kins) A group of cytokines (signaling molecules) produced mainly by macrophages and lymphocytes.

interneuron A neuron that links sensory and motor neurons within the central nervous system.

interoceptor (in'-ter-o-**sep'**-tor) A sensory receptor that transmits information from the viscera to the central nervous system.

interphase (**in'**-ter-faze) The stage in the life of a cell between mitotic divisions.

interstitial (in'-ter-**stish'**-al) Located between parts or cells.

interstitial cells Cells located in groups between the seminiferous tubules in the testes; produce the male hormone *testosterone.* Also called the *interstitial cells of Leydig.*

interstitial fluid Fluid located between cells or body parts; tissue fluid.

interventricular (in'-ter-ven-**trik'**-yoo-lar) **septum** That portion of the heart wall located between the two ventricles.

intervertebral (in'-ter-**ver'**-teh-brahl) **disk** Fibrocartilaginous disk located between two adjacent vertebral bodies.

intracellular (in-trah-**sell'**-yoo-lar) Located within the cell, as in the case of intracellular fluid.

intramembranous bone formation One type of bone formation in which bone develops in a noncartilage connective tissue. As in endochondral bone formation, the connective tissue is replaced by bone itself.

inversion (in-**ver'**-zhun) Movement of the medial border of the foot such that the sole or planter aspect is directed medially; opposite of eversion.

ion (**eye'**-on) A charged atom or group of atoms. (The electric charge results from gain or loss of electrons.)

ionic bond Type of bond formed when one atom donates an electron to another atom. Also called an *electrovalent bond.*

ionization (eye'-on-eye-**zay'**-shun) The dissociation of a substance (acid, base, salt) in solution into ions.

ipsilateral (ip'-sih-**lat'**-er-al) Pertaining to the same side of the body.

iris (**eye'**-ris) The visible, colored, circular disc of the eye that controls the amount of light entering the eye.

ischemia (is-**kee'**-me-ah) Deficiency of blood to a body part as a result of functional constriction or actual obstruction of a blood vessel.

ischemic heart disease Heart disease resulting from deficiency of blood to the heart muscle; can result from narrowing of a coronary artery.

ischium (**is'**-kee-um) The dorsal and inferior portion of the hip bone.

islets of Langerhans (**eye'**-lits of **Lahng'**-er-hanz) The endocrine portion of the pancreas; alpha cells of the islets release glucagon, and beta cells secrete insulin. These hormones regulate the concentration of glucose in the blood.

isometric (cyc-so-**met'**-rik) Maintaining the same measure or length. In muscle physiology, a contraction in which muscle length does not change much but muscle tension may increase greatly.

isotonic (eye-so-**ton'**-ik) (1) Refers to a solution having the same solute concentration or osmotic pressure as some other solution to which it is compared. Also a solution in which body cells can be immersed without a net flow of water across the semipermeable plasma membrane. (2) A form of muscle contraction in which the muscles shorten and thicken as they contract.

jejunum (jeh-**joo'**-num) The middle portion of the small intestine; located between the duodenum and the ileum.

joint The junction between two or more bones of the skeleton. Also called an *articulation.*

juxtaglomerular (jux'-tah-glow-**mer'**-you-lar) **apparatus** A group of specialized cells in the kidney that secrete renin; helps regulate blood pressure.

keratin (**ker'**-ah-tin) An insoluble protein found in epidermis, hair, nails, and other horny tissues.

ketone (**key'**-tone) **bodies** Compounds such as acetone, beta hydroxybutyric acid, and acetoacetic acid that are produced during fat metabolism.

ketosis (kee-**tow'**-sis) Abnormal condition marked by an elevated concentration of ketone bodies in the body fluids and tissues; a complication of diabetes mellitus and of starvation.

kidney (**kid'**-nee) One of the paired organs of the urinary system responsible for the production of urine. Functions in the regulation of fluid volume and composition.

kilocalorie (**kil'**-oh-kal'-oh-ree) Quantity of heat required to elevate the temperature of 1 kg of water 1° C; the unit of measurement of basal metabolic rate.

labia (**lay'**-be-ah) The liplike borders of the vulva.

labor Strong contractions of the uterus that occur with increasing frequency and intensity during the latter part of pregnancy and that lead to delivery of the baby.

labyrinth (**lab'**-ih-rinth) The system of intercommunicating canals and cavities that make up the inner ear.

lacteal (**lak'**-tee-al) One of the many lymphatic vessels in the intestinal villi that absorb fat.

lactic (**lak'**-tik) **acid** Compound produced from pyruvic acid during anaerobic energy metabolism. Its accumulation in muscle causes fatigue, and oxygen is required for its elimination.

lactose (**lak'**-tose) A disaccharide composed of one molecule of glucose and one molecule of galactose.

lacunae (la-**koo'**-nee) Small spaces or cavities; spaces in bone and cartilage that contain cartilage cells or bone cells.

laryngopharynx (lah-ring'-oh-**far'**-inks) One of three divisions of the pharynx.

larynx (**lar'**-inks) The organ at the superior end of the trachea that contains the vocal cords; located between the pharynx and trachea.

lateral (**lat'**-er-al) Positional term designating a location away from the midline of the body or one of its organs or parts.

leg That portion of the lower limb located between the knee and the ankle.

lens Transparent structure responsible for focusing images on the retina. Differential focusing of near and far objects is related to the lens's ability to alter its shape.

lesion (**lee'**-zhun) Any local damage to tissue or loss of function of a part; may be the result of injury or disease.

lesser omentum (oh-**men'**-tum) The peritoneal fold connecting the liver with the lesser curvature of the stomach and the duodenum.

lesser vestibular (ves-**tib'**-yoo-lar) **glands** Mucus-producing glands whose ducts open into the female vestibule near the external urethral orifice.

leukemia (loo-**key'**-mea-ah) A form of cancer in which any one of the kinds of white blood cells proliferates wildly in the bone marrow; may be of either an acute or chronic nature.

leukocyte (**loo'**-koe-site) A white blood cell (WBC).

ligament (**lig'**-ah-ment) Strong connective tissue cord, or band, that unites bones.

limbic system An action system of the brain involved in motivation, learning, and the emotional aspects of behavior.

lipid (**lip'**-id) A class of organic compounds that includes fats and steroids (including several hormones); insoluble in water but soluble in fat solvents such as alcohol; serves as a storage form of fuel and an important component of cellular membranes.

lobe A well-defined portion of any organ, especially of the brain, lungs, and glands.

lumen (**loo'**-men) The space within a tubelike structure such as the intestine or a blood or lymphatic vessel.

luteinizing (**loo'**-tee-in-eye'-zing) **hormone (LH)** Hormone secreted by the anterior lobe of the pituitary gland that stimulates ovulation and progesterone secretion by the corpus luteum. In males, LH stimulates the testes to secrete testosterone.

lymph (limf) The fluid within the lymphatic vessels that is collected from the interstitial fluid and ultimately returned to the circulatory system.

lymphatic (lim-**fat'**-ik) Of or pertaining to lymph. Also, one of several large lymph vessels that unite to form the right and left lymphatic ducts.

lymph node A mass of lymphatic tissue surrounded by a connective tissue capsule; filters lymph and produces lymphocytes.

lymph nodules Small masses of lymphatic tissue that produce lymphocytes; lack a connective tissue capsule. Found scattered throughout loose connective tissue, especially beneath moist epithelial membranes.

lymphocyte (**lim'**-foe-site) A type of agranular white blood cell. This class of cells includes the T and B lymphocytes and natural killer (NK) cells.

lysosome (**lye'**-so-sowm) A membrane-enclosed cytoplasmic organelle containing digestive enzymes.

macrophage (**mak'**-row-faje) A large phagocytic cell capable of ingesting and digesting bacteria and cellular debris.

malnutrition Poor nutritional status; can result from dietary intake that is either above or below required needs.

mammary (**mam'**-er-ee) **glands** Organs in the breasts that produce and secrete milk, providing nutrition for the young; develop as modified sweat glands.

mammography (mam-**og'**-rah-fee) A soft-tissue radiological study of the breast.

manubrium (mah-**noo'**-bree-um) Superior portion of the sternum.

mast cell A type of cell present in connective tissue; contains histamine and is important in inflammation and in allergic reactions.

meatus (me-**a'**-tus) A passageway or opening.

mechanoreceptor (meh-**kan'**-oh-re-sep'-tor) A sensory receptor that responds to mechanical stimuli such as bending or deforming the cell; examples include receptors for touch, pressure, and hearing.

medial (**me'**-dee-al) Directional term meaning nearer to the midline of the body or structure.

median plane A vertical plane situated at a right angle to a frontal or coronal plane and dividing the body into right and left halves.

mediastinum (me'-dee-as-**tie'**-num) Region between the lungs that holds several organs.

medulla (meh-**dul'**-ah) The inner portion of an organ such as the kidney.

medulla oblongata (ob-long-**gah'**-tuh) The most inferior aspect of the brainstem; connects the brain with the spinal cord.

meiosis (my-**oh'**-sis) Reduction division; the special type of nuclear and cell division by which gametes are produced.

melanin (**mel'**-ah-nin) A group of dark pigments produced by certain cells (melanocytes) in the epidermis of the skin.

membrane A sheet of tissue that covers or lines a body surface.

membrane bones Bones that develop by intramembranous formation, for example, the parietal bones of the cranium.

memory B cells Activated B cells that continue to produce small quantities of antibody long after an infection has been overcome.

meninges (meh-**nin'**-jeez) The three membranes that envelop the brain and spinal cord: the dura mater, arachnoid, and pia mater.

meniscus (meh-**nis'**-kus) Articular disk composed of fibrocartilage; found in certain types of synovial joints.

menopause (**men'**-oh-pawz) The period during which menstruation ceases in the human female, usually at about age 50.

menstrual (**men'**-stroo-al) **cycle** Monthly cycle of physiological changes that prepare the uterine lining for the reception of a fertilized ovum.

menstruation (men-stroo-**ay'**-shun) The monthly discharge of blood and degenerated uterine lining in the female; marks the beginning of each menstrual cycle.

mesentery (**mez'**-en-ter-ee) A fold attaching various organs to the body wall, especially the peritoneum connecting the intestine to the posterior abdominal wall.

mesocolon (mez-oh-**ko'**-lon) A fold of peritoneum connecting a portion of the colon to the posterior abdominal wall.

metabolism (meh-**tab'**-oh-liz-um) All the chemical processes that take place within the body.

metaphase (**met'**-ah-faze) Stage of mitosis characterized by pairs of chromatids lining up along the equator of the cell.

metaphysis (meh-**taf'**-ih-sis) Region of growing long bone between the epiphyses and the diaphysis.

metastasis (meh-**tas'**-tah-sis) The transfer of a disease such as cancer from one organ or part to another not directly connected to it.

microvilli (my-krow-**vill'**-ee) Minute projections of the plasma membrane that increase the surface area of the cell; present mainly in cells concerned with absorption and secretion, such as those lining the intestine.

micturition (mik-tyoo-**rish'**-un) Urination; the passage of urine from the urinary bladder.

midbrain The portion of the brain located between the pons and the diencephalon. Also referred to as the *mesencephalon.*

mineralocorticoids (min'-er-al-o-**kor'**-tih-koyds) A class of hormones produced by the adrenal cortex that regulates mineral metabolism and, indirectly, fluid balance. The principal mineralocorticoid is aldosterone.

mitochondria (my'-tow-**kon'**-dree-ah) Cellular organelles that are the site of most cellular respiration; sometimes referred to as the *power plants of the cell.*

mitosis (my-**tow'**-sis) Division of the cell nucleus resulting in the distribution of a complete set of chromosomes to each end of the cell. Cytokinesis (actual division of the cell itself) usually occurs during the telophase stage of mitosis, giving rise to two daughter cells.

mitral (**my'**-tril) **valve** Alternative term for the left atrioventricular (bicuspid) valve.

molecule (**mol'**-eh-kewl) A chemical combination of two or more atoms that form a specific chemical compound.

monocyte (**mon'**-oh-site) A type of white blood cell; a large, phagocytic, nongranular leukocyte that enters the tissues and differentiates into a macrophage.

monoglyceride (mon-oh-**gliss'**-er-ide) A fat that contains only one fatty acid per molecule.

motor neuron An efferent neuron that transmits impulses away from the central nervous system to skeletal muscle.

mucosa (mew-**koe'**-sah) See mucous membrane.

mucous membrane An epithelial membrane that lines a body cavity that opens to the outside of the body, for example, the lining of the digestive tract.

mucus (**mew'**-kus) A sticky secretion produced by certain gland cells (e.g., goblet cells), especially in the lining of the gastrointestinal and respiratory tracts. It serves to lubricate body parts and trap particles of dirt. The adjectival form is spelled *mucous.*

muscle (**mus'**-ul) An organ that produces movement by contraction.

muscle tissue A tissue composed of cells specialized for contraction; three main types are skeletal, smooth, and cardiac.

muscle tone The incomplete but sustained contraction of a portion of a skeletal muscle.

mutation A change in one of the bases of DNA, resulting in an alteration of genetic information.

myelin (**my'**-eh-lin) The white fatty substance forming a sheath around certain nerve fibers, which are then called *myelinated fibers.*

myocardial infarction (my'-oh-**kar'**-dee-al in-**fark'**-shun) Heart attack; serious condition that occurs when the heart muscle does not receive sufficient oxygen.

myocardium (my'-oh-**kar'**-dee-um) Middle layer of the heart wall; composed of cardiac muscle.

myofibrils (my-oh-**fye'**-brills) Threadlike structures in the cytoplasm of striated and cardiac muscle that are responsible for contraction.

myofilament (my'-oh-**fil'**-ah-ment) One of the filaments making up the myofibril; the structural unit of muscle proteins in a muscle cell.

myosin (**my'**-oh-sin) A protein that, together with actin, is responsible for muscle contraction.

myosin filaments Thick filaments composed mainly of the protein *myosin;* actin and myosin filaments make up the myofibrils of muscle fibers.

nail The hard cutaneous plate situated on the dorsal aspect of the distal region of each digit of the hand or foot.

nares (**nay'**-reez) The external openings of the nose; also referred to as the *nostrils.*

nasopharynx (nay′-zo-**far**′-inks) The division of the pharynx that is posterior to the nasal cavity.

natural killer (NK) cell A type of lymphocyte that recognizes and destroys cancer cells and cells infected by viruses or other pathogens.

negative feedback system A homeostatic system in which a change in some condition triggers a response that reverses the changed condition, thus restoring the steady state (homeostasis); the response of the regulator is opposite (negative) to the output.

neonate (**nee**′-oh-nate) Pertaining to the newborn infant during the first 4 weeks after birth.

neoplasm (**nee**′-oh-plazm) A tumor; new and abnormal growth of cells or tissues.

nephron (**nef**′-ron) The functional microscopic unit of the kidney.

nerve (nerv) A large bundle of axons (or dendrites), wrapped in connective tissue, that conveys impulses between the central nervous system and some other part of the body.

neuron (**new**′-ron) A nerve cell; an impulse-conducting cell of the nervous system that typically consists of a cell body, dendrites, and an axon.

neurotransmitter A chemical signal used by neurons to send signals across a synapse.

neutrophil (**noo**′-trow-fil) A type of granular leukocyte that engulfs and destroys bacteria and other foreign matter.

nitric oxide (NO) A gaseous signaling molecule; a neurotransmitter.

nociceptors (**no**′-sih-sep-tors) Pain receptors; free endings of certain sensory neurons whose stimulation is perceived as pain.

norepinephrine (nor′-ep-ih-**nef**′-rin) (1) A neurotransmitter. (2) A hormone produced by the adrenal medulla.

nucleic (new-**klee**′-ik) **acids** Deoxyribonucleic acid (DNA) or ribonucleic acid (RNA); very large compounds composed of carbon, oxygen, hydrogen, nitrogen, and phosphorus arranged in molecular subunits called *nucleotides.* Nucleic acids code information specifying the structure and function of the organism.

nucleolus (new-**klee**′-oh-lus) Spherelike organelle located within the nucleus; site where the subunits of ribosomes are assembled.

nucleotide (**new**′-klee-oh-tide) A subunit of nucleic acids (DNA and RNA); consists of a phosphate group, a pentose (5-carbon) sugar, and a nitrogen-containing base.

nucleus (**new**′-klee-us) (1) The core of an atom that contains the protons and neutrons. (2) A cellular organelle that contains DNA and serves as the control center of the cell. (3) A mass of nerve cell bodies in the central nervous system.

nutrients (**new**′-tree-ents) The chemical substances present in food that are utilized by the body as components for synthesizing needed materials and for fuel.

nutrition (new-**trish**′-un) The process of taking in and using food; nourishment.

obesity (oh-**bees**′-ih-tee) The condition of being extremely overweight (body mass index of 30 or higher).

oocyte (**oh**′-oh-site) A developing egg cell in either the primary or secondary stage.

opposition Type of movement unique to the thumb. This movement is a combination of rotation and adduction.

optic (**op**′-tik) Of or pertaining to the eye or vision.

optimum (**op**′-ti-mum) Most favorable; optimum conditions are the most favorable conditions under which a particular function can occur.

orbit (**or**′-bit) The bony cavity that houses the eyeball.

organ (**or**′-gan) A specialized structure, such as the heart or stomach; composed of tissues and adapted to perform a specific function or group of functions.

organelle (or-gah-**nell**′) One of many specialized parts of a cell, such as the nucleus, mitochondria, Golgi apparatus, and plasma membrane.

organ of Corti The organ that contains the sensory receptors for hearing.

orgasm (**or**′-gazm) The climax of sexual excitement; includes ejaculation in the male and involuntary rhythmic contraction of the perineal muscles in both sexes.

orifice (**or**′-ih-fis) The entrance or outlet of any body cavity.

origin (**or**′-ih-jin) The more fixed end of attachment of a muscle to a bone; the end opposite the insertion.

oropharynx (or-oh-**far**′-inks) The part of the pharynx between the soft palate and the upper edge of the epiglottis.

osmosis (oz-**mow**′-sis) The net movement of water molecules by diffusion through a selectively permeable membrane in response to solute concentrations.

osmotic pressure A measure of the tendency of a solution to take up water when separated by a selectively permeable membrane from a solution of lower solute concentration.

osseous (**os**′-ee-us) Bony.

ossicle (**os**′-ih-kul) A small bone, especially one of the three bones of the middle ear (malleus, incus, stapes).

ossification (**os**′-ih-fih-**kay**′-shun) Formation of bone; also called *osteogenesis.*

osteoblast (**os**′-tee-oh-blast′) A cell that produces bone.

osteoclast (**os**′-tee-oh-klast′) A large, multinuclear cell that helps sculpt and remodel bones by dissolving and removing part of the bony substance.

osteocyte (**os**′-tee-oh-site′) A mature bone cell; an osteoblast that has become embedded within the bone matrix and occupies a lacuna.

osteon (**os**′-tee-on) The basic unit of structure of compact bone consisting of concentric rings of lamellae arranged around a central (haversian) canal. Also called a *haversian system.*

osteoporosis (**os**′-tee-oh-poe-**row**′-sis) A disease in which there is a severe reduction in bone mass; most common bone disease.

oval window (of ear) Opening between the middle and inner ear on which the stapes rests.

ovarian ligament The cord of connective tissue that attaches the ovary to the uterus.

ovary (oh′-var-ee) The female gonad; produces ova and sex hormones, principally estrogens and progesterone.

ovulation (oh-vu-**lay′**-shun) The release of an ovum (actually a secondary oocyte) from the ovary into the pelvic cavity.

ovum (oh′-vum) Egg cell; female gamete.

oxidants Highly reactive molecules that can damage DNA and other cell molecules by snatching electrons; produced during normal cell activities.

oxidation (oks-ih-**day′**-shun) The removal of electrons, or loss of hydrogen, from a compound; for example, cellular respiration is the oxidation of glucose.

oxygen debt The amount of oxygen needed to oxidize the lactic acid produced during exercise.

oxyhemoglobin (ok′-see-**he′**-mow-glow-bin) Hemoglobin combined with oxygen; the form in which oxygen is transported in the body.

oxytocin (ok -see-**tow′**-sin) A hormone produced by the hypothalamus and released by the posterior lobe of the pituitary gland; stimulates contraction of the uterus and release of milk from the lactating breast.

pacinian corpuscle Encapsulated, onion-shaped tactile receptor that responds to pressure.

palate (pal′-at) The roof of the mouth; the horizontal partition separating the oral and nasal cavities.

pancreas (pan′-kree-as) The large, elongated gland located behind the stomach, between the spleen and duodenum. Composed of both exocrine tissue (secretes pancreatic juice) and endocrine tissue (secretes insulin and glucagon).

pancreatic duct A single tube that joins the common bile duct, forming a single duct that passes into the wall of the duodenum.

papilla (pah-**pil′**-ah) A small, nipplelike mound, for example, the papilla at the base of each hair follicle.

parasympathetic (par′-ah-sim′-pah-**thet′**-ik) **system** One of the two subdivisions (the craniosacral portion) of the autonomic nervous system; its general effect is to conserve and restore energy.

parathyroid (par-ah-**thy′**-royd) **glands** Small endocrine glands located within the connective tissue surrounding the thyroid gland; secrete parathyroid hormone, which regulates calcium and phosphate metabolism.

parathyroid hormone (PTH) A hormone secreted by the parathyroid glands that regulates calcium and phosphate concentrations in the blood.

parietal (pah-**rye′**-eh-tal) (1) Pertaining to the walls of an organ or cavity. (2) Pertaining to the parietal bone of the skull.

parotid (pah-**rot′**-id) **glands** The largest of the three main pairs of salivary glands, located on either side of the face, just inferior and anterior to the ears.

parturition (par′-too-**rish′**-un) The process of giving birth to a child; delivery of a baby.

passive immunity Temporary immunity that depends on the presence of antibodies produced by another person or animal.

patellar (pah-**tell′**-ar) **reflex** Involuntary contraction of the quadriceps muscle and jerky extension of the leg when the patellar ligament is sharply tapped.

pathogen (path′-o-jen) Any disease-producing organism or agent.

pectoral (pek′-ter-il) Pertaining to the chest or breast.

pelvic (pel′-vik) **cavity** Inferior portion of the abdominopelvic cavity; contains the urinary bladder, sigmoid colon, rectum, and internal female and male reproductive structures.

pelvis (pel′-vis) Any basinlike structure, for example, the basinlike structure formed by the hip bones, the sacrum, and the coccyx.

penis (pee′-nis) The external male organ that functions in urination and in copulation.

pepsin (pep′-sin) A protein-digesting enzyme that is the main digestive component of gastric juice.

peptide (pep′-tide) A compound composed of two or more amino acids; components of proteins.

pericardial (per′-ih-**kar′**-dee-al) **cavity** Potential space between the visceral and parietal layers of the pericardium.

pericardium (per′-ih-**kar′**-dee-um) The sac enclosing the heart; composed of an outer fibrous layer and an inner serous layer.

perilymph (per′-ih-limf) The fluid contained between the bony and membranous labyrinths of the inner ear.

perimysium (per-ih-**mis′**-ee-um) Connective tissue that surrounds the fascicles (bundles) of skeletal muscle fibers.

perineum (per′-ih-**nee′**-um) The pelvic floor and associated structures; diamond-shaped region bounded by the coccyx, symphysis pubis, and ischial tuberosities.

periosteum (per′-ee-**os′**-tee-um) The connective tissue membrane covering bones; important in bone growth and repair.

peripheral nervous system (PNS) That portion of the nervous system consisting of the receptors, the nerves that link receptors with the central nervous system (CNS), and the nerves that link the CNS with the effectors (muscles and glands).

peripheral resistance The resistance to blood flow caused by the viscosity of blood and by the friction between the blood and the wall of the blood vessels.

peristalsis (per-ih-**stal′**-sis) Waves of muscle contractions along the wall of a tube such as the digestive tract.

peritoneum (per′-ih-tow-**nee′**-um) The largest serous membrane of the body; lines the walls of the abdominal and pelvic cavities (parietal peritoneum) and covers the contained viscera (visceral peritoneum).

peritonitis (per-ih-tow-**nie**′-tis) Inflammation of the peritoneum.

pH A measure of the acidity or alkalinity of a solution. The pH scale extends from 0 to 14, with 7 being neutral; values lower than 7 indicate increasing acidity, and values higher than 7 indicate increasing alkalinity.

phagocyte (**fag**′-o-site) A cell that engulfs bacteria, foreign matter, and dead cells, for example, certain white blood cells and macrophages.

phagocytosis (fag′-oh-sigh-**tow**′-sis) The process by which a cell engulfs and ingests microorganisms, other cells, or foreign particles.

phalanx (**fay**′-lanks) The bone of a toe or finger. (Plural— *phalanges* [fay-**lan**′-jeez].)

pharynx (**far**′-inks) The throat; passageway for food and air; begins at the internal nares and extends partway down the neck, communicating with the mouth and opening into the esophagus posteriorly and into the larynx anteriorly.

photoreceptor (fo′-tow-re-**sep**′-tor) A sensory receptor sensitive to light.

physiology (fiz′-ee-**ol**′-oh-jee) Science that deals with the functions of the body and its parts.

phytochemicals (**fye**′-tow-kem-ih-kals) Compounds found in plants that promote health.

pia mater (**pee**′-ah **may**′-ter) The inner of the three meninges (membranes) covering the brain and spinal cord.

pineal (**pin**′-ee-al) **gland** Endocrine gland attached by a stalk to the posterior wall of the third ventricle; helps regulate biological rhythms.

pinna (**pin**′-ah) The projecting part of the external ear; composed of elastic cartilage and covered with skin.

pituitary (pih-**too**′-ih-terr′-ee) **gland** An endocrine gland attached by a stalk to the hypothalamus of the brain; secretes a variety of hormones influencing a wide range of physiologic processes. Sometimes called the *master gland.* Also called the *hypophysis.*

placenta (plah-**sen**′-tah) The organ of exchange between mother and developing fetus; provides for exchange of nutrients, gases, and waste products between fetal and maternal circulations.

plasma (**plaz**′-muh) The fluid portion of blood consisting of a pale yellowish fluid containing proteins, salts, and other substances.

plasma cell A differentiated, functioning B lymphocyte; produces antibodies.

plasma membrane Cell membrane; outer, limiting membrane of the cell that separates the cell from its external environment.

platelet (**plate**′-let) A blood platelet or thrombocyte; a cell fragment suspended in the plasma that functions in blood clotting.

pleura (**ploor**′-ah) The serous membrane that surrounds the lungs (visceral pleura) and lines the walls of the thoracic cavity (parietal pleura).

pleural cavity Potential space between the visceral and parietal pleura.

plexus (**plex**′-us) A network of veins or nerves.

polypeptide (pol′-ee-**pep**′-tide) A chain of many amino acids linked together by peptide bonds; proteins consist of polypeptide units.

polysaccharides (pol′-ee-**sak**′-uh-rides) Carbohydrates consisting of three or more, usually many, sugar units chemically combined to form a large molecule.

polyunsaturated fat A fat that contains two or more double bonds between its carbon atoms. Most vegetable oils are polyunsaturated.

polyuria (pol-ee-**yoo**′-ree-ah) Excessive excretion of urine.

pons (ponz) That part of the brainstem that forms a bridge between the medulla and the midbrain, anterior to the cerebellum; connects various other parts of the brain.

portal vein A vein that delivers blood to a second set of exchange vessels (capillaries or sinusoids), for example, the hepatic portal vein.

positive feedback system A homeostatic system in which a change in some condition that varies from the steady state sets off a series of events that intensify the change.

positron emission tomography (PET) A nuclear medicine imaging technique that produces a cross-sectional image of the distribution of radioactivity in a slice through the subject a few centimeters thick.

posterior (pos-**teer**′-ee-or) Toward or at the back of the body; dorsal.

postganglionic (post′-gang-glee-**on**′-ik) **neuron** Neuron located distal to a ganglion. The second efferent neuron in an autonomic pathway.

postovulatory phase (post-**ov**′-u-lah-tor-y) The period of the menstrual cycle from ovulation until the beginning of the next menstrual cycle.

postsynaptic (post′-sin-**ap**′-tik) **neuron** A neuron that transmits action potentials away from a synapse. Compare with presynaptic neuron.

preganglionic (pre′-gang-glee-**on**′-ik) **neuron** Neuron located proximal to a ganglion. The first efferent neuron in an autonomic pathway; synapses with a postganglionic neuron.

pregnancy The condition of having a developing embryo or fetus in the body.

preovulatory phase (pre-**ov**′-u-lah-tor-y) The first 2 weeks or so of the menstrual cycle; the time from the first day of the menstrual cycle until after ovulation.

prepuce (**pre**′-pyoos) The loose-fitting skin covering the glans of the penis or clitoris. Also referred to as the *foreskin.*

presynaptic (pre′-sin-**ap**′-tik) **neuron** A neuron that transmits action potentials toward a synapse.

prevertebral (pre-**vert**′-eh-bral) **ganglion** A mass of cell bodies of postganglionic sympathetic neurons located close to blood vessels. Also called *collateral ganglion.*

primary motor area A region within the precentral gyrus of the frontal lobe of the cerebrum that controls skeletal muscles. Also called the *motor cortex.*

progesterone (pro-**jes'**-ter-own) A steroid sex hormone secreted by the corpus luteum (in the ovary) and by the placenta; stimulates thickening of the endometrium of the uterus and helps prepare the mammary glands for milk secretion.

prolactin (pro-**lak'**-tin) A hormone secreted by the anterior lobe of the pituitary gland that stimulates lactation (milk production). Also called *lactogenic hormone.*

prolapse (**pro'**-laps) The downward displacement, or falling down, of a part or organ.

proliferation (pro-lif-er-**a'**-shun) Multiplication of new parts, especially cells.

pronation (pro-**nay'**-shun) The act of assuming the prone (lying face downward) position. Applied to the hand, the turning of the palm of the hand backward (posteriorly) or downward.

prophase (**pro'**-faze) The first stage of mitosis or meiosis.

proprioceptors (pro'-pre-o-**sep'**-ters) Mechanoreceptors located within the skeletal muscles, tendons, joints, and inner ear that send sensory information to the brain, allowing us to know the location of one body part in relation to another.

prostaglandins (pros'-tah-**glan'**-dins) **(PG)** A group of fatty acids released by many different tissues; act as local hormones; prostaglandins interact with other hormones to regulate various metabolic activities.

prostate (**pros'**-tate) **gland** A gland in the male that surrounds the neck of the bladder and the urethra and secretes an alkaline fluid that is a component of semen.

protein (**pro'**-teen) A complex organic compound composed of chemically linked amino acid subunits; contains carbon, hydrogen, oxygen, nitrogen, and sulfur.

prothrombin (pro-**throm'**-bin) An inactive protein synthesized by the liver and released into the blood; converted to thrombin during blood clotting.

proximal (**prok'**-sih-mal) Nearer to the center of the body or to the point of attachment or origin.

pseudostratified (soo'-dow-**strat'**-ih-fide) **epithelium** An epithelial tissue that appears to be stratified (layered) but is not.

puberty (**pyoo'**-ber-tee) The period of sexual maturation during which the secondary sex characteristics begin to develop and the individual becomes capable of sexual reproduction.

pudendum (poo-**den'**-dum) The female external reproductive structures. Also called *vulva.*

pulmonary (**pul'**-mon-air-ee) Pertaining to the lungs.

pulmonary circulation The circuit of blood flow between the heart and lungs. The flow of oxygen-poor blood from the right ventricle to the lungs where it is oxygenated and the return of the oxygen-rich blood from the lungs to the left atrium. Compare with systemic circulation.

pulp cavity A cavity within the tooth filled with pulp—a connective tissue containing blood vessels, nerves, and lymphatics.

pulse The rhythmic expansion and recoil of the elastic arteries each time the left ventricle pumps blood into the aorta. The pulse rate corresponds to the heart rate.

pupil The opening in the center of the iris through which light enters the eye.

Purkinje (per-**kin'**-jee) **fibers** Modified cardiac muscle fibers concerned with conducting impulses through the heart.

pus The liquid product of inflammation that contains white blood cells and debris of dead cells.

pyloric sphincter (pie-**lor'**-ik **sfink'**-ter) A thick ring of muscle that serves as a gate; opens to allow food to pass from the stomach into the duodenum.

pyramid (**pir'**-a-mid) A pointed or cone-shaped structure. (1) Pyramids of the medulla oblongata are two prominent bulges of white matter on the ventral side of the medulla containing descending fibers of the pyramidal tracts that pass from the cerebrum to the spinal cord. (2) Renal pyramids are conical masses that make up the medulla of the kidney.

pyramidal (pih-**ram'**-i-dal) **tracts** Groups of descending tracts arising in the cerebral cortex, crossing in the pyramids of the medulla, and extending into the spinal cord; provide for control of skilled voluntary movement.

ramus (**ray'**-mus) A general term for a branch of a nerve, artery, or vein.

rapid eye movement (REM) sleep A stage of sleep characterized by rapid movement of the eyes, dreams, and a brainwave pattern similar to that of an awake individual.

reception Process of detecting a stimulus.

receptor (re-**sep'**-tor) (1) A sensory structure that responds to specific stimuli such as light, sound, touch, pressure, or change in position. (2) A specific chemical grouping (usually a protein) on a cell surface (or sometimes inside the cell) that may combine with a specific signaling molecule such as a neurotransmitter or hormone.

rectum (**rek'**-tum) The distal portion of the large intestine, extending from the sigmoid colon to the anus.

reflex (**re'**-flex) A predictable, automatic sequence of stimulus-response usually involving a reflex pathway consisting of at least three neurons: a sensory neuron, an association neuron, and a motor neuron.

refractory (re-**frak'**-to-ree) **period** The time period during which a neuron cannot respond to a stimulus that is usually sufficient to result in an action potential.

releasing hormones Chemical messengers secreted by the hypothalamus; regulate the anterior lobe of the pituitary gland.

renal (**ree'**-nul) Pertaining to the kidney.

renal pelvis The funnel-shaped expansion of the upper end of the ureter into which the renal calices open.

renin (**reh'**-nin) An enzyme synthesized by the juxtaglomerular cells of the kidney; it plays a role in the regulation of blood pressure by stimulating formation of angiotensin.

repolarization (re-pole′-ur-ih-**za**′-shun) The process of returning membrane potential to its resting level.

respiration (res′-pih-**ray**′-shun) The exchange of oxygen and carbon dioxide between the atmosphere and the body cells, including inspiration and expiration, diffusion of gases between the alveoli and blood, transport of oxygen and carbon dioxide, and cellular respiration.

response The change in cell (or body) activity that is the effect of some signal.

resting potential The membrane potential (difference in electrical charge between the two sides of the plasma membrane) of a resting neuron; the inside of the cell is negative relative to the outside.

reticular (reh-**tik**′-yoo-lur) **activating system (RAS)** A diffuse network of neurons in the brainstem responsible for maintaining consciousness and alertness; the system of neurons of the reticular formation that project to higher centers.

retina (ret′-ih-nah) The inner coat of the eyeball; composed of light-sensitive neurons including the rods and cones.

retroperitoneal (reh′-trow-per′-ih-tow-**nee**′-al) External to the peritoneal lining of the abdominal cavity; behind the peritoneum.

rhodopsin (row-**dop**′-sin) A photosensitive pigment in the retinal rods.

Rh system A system of blood types with more than 40 different kinds of Rh antigens, each referred to as an *Rh factor*.

ribonucleic acid (RNA) Functions mainly in the expression of the cell's genetic information. It is a single-stranded nucleic acid whose pentose sugar is ribose and whose bases are adenine, uracil, guanine, and cytosine. (Varieties are messenger RNA, transfer RNA, and ribosomal RNA.)

ribosome (**rye**′-bow-sowm) Organelle containing RNA that may be attached to the endoplasmic reticulum (ER) and that functions in protein synthesis.

rickets (**rik**′-ets) A condition affecting children in which vitamin D deficiency leads to altered calcium metabolism and disturbance of ossification of bone; bones become soft and deformed.

right lymphatic duct A lymphatic vessel that drains lymph from the upper right side of the body and empties it into the right subclavian vein.

rods Photoreceptors in the retina that are stimulated by low light intensities. There are more than 100 million rods in each eye.

roentgenogram (**rent**′-gen-oh-gram′) An x-ray; a film produced by taking pictures of internal structures by passage of x-rays through the body.

root canal The narrow extension of the pulp cavity that lies within the root of a tooth.

rotation The process of turning around an axis; moving a bone around its own axis.

rugae (**roo**′-jee) Folds, such as those in the lining of the stomach.

saccule (**sak**′-yool) The sac within the vestibule of the inner ear that along with the utricle houses the receptors for static equilibrium.

sacral (**say**′-kral) **plexus** The network formed by the anterior branches of spinal nerves L4 through S3.

saddle joint A synovial joint in which the articular surfaces of both bones are saddle shaped.

sagittal (**sadj**′-ih-tul) **plane** A vertical section or plane that divides the body (or an organ) into right and left parts.

saliva The secretion of the salivary glands; contains the enzyme salivary amylase.

salivary amylase (**sal**′-ih-ver-ee **am**′-ih-lase) An enzyme in saliva that initiates the digestion of starch.

salivary glands Accessory digestive glands that secrete saliva into the mouth. The major ones are the paired parotid, submaxillary, and sublingual glands.

saltatory conduction Transmission of a neural impulse along a myelinated neuron; ion activity at one node depolarizes the next node along the axon.

sarcolemma (sar-koe-**lem**′-ma) The plasma membrane of a muscle cell, especially of a skeletal muscle cell.

sarcomere (**sar**′-koe-mere) A segment of a muscle fiber extending from one Z line to the next that serves as a unit of contraction.

sarcoplasm (**sar**′-koe-plazm) The cytoplasm of a muscle cell.

saturated fat A fat that contains no double bonds between any of its carbon atoms; each carbon is bonded to the maximum number of hydrogen atoms. Saturated fat is found in animal foods such as meat, milk, dairy products, and eggs.

Schwann (shvon) **cell** A type of glial cell found in the peripheral nervous system that forms the myelin sheath and cellular sheath of a nerve fiber by wrapping itself around the fiber.

sclera (**skleh**′-rah) The tough, white outer coat of the eyeball that protects the inner structures; continuous anteriorly with the cornea and posteriorly with the covering of the optic nerve.

scrotum (**skrow**′-tum) The external, skin-covered pouch that contains the testes and their accessory structures.

sebaceous (see-**bay**′-shus) **gland** An exocrine gland in the dermis of the skin that secretes sebum, an oily material that lubricates the skin surface; its duct opens into a hair follicle. Also called *oil gland*.

sebum (**see**′-bum) The oil secretion of the sebaceous glands.

secondary sex characteristics Characteristic male or female features that develop at puberty in response to sex hormones; for example, shape of body, muscle development, pubic hair, and pitch of voice.

secretion (se-**kree**′-shun) (1) The process by which a cell releases a specific product. (2) Any substance produced by secretion, for example, saliva produced by the cells of the salivary glands.

sella turcica (**sel**′-ah **tur**′-sih-kah) The depression on the upper surface of the sphenoid bone that houses the pituitary gland.

semen (**see**′-men) Fluid discharged at ejaculation in the male, consisting of sperm suspended in the secretions of the seminal vesicles, prostate gland, and bulbourethral glands.

semicircular canals The three curved channels located in the bony labyrinth of the inner ear that contain receptors (cristae) for dynamic equilibrium (balance).

semilunar (sem′-ee-**loo**′-nar) **valve** A valve between each ventricle and the great artery into which it pumps blood; consists of flaps shaped like half moons.

seminal vesicles (sem′-ih-nul **ves**′-ih-kuls) Glands that secrete a major portion of the semen into the ejaculatory ducts.

seminiferous (sem′-ih-**nif**′-er-us) **tubules** The coiled tubules within the testes where sperm cells are produced.

sensation A feeling; awareness of sensory input.

sensory adaptation The decrease in frequency of action potentials in a sensory neuron even when the stimulus is maintained; results in decreased response to that stimulus.

sensory areas of cerebrum Areas in the cerebrum that receive and interpret information from the sensory receptors.

sensory neuron An afferent neuron that transmits impulses from a receptor to the central nervous system.

septum (**sep**′-tum) A wall dividing a body cavity.

serosa (ser-**oh**′-sah) Any serous membrane. Serous membranes line the pleural, pericardial, and peritoneal cavities.

serotonin (ser-uh-**tow**′-nin) A neurotransmitter of the biogenic amine group.

serum (**see**′-rum) The fluid part of blood that remains after the solid components (cells and platelets) and proteins involved in clotting have been removed.

sesamoid (**ses**′-ah-moyd) **bone** A small bone that typically occurs in a tendon subject to stress or pressure; it does not form a joint directly.

sex chromosomes The X and Y chromosomes. Females have two X chromosomes, whereas males have one X and one Y chromosome.

sigmoid colon (**sig**′-moyd **koe**′-lon) The distal S-shaped part of the colon from the level of the iliac crest to the rectum.

signal transduction The process by which a cell receptor converts a signal outside the cell into a signal inside the cell that affects some cellular process.

sinoatrial (sigh′-no-**ay**′-tree-al) **(SA) node** Pacemaker of the heart; a mass of specialized cardiac muscle in which the impulse triggering the heartbeat originates; located in the posterior wall of the right atrium near the opening of the superior vena cava.

sinus (**sigh**′-nus) A cavity or channel such as the air cavities in the cranial bones (paranasal sinuses) or dilated channels for venous blood.

sinusoids (**sigh**′-nuh-soyds) Tiny blood vessels (slightly larger than capillaries) found in certain organs such as the liver and spleen.

skeletal muscle An organ specialized for contraction that is characterized by striated (striped) muscle fibers and is under voluntary control; stimulated by somatic efferent (motor) neurons.

skin The outer covering and the largest organ of the body; the skin and its associated structures, such as hair and sweat glands, make up the integumentary system.

skull The bony framework of the head consisting of the cranium and facial skeleton.

small intestine The region of the digestive tract that extends from the stomach to the large intestine; it is a long, coiled tube consisting of the duodenum, jejunum, and ileum.

smooth muscle Involuntary muscle composed of smooth (nonstriated) muscle fibers; located in the walls of hollow organs such as the intestine or uterus.

sodium-potassium pump An active transport system located in the plasma membrane; uses the energy from adenosine triphosphate (ATP) to transport sodium ions out of the cell and potassium ions into the cell; maintains the concentrations of these ions at homeostatic levels.

soft palate (**pal**′-at) The posterior portion of the roof of the mouth; a muscular partition lined with mucous membrane that extends from the palatine bones to the uvula.

solute (**sol**′-yoot) The substance that is dissolved in a liquid (solvent) to form a solution.

solution A liquid (solvent) in which one or more substances (solutes) is dissolved.

solvent (**sol**′-vent) A liquid that dissolves another substance (solute) to form a solution without chemical change in either.

somatic (so-**mat**′-ik) **division (of the nervous system)** The part of the peripheral nervous system that keeps the body in adjustment with the external environment; includes the sensory receptors on the body surface and within the muscles, the nerves that link them with the central nervous system (CNS), and the efferent nerves that link the CNS with the skeletal muscles.

sperm Male gamete (sex cell) that combines with an ovum in sexual reproduction to produce a new individual. Also called *spermatozoon.*

spermatic (sper-**mat**′-ik) **cord** The male reproductive structure extending from the abdominal inguinal ring to the testis; includes the vas deferens, testicular artery, veins, nerves, cremaster muscle, and connective tissue.

sphincter (**sfink**′-ter) A circular muscle that constricts a passageway or orifice.

sphygmomanometer (sfig′-mow-mah-**nom**′-eh-ter) An instrument for measuring arterial blood pressure.

spinal (**spy**′-nal) **cord** The part of the central nervous system located in the vertebral canal and extending from the foremen magnum to the upper part of the lumbar region; the dorsal, tubular nerve cord.

spinal ganglion Dorsal root ganglion; consists of the cell bodies of sensory neurons and is located along the dorsal root just before it joins the spinal cord.

spinal nerve Any of the 31 pairs of nerves that arise from the spinal cord and pass out between the vertebrae.

spleen The largest organ of the lymphatic system, located in the upper part of the abdominal cavity on the left side; filters blood, and plays a role in immunity.

sprain Wrenching or twisting of a joint with partial rupture of its ligaments.

squamous (skway′-mus) epithelium Epithelium consisting of flat, scalelike cells.

stem cells Immature cells that give rise to various types of cells; for example, stem cells in the bone marrow give rise to blood cells.

stenosis (steh-no′-sis) Narrowing or contraction of a body passage or opening.

stereocilia Hairlike projections of hair cells; microvilli that contain actin filaments.

sterile (ster′-il) (1) Not fertile; not producing young. (2) Aseptic; free from living microorganisms.

sterilization (ster′-il-ih-zay′-shun) The process of rendering an individual incapable of producing offspring; the most common surgical procedures are vasectomy in the male and tubal ligation in the female.

stimulus Any change in the environment that produces a response in a receptor or irritable tissue.

stomach (stum′-ak) The curved, muscular, saclike part of the digestive tract between the esophagus and the small intestine; occupies the abdominal cavity just below the diaphragm.

stratum (stray′-tum) A sheetlike mass of tissue of fairly uniform thickness; used to designate distinct sublayers making up various tissues or organs; for example, the strata of the skin. (Plural—*strata*.)

stressor Any factor that disturbs homeostasis, producing stress.

stroke volume The volume of blood pumped by one ventricle during one contraction.

subarachnoid (sub′-ah-rak′-noyd) space The space between the arachnoid and pia mater through which cerebrospinal fluid circulates.

subcutaneous (sub′-koo-tay′-nee-us) Beneath the skin.

subcutaneous layer The layer of loose connective tissue and adipose tissue beneath the skin.

subdural (sub-doo′-ral) space The space between the dura mater and arachnoid.

sublingual (sub-ling′-gwal) glands The paired salivary glands located in the floor of the mouth under the tongue.

submandibular (sub′-man-dib′-you-lar) glands The paired salivary glands located in the posterior region of the floor of the mouth, posterior to the sublingual glands.

submucosa (sub′-myoo-koe′-sah) A layer of connective tissue located beneath a mucous membrane, as in the digestive tract.

substance P A neurotransmitter released by certain sensory neurons in pain pathways; signals the brain about painful stimuli.

substrate (sub′-strate) Any substance on which an enzyme acts.

sulcus (sul′-kus) A groove or furrow; a linear depression as is found between the gyri of the brain.

superficial (soo′-per-fish′-al) Located on or near the body surface.

superior (sue-peer′-ee-ur) Higher; refers to structures nearer the head than the feet.

superior vena cava (vee′-nah kay′-vah) Large vein that receives blood from parts of the body superior to the heart and returns it to the right atrium.

supination (soo′-pih-nay′-shun) The act of assuming the supine position, that is, lying on the back. Applied to the hand, the act of turning the palm upward.

suture (soo′-cher) The fibrous joint between adjoining bones in the skull.

sweat (swet) Perspiration; the salty fluid, consisting mainly of water, excreted by the sweat glands in the skin.

sympathetic (sim′-pah-thet′-ik) system The thoracolumbar portion of the autonomic nervous system; its general effect is to mobilize energy, especially during stressful situations; prepares body for fight-or-flight response.

symphysis (sim′-fih-sis) A slightly movable type of joint in which the two joining bones are firmly united by a plate of fibrocartilage.

symphysis pubis (pyoo′-bis) A slightly movable cartilaginous joint between the pubic bones.

symptom (simp′-tum) Any sign or indication of disease perceived by the patient.

synapse (sin′-aps) Junction between two neurons or between a neuron and an effector (muscle or gland).

synaptic (sin-ap′-tik) cleft The narrow gap that separates the axon terminal of one neuron from another neuron or from a muscle fiber. Neurotransmitter diffuses across the cleft to affect the postsynaptic cell.

synaptic plasticity The ability of synapses to change in response to certain types of stimuli; allows learning and remembering to occur.

synaptic terminals Tiny enlargements in the distal ends of axons that contain synaptic vesicles that store neurotransmitter. Also called *synaptic knobs.*

synaptic vesicle Membrane-enclosed sac containing neurotransmitter; found in the synaptic terminals of axons.

synarthrosis (sin′-ar-throw′-sis) An immovable joint; a joint in which the bones are tightly united by fibrous tissue.

syndrome (sin′-drome) A combination of symptoms that occur together forming a pattern characteristic of a particular disorder.

synovial (sih-**no′**-vee-al) **fluid** The transparent, viscous fluid secreted by the synovial membrane and found in joint cavities, bursae, and tendon sheaths.

synovial joint A fully movable or diarthrotic joint in which a synovial cavity is present between the two articulating bones.

systemic (sis-**tem′**-ik) Affecting the body as a whole.

systemic circulation The circuit of blood vessels through which oxygen-rich blood is delivered to all of the tissues and organs of the body and oxygen-poor blood is returned to the right atrium.

systole (**sis′**-tow-lee) The contraction phase of the cardiac cycle during which blood is forced into the aorta and pulmonary artery.

systolic (sis-**tol′**-ik) **blood pressure** The force exerted by the blood on arterial walls during ventricular contraction; about 110 mm Hg under normal conditions for a young adult.

tachycardia (tak′-ee-**kar′**-dee-ah) An abnormally rapid heart rate, usually defined as more than 100 beats per minute.

tactile (**tak′**-tile) Pertaining to the sense of touch.

target cell A cell with receptors that combine with a particular hormone or other signaling molecule.

tarsus (**tar′**-sus) The seven bones that make up the ankle.

T cell A T lymphocyte; responsible for cell-mediated immunity.

telophase (**tel′**-oh-faze) The last of the four stages of mitosis and of the two divisions of meiosis; the cytoplasm usually divides during telophase, giving rise to two daughter cells.

tendinitis (ten′-din-**i′**-tis) Inflammation of tendons and tendon-muscle attachments; frequently associated with calcium deposits and may also involve the bursa around the tendon, causing bursitis.

tendon (**ten′**-don) A cord of strong, white fibrous tissue that connects a muscle to a bone.

testis (**tes′**-tis) The male gonad; either of the paired glands located in the scrotum that produce sperm and the male sex hormone *testosterone*. Also called *testicle*. (Plural—*testes*.)

testosterone (tes-**tos′**-teh-rone) The principal male sex hormone (androgen); produced by the interstitial cells in the testes; stimulates development of the male reproductive organs and secondary sex characteristics.

tetany (**tet′**-ah-nee) (1) Steady contraction of a muscle without distinct twitching. (2) A syndrome characterized by muscle twitchings, cramps, and convulsions, caused by abnormal calcium metabolism.

thalamus (**thal′**-ah-mus) A region of the brain composed of gray matter covered by a thin layer of white matter and located at the base of the cerebrum. The thalamus serves as a main relay center transmitting information between the spinal cord and the cerebrum.

thermoreceptor (ther′-mow-ree-**sep′**-tor) A receptor that detects changes in temperature.

thigh The part of the lower limb between the hip and the knee.

thoracic (thow-**ras′**-ik) **cavity** The superior part of the ventral body cavity; contains the two pleural cavities, pericardial cavity, and mediastinum.

thoracic duct A lymphatic vessel that receives lymph from all regions of the body except the upper right quadrant and empties it into the left subclavian vein.

thorax (**thow′**-rax) The chest.

threshold level The electrical potential that a neuron or other excitable cell must reach for an action potential to be initiated.

thrombin (**throm′**-bin) An enzyme formed by the activation of prothrombin; catalyzes the conversion of fibrinogen to fibrin.

thrombus (**throm′**-bus) A blood clot formed within a blood vessel or within the heart.

thymus (**thy′**-mus) **gland** A gland located in the upper mediastinum beneath the sternum that plays a key role in immunologic function.

thyroid (**thy′**-royd) **gland** An endocrine gland located in the front and sides of the neck just below the thyroid cartilage; its hormones are essential for normal growth and metabolism.

thyroid-stimulating hormone (TSH) A tropic hormone secreted by the anterior lobe of the pituitary gland that stimulates the synthesis and secretion of hormones produced by the thyroid gland.

thyroxine (thy-**rok′**-sin) (T_4) One of the hormones secreted by the thyroid gland; essential for normal growth and metabolism.

tissue (**tiss′**-yoo) A group of closely associated similar cells that work together to carry out specific functions.

tongue A large muscular organ on the floor of the mouth that functions in chewing, swallowing, and speech.

tonsil Aggregate of lymph nodules embedded in the mucous membrane in the throat region. The tonsils are located strategically to defend against pathogens that enter through the mouth or nose.

toxic (**tok′**-sik) Poisonous; pertaining to poison.

trachea (**tray′**-kee-ah) The air passageway extending from the larynx to the main bronchi. Also called *windpipe*.

tract A bundle of nerve fibers in the central nervous system.

transduction Conversion of energy of a stimulus to electrical signals.

transmission (trans-**mish′**-un) Conduction of an action potential (neural impulse) along a neuron or from one neuron to another.

transverse colon (trans-**verse′ koe′**-lon) The portion of the large intestine extending across the abdomen from the ascending to the descending colon.

trauma (**traw′**-mah) A wound or injury, especially damage caused by external force.

tricuspid (try-**kus′**-pid) **valve** The valve consisting of three flaps that guards the opening between the right atrium and right ventricle.

triiodothyronine (tri′-i-o-doe-**thy**′-row-nene) (**T₃**) One of the thyroid hormones; essential for normal growth and metabolism.

tropic (**trow**′-pik) **hormone** A hormone that helps regulate another endocrine gland; for example, thyroid-stimulating hormone secreted by the pituitary gland regulates the thyroid gland.

trunk (1) The main part of the body to which the head and limbs are attached. (2) A large structure, such as a nerve or blood vessel, from which smaller branches arise or which is formed by small branches.

tubular reabsorption In the kidneys, the movement of a substance out of the renal tubule and into the peritubular capillaries.

tubular secretion In the kidneys, the movement of a substance out of the peritubular capillaries and into the renal tubule.

tumor (**too**′-mor) Neoplasm; a new growth of tissue in which cell multiplication is unregulated and progressive.

twitch Rapid, brief, jerky contraction of a muscle in response to a single stimulus.

tympanic (tim-**pan**′-ik) **membrane** Thin, semitransparent membrane that stretches across the ear canal, separating the outer ear from the middle ear.

ulcer (**ul**′-ser) An open lesion, or excavation, of a tissue produced by the sloughing of inflamed, dying tissue.

umbilical (um-**bil**′-ih-kal) Refers to the navel; middle region of the abdomen.

umbilical cord The long, ropelike structure that connects the fetus to the placenta; contains the umbilical arteries and vein.

uremia (yoo-**ree**′-me-ah) An excess in the blood of urea and other nitrogenous wastes, generally resulting from kidney malfunction. A sign of renal failure.

ureter (yoo-**ree**′-ter) One of the paired tubes that conduct urine from the kidneys to the bladder.

urethra (yoo-**ree**′-thruh) A muscular tube that conducts urine from the bladder to the exterior surface of the body.

urinalysis (yoo′-rih-**nal**′-ih-sis) Examination of the physical, chemical, and microscopic characteristics of urine used as an aid in the diagnosis of disease.

urinary bladder A muscular sac in the anterior floor of the pelvic cavity that serves as a storage sac for urine.

urine (**yoo**′-rin) The fluid containing water, nitrogenous wastes, salts, and traces of other substances that is produced and excreted by the kidneys.

uterine (**yoo**′-tur-in) **tube** One of the paired tubes attached to each end of the uterus; site of fertilization and passageway through which the fertilized ovum reaches the uterus. Also called *fallopian tube* or *oviduct*.

uterus (**yoo**′-tur-us) The womb; the organ that houses the embryo and fetus during development.

utricle (**yoo**′-trih-kul) The larger of the two divisions of the membranous labyrinth of the inner ear; along with the saccule, responsible for static equilibrium.

uvula (**yoo**′-vue-lah) A fleshy mass of tissue, especially the structure extending from the soft palate.

vacuole (**vac**′-yoo-ole) A membrane-enclosed sac located in the cytoplasm; may function in storage or digestion.

vagina (vah-**jye**′-nuh) The elastic, muscular tube extending from the cervix to the vestibule; receives the penis during sexual intercourse and serves as the birth canal.

vagus (**vay**′-gus) **nerve** The tenth cranial nerve; each vagus nerve emerges from the medulla and innervates thoracic and abdominal organs; the main nerve of the parasympathetic system.

valve A structure that prevents fluid from flowing backward; for example, valves prevent blood from flowing backward in the heart and veins.

varicose (**var**′-ih-kose) **veins** Swollen, distended veins usually located in the subcutaneous tissues of the leg.

vascular (**vas**′-kyoo-lar) Pertaining to or containing many blood vessels.

vas deferens (**def**′-ur-enz) One of the paired ducts that conveys semen from the epididymis to the ejaculatory duct.

vasectomy (vah-**sek**′-tow-me) A sterilization procedure in the male in which each vas deferens is cut and the ends cauterized so that sperm cannot be ejaculated as part of the semen.

vasoconstriction (vas′-o-kon-**strik**′-shun) The narrowing of the lumen of blood vessels; refers especially to the narrowing of the arterioles.

vasodilation (vas′-o-die-**lay**′-shun) The widening of the lumen of blood vessels; refers especially to the widening of arterioles.

vein (vane) A vessel that conducts blood from tissues back to the heart.

vena cava (**vee**′-nah **kay**′-vah) The superior or inferior vein that opens into the right atrium; returns oxygen-poor blood to the heart.

ventral (**ven**′-tral) Pertaining to the abdomen or anterior (front side) of the body; opposite of dorsal.

ventricle (**ven**′-tri-kul) A cavity or chamber, such as one of the cavities of the brain or heart.

venule (**ven**′-yule) A small vein that collects blood from capillaries and delivers it to a larger vein.

vermiform (**ver**′-mih-form) **appendix** A small appendage attached to the cecum.

vertebra (**ver**′-teh-brah) A bone of the spine. (Plural—*vertebrae.*)

vertebral (**ver**′-teh-bral) **canal** The canal formed by the series of vertebral foramina together; contains the spinal cord.

vertebral column The spine; the rigid structure in the midline of the back, composed of the vertebrae.

vesicle (**ves**′-ih-kul) A small, membrane-enclosed sac in the cytoplasm of a cell that contains various materials.

vestibule (**ves**′-tih-byool) A small space or region at the entrance of a canal; for example, the vagina opens into a vestibule.

villus (**vil′**-us) A small vascular projection from the free surface of a membrane; for example, intestinal villi project from the surface of the small intestine.

viscera (**vis′**-ur-uh) The organs located within the body cavities.

visceral (**vis′**-er-al) Pertaining to the organs or to the covering of an organ.

visceral peritoneum The inner layer of the serous membrane that covers the abdominal viscera.

vitamin (**vie′**-tah-min) An organic compound essential in the diet in small amounts; acts as a coenzyme in metabolic reactions and is essential for normal growth and health.

vitreous humor (**vit′**-ree-us **hyoo′**-mor) In the eye, a clear, jellylike fluid that fills the posterior cavity lying between the lens and retina.

vocal cords The folds of mucous membranes in the larynx that vibrate to make vocal sounds during speaking. The inferior folds are called *true vocal cords.*

vulva (**vul′**-vah) The external genital organs in the female. Also called *pudendum.*

white blood cell (WBC) Leukocyte.

white matter Nervous tissue of the brain and spinal cord; composed mainly of myelinated nerve fibers.

wound A bodily injury caused by physical means, with disruption of the normal continuity of structures.

zygote (**zy′**-goat) Fertilized ovum; the cell resulting from the fusion of male and female gametes.

Page numbers followed by *f* indicate figures; *t,* tables; boldface page numbers indicate definitions.

SCIENTIFIC MEASUREMENT

STANDARD METRIC UNITS

		Abbreviation
Standard unit of mass	Gram	g
Standard unit of length	Meter	m
Standard unit of volume	Liter	L

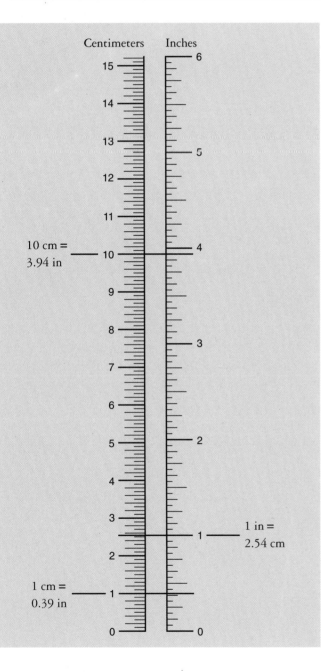

10 cm = 3.94 in

1 in = 2.54 cm

1 cm = 0.39 in

SOME COMMON PREFIXES

		Examples
kilo	1000	A kilogram is 1000 grams.
centi	0.01	A centimeter is 0.01 meter.
milli	0.001	A milliliter is 0.001 liter.
micro (µ)	One millionth	A micrometer is 10^{-6}, or 0.000001 (one millionth) of a meter.
nano (n)	One billionth	A nanogram is 10^{-9} (one billionth) of a gram.
pico (p)	One trillionth	A picogram is 10^{-12} (one trillionth) of a gram.

SOME COMMON UNITS OF LENGTH

Unit	Abbreviation	Equivalent
Meter	m	Approximately 39 in
Centimeter	cm	10^{-2} m
Millimeter	mm	10^{-3} m
Micrometer	µm	10^{-6} m
Nanometer	nm	10^{-9} m

Length Conversions

1 in = 2.5 cm	1 mm = 0.039 in
1 ft = 30 cm	1 cm = 0.39 in
1 yd = 0.9 m	1 m = 39 in
1 mi = 1.6 km	1 m = 1.094 yd
	1 km = 0.6 mi

To convert	Multiply by	To obtain
Inches	2.54	Centimeters
Feet	30	Centimeters
Centimeters	0.39	Inches
Millimeters	0.039	Inches